New Techniques and Concepts in Maternal and Fetal Medicine

Van Nostrand Reinhold Semmelweis Memorial Series

Edited by

Harold A. Kaminetzky, M.D.
and
Leslie Iffy, M.D.

Associate Editor

Joseph J. Apuzzio, M.D.

NEW TECHNIQUES AND CONCEPTS IN MATERNAL AND FETAL MEDICINE, edited by Harold A. Kaminetzky and Leslie Iffy. Associate editor, Joseph J. Apuzzio

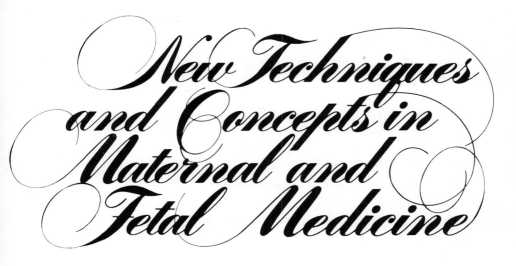

New Techniques and Concepts in Maternal and Fetal Medicine

EDITED BY

HAROLD A. KAMINETZKY, M.D.
LESLIE IFFY, M.D.
ASSOCIATE EDITOR
JOSEPH J. APUZZIO, M.D.

College of Medicine and Dentistry of New Jersey
New Jersey Medical School
Newark, New Jersey

VAN NOSTRAND REINHOLD SEMMELWEIS MEMORIAL SERIES

 VAN NOSTRAND REINHOLD COMPANY
NEW YORK   CINCINNATI   ATLANTA   DALLAS   SAN FRANCISCO
LONDON   TORONTO   MELBOURNE

Van Nostrand Reinhold Company Regional Offices:
New York Cincinnati Atlanta Dallas San Francisco

Van Nostrand Reinhold Company International Offices:
London Toronto Melbourne

Copyright © 1979 by Litton Educational Publishing, Inc.

Library of Congress Catalog Card Number: 79-9517
ISBN: 0-442-26244-2

Manufactured in the United States of America

Published by Van Nostrand Reinhold Company
135 West 50th Street, New York, N.Y. 10020

Published simultaneously in Canada by Van Nostrand Reinhold Ltd.

15 14 13 12 11 10 9 8 7 6 5 4 3 2 1

Library of Congress Cataloging in Publication Data
Main entry under title:

New techniques and concepts in maternal and fetal
medicine.

   (Van Nostrand Reinhold Semmelweis memorial series)
   Includes bibliographical references and index.
   1. Obstetrics—Congresses. 2. Pregnancy,
Complications of—Congresses. 3. Fetus—Diseases—
Congresses. I. Kaminetzky, Harold A. II. Iffy,
Leslie. III. Apuzzio, Joseph J. IV. Series.
RC31.N48   618.3   79-9517
ISBN 0-447-26244-2

Contributors And Editors

Raja W. Abdul-Karim, M.D. Professor of Obstetrics and Gynecology, State University of New York, College of Medicine, Upstate Medical Center, Syracuse, New York.

V. P. Aggarwal, M.D. Department of Obstetrics and Gynecology, University of Nairobi, Faculty of Medicine, Nairobi, Kenya.

Joseph Apuzzio, M.D. Assistant Professor of Obstetrics and Gynecology, College of Medicine and Dentistry of New Jersey, New Jersey Medical School, Newark, New Jersey.

Andrew J. Baeder, M.D. President, Semmelweis Scientific Society. Director, Emeritus, National School of Nurse/Midwifery, Budapest, Hungary.

Gad Barkai, M.D. Department of Obstetrics and Gynecology, The Chaim Sheba Medical Center, Tel-Hashomer, Tel-Aviv University, School of Medicine, Israel.

Franklin C. Behrle, M.D. Professor and Chairman, Department of Pediatrics, CMDNJ-New Jersey Medical School, Newark, New Jersey.

Anne Boyce, M.D. Consultant, Institute National de la Sante, Et de la Recherche Medicale, Unite de Recherches Statistiques, Villejuif, France.

R. Clay Burchell, M.D. Professor and Director, Department of Obstetrics and Gynecology, Hartford Hospital, University of Connecticut, Hartford, Connecticut.

Leon C. Chesley, Ph.D. Professor of Obstetrics and Gynecology, State University of New York, Downstate Medical Center, Brooklyn, New York.

Sir Cyril A. Clarke, KBE, M.D., FRCOG, FRS. President, Emeritus, Royal College of Physicians. Professor, Emeritus, Department of Medicine, Nuffield Unit of Medical Genetics, Liverpool, England.

Garry Frisoli, M.D. Fellow in Maternal/Fetal Medicine, Clinical Assistant Professor of Obstetrics and Gynecology, CMDNJ-New Jersey Medical School, Newark, New Jersey.

Boleslav Goldman, M.D. Department of Obstetrics and Gynecology, The Chaim Sheba Medical Center, Tel-Aviv University, Tel-Hashomer, Israel.

Robert C. Goodlin, M.D. Professor of Obstetrics and Gynecology, University of California, Sacramento Medical Center, Sacramento, California.

Edward Gordon, M.D. Department of Obstetrics and Gynecology, Cedars Sinai Medical Center, Los Angeles, California.

William J. Hartko, M.D. Assistant Professor of Obstetrics and Gynecology, CMDNJ-Rutgers Medical School, Piscataway, New Jersey.

Leslie Iffy, M.D. Professor of Obstetrics and Gynecology, Director of Perinatology, College of Medicine and Dentistry of New Jersey, New Jersey Medical School, Newark, New Jersey.

György Illei, M.D. Director, Department of Obstetrics and Gynecology, Markusovszky Teaching Hospital, Szombaphely, Hungary.

Antal Jakobovits, M.D., Ph.D.   Associate Professor of Obstetrics and Gynecology, University of Szeged, Chairman, Department of Obstetrics and Gynecology, Hetényi Géza Hospital, Szolnok, Hungary.

James R. Jones, M.D.   Professor and Chairman, Department of Obstetrics and Gynecology, Rutgers Medical School, Piscataway, New Jersey.

Harold Kaminetzky, M.D.   Professor and Chairman, Department of Obstetrics and Gynecology, College of Medicine and Dentistry of New Jersey, New Jersey Medical School, Newark, New Jersey.

Theodore Kushnick, M.D.   Professor of Pediatrics, CMDNJ-New Jersey Medical School, Newark, New Jersey.

Alvin Langer, M.D.   Professor of Obstetrics and Gynecology, Northeastern Ohio Universities, College of Medicine, Academic Director, Department of Obstetrics and Gynecology, Aultman Hospital, Canton, Ohio.

Lula O. Lubchenco, M.D.   Professor of Pediatrics, Co-Director, Newborn Service, University of Colorado Medical Center, Denver, Colorado.

Alfonso Madrazo, M.D.   Associate Director of Pathology, St. Vincent's Hospital and Medical Center of New York, New York, New York.

Shlomo Mashiach, M.D.   Department of Obstetrics and Gynecology, The Chaim Sheba Medical Center, Tel-Hashomer, Tel-Aviv University School of Medicine, Israel.

J. K. G. Mati, M.D.   Professor and Chairman, Department of Obstetrics and Gynecology, University of Nairobi, Nairobi, Kenya.

Gail A. McGuinness, M.D.   Fellow in Clinical Neonatology, Newborn Service, University of Colorado Medical Center, Denver, Colorado.

Milivoje Milosevic, M.D.   Fellow in Maternal/Fetal Medicine, Department of Obstetrics and Gynecology, CMDNJ-New Jersey Medical School, Newark, New Jersey.

Audrey H. Nora, M.D. Associate Clinical Professor of Pediatrics, University of Colorado Medical Center. Director of Genetics, Children's Hospital, Denver, Colorado.

James J. Nora, M.D. Professor of Pediatrics, University of Colorado Medical Center, Denver, Colorado.

Paul Pedowitz, M.D. Professor of Obstetrics and Gynecology, CMDNJ-New Jersey Medical School. Director, Department of Obstetrics and Gynecology, Newark Beth Israel Medical Center, Newark, New Jersey.

R. J. Pepperell, M.D. Professor and Chairman, Department of Obstetrics and Gynecology, University of Melbourne, Royal Women's Hospital, Parkville, Victoria, Australia.

Douglas P. Pugh, M.D. Fellow in Clinical Neonatology, Department of Pediatrics, University of Colorado Medical Center, Denver, Colorado.

Elizabeth M. Ramsey, M.D. Research Associate, Department of Embryology, Carnagie Institution of Washington, Baltimore, Maryland.

Clyde L. Randall, M.D. Professor and Chairman, Emeritus Department of Obstetrics and Gynecology, State University of New York. Director of Education, Johns Hopkins Program of International Education, Gynecology and Obstetrics, Baltimore, Maryland.

Joseph F. Russo, M.D. Assistant Professor, Department of Obstetrics and Gynecology, CMDNJ-New Jersey Medical School, Newark, New Jersey.

Barry S. Schifrin, M.D. Associate Professor, Department of Obstetrics and Gynecology, Director, Maternal/Fetal Medicine, Cedars Sinai Medical Center, Los Angeles, California.

D. Schwartz, M.D. Professor, Institute National de la Sante, Et de la Recherche Medicale Unite de Recherches Statistiques, Villejuif, France.

David M. Serr, M.D. Director and Professor of Obstetrics and Gynecology, The Chaim Sheba Medical Center, Tel-Hashomer. Vice Dean, Sackler School of Medicine, Tel-Aviv University, Tel-Hashomer, Israel.

Leo Stern, M.D. Professor and Chairman, Department of Pediatrics, Brown University, Providence, Rhode Island.

Shirazali G. Sunderji, M.D. Department of Obstetrics and Gynecology, State University of New York, Upstate Medical Center, Syracuse, New York.

Howard C. Taylor, Jr., M.D. Professor and Chairman, Emeritus, Department of Obstetrics and Gynecology, Columbia University, New York, New York.

Alan Tomlinson, M.D. Division of Perinatal Medicine University of Colorado Medical Center Denver, Colorado.

Ilona R. Toth, M.D. Consultant Pathologist, St. Vincent's Hospital and Medical Center, New York, New York.

Sir Lance Townsend, M.D. Professor and Chairman, Emeritus, Department of Obstetrics and Gynecology, University of Melbourne, Royal Women's Hospital, Parkville, Victoria, Australia.

Martin B. Wingate, M.D. Professor and Vice Chairman, Department of Obstetrics and Gynecology, State University of New York at Buffalo, Buffalo, New York.

Preface

The yearly Ignatz Semmelweis Seminars established in 1975 have featured outstanding perinatologists. Their presentations, attended by hundreds of physicians and almost as many nurses, have had a profound impact each year upon prevailing philosophies in the specialty. In view of the unprecedented interest that this yearly parade of prominent authorities has evoked, it seems appropriate to present this volume, which, under the authorship of the same speakers who attracted great interest in the 3rd and 4th Memorial Semmelweis Seminars, includes some of the most interesting subjects of the meetings.

Those who attended the lectures by these authorities found them enlightening and thought-provoking. Hopefully, the updated and written versions of their discussions of a broad variety of subjects will be equally instructive and enjoyable for all readers of this volume, whether experts or students in the field of maternal-fetal medicine.

Harold A. Kaminetzky, M.D.
Leslie Iffy, M.D.

Acknowledgments

The Editors wish to record their gratitude to Mrs. Margot Stickley for her invaluable help in correcting and improving the manuscripts. Our thanks are also due to Ms. Sheila Kalinoski and Ms. Shawna Williams for their deligent help in keeping in contact with the contributors and transcribing the manuscripts.

Contents

New Techniques and Concepts in Maternal and Fetal Medicine

SCOPE OF MATERNAL AND FETAL MEDICINE

I. Teratology
- a) Embryology.
- b) Effect of drugs on the fetus.
- c) Fetal effects of viral and other infections.
- d) The effect of radiation on the embryo and the fetus.
- e) Miscellaneous teratogenic factors.

II. Genetics
- a) Biochemistry of genes and chromosomes.
- b) Gene transformations in man.
- c) Cytogenetics and karyotyping.
- d) Population genetics.
- e) Genetic counseling.
- f) Inborn errors of metabolism.

III. Maternal Physiology
- a) Biological changes secondary to pregnancy.
- b) Pathophysiology of diseases of pregnancy.
- c) Maternal nutrition.

IV. Fetal Physiology
- a) Fetal growth and development.
- b) Pathophysiology of intrauterine disease.
- c) Placental function and dysfunction.
- d) Evaluation of fetal well being.
- e) Fetal pathology.

V. Immunology of Pregnancy
- a) Considerations relevant to physiology.
- b) Immune pathology: clinical manifestations.

VI. Endocrinology of Pregnancy and Labor
- a) Hormonal physiology.
- b) Pathology of endocrine function.
- c) Coincidental endocrine disorders.

VII. Complications of Pregnancy
- a) Complications intrinsic to gestation.
- b) Incidental medical complications.

VIII. Physiology and Pathology of Labor
- a) Basic concepts.
- b) Clinical considerations.

IX. Perinatal Infections
- a) Maternal disease.
- b) Fetal effects of maternal infection.
- c) Bacteriology of obstetrical infection.
- d) Choice of antibiotics in obstetrics.

X. Obstetrical Anesthesia

XI. Operative Obstetrics

XII. Physiology and Pathology of the Puerperium

XIII. Psychosomatic Effects of Pregnancy
- a) Physiology.
- b) Pathology.

XIV. Neonatology
- a) Adjustments and adaptations.
- b) Pathological conditions.

XV. Organization and Delivery of Perinatal Care (Preventive Perinatology)

XVI. Medicolegal Perinatology

XVII. Educational Aspects of Maternal-Fetal Medicine

XVIII. The History of Obstetrics

1

Physician Education for the Problems of Reproductive Health

CLYDE L. RANDALL, M.D.

Let's look at ourselves as other health care professionals see us. Obstetricians and gynecologists do have reasons for satisfaction in the dramatically reduced numbers of maternal mortalities, in the decreasing numbers of fetal and newborn deaths, in the effectiveness of the current management of endocrinologic dysfunctions, and especially in the earlier detection of gynecologic malignancies and their more effective management in an earlier, curable stage.

Yet why, if we are doing so many things well, are some of our colleagues in other specialties, professionals in public health services and particularly those who claim they are speaking for the consumers of health care, dissatisfied with the practicing obstetricians and gynecologists? Why are so many professionals in international health so critical of what they term "maternity care in the Western World," particularly since such care is being provided by specialists in the U.S.? The answer relates to the conviction that these services are being provided within the framework of private practice and are not available to the very large numbers of medically indigent women who are also in need of maternity and gynecologic care. There is no doubt that we are doing a good job of taking care of the women we do care for; however, we are not providing, nor do we seem to be preparing to provide, for the much greater volume of obstetric and gynecologic services that are, and will continue to be, needed in the future in this country.

During the past decade there has been an increasingly evident need in the U.S. to establish reliable data from which estimates can be made of the number and types of physicians necessary to provide improved and more generally available health care. Obstetricians and gynecologists in particular have not yet developed the data base necessary to determine (1) what health services are essential to the maintenance of womens' health; (2) to what extent these services can be provided by obstetric and gynecologic nurses in public health roles, by non-specialist physicians and by other professional personnel; (3) what additional health services could contribute to improving the health of the women of this country. Reliable data are needed before anyone can answer the all-important question of how many physician specialists, family physicians and assisting health personnel will be needed in the U.S. during the next decade to provide the required health services for women.

Significant information in this regard is just beginning to be developed. Dr. Warren Pearse,[1] Executive Director of the American College of Obstetricians and Gynecologists has recently reported the results of the first comprehensive study of the current practices of an adequate sample of U.S. obstetricians and gynecologists. The objective was to determine the numbers of patients being cared for by the average U.S. specialist and the nature of the services being provided to these patients during the period studied. The findings to date indicate that the average obstetrician-gynecologist in the United States is counseling, examining or providing treatment for an average of 51 hours of every week in the year. This figure is an average and takes into account the half-days and weekends not on call, as well as vacation periods and time taken for out-of-town meetings. During the 51 hour period per week the average U.S. specialist is now caring for the obstetric and gynecologic health needs of approximately 500 women per year. These data can be presumed to be reasonably reliable, since they tend to be supported by the findings in another survey Pearse reports on practices of obstetricians and gynecologists in Canada,[2] which indicates that the average specialist was observed to be providing patient services for an average of 52 hours per week.

Although these data are important, they fail to provide insight into a major issue. We must decide if we need two or three times as many obstetric and gynecologic specialists in the U.S. to provide the needed services for all the women in the U.S. who might seek them if they were made available. In addition, we need to decide if the physician specialist should fulfill the role of consultant in a practice pattern based on nurse practitioners, nurse midwives and assisting technical and professional personnel who will provide more routine health services and who will refer those with signs of a health problem to the consultant.

A look at the practice patterns of physicians in other developed countries with economies not unlike our own now suggests that U.S. physicians and others of our health professions must soon agree upon the desirability of a practice pattern that will meet the needs for health services in this country. This decision and agreement must occur before anyone (or any computer) can calculate what type and what numbers of health personnel are needed to make adequate health care readily available to all Americans. We can be certain that legislative bodies in the U.S. are now being advised by representatives of the consumer, as well as by providers of current health services. I suspect that the chances of spontaneous voluntary agreement among the health professions are not bright and that unfortunately, we can expect competition rather than cooperation which will not necessarily be in the best interests of those who need health services. If I were asked to predict likely developments, I would suggest that the care of the ill and the injured will, in all probability, remain the responsibility of the physician. On the other hand, activities involved in the maintenance of health are likely to become the responsibility of non-physician health professionals. Just how much of the care of pregnant women would then be considered the "maintenance of health" and when during pregnancy the attention of the physician specialist is required is likely to remain an unresolved question in this country, one resolved most frequently by the local availability of the type of health personnel desired by the patient. In the United States, however, there are certain to be many communities in which the obstetrician-gynecologist must soon participate among a group of professionals, including nurses and allied health personnel, organized to provide adequate, even optimal obstetric and gynecologic care for a much greater number of women than a physician specialist can now provide even in a well-organized solo practice.

Thus, while benefiting from the stimulation and information generated during the Third Semmelweis Conference, should it not also be our purpose to consider the ways in which the specialty of obstetrics and gynecology could do a better job? Let us then consider some of the factors that affect reproductive health, including some of the problems evident in the educational programs of the health professions, particularly the preparation required to practice as an obstetrician-gynecologist. First, what do we mean by reproductive health? Under what circumstances would we say that reproductive health has been achieved? Simply, when people— represented by family units—realize a desired and altogether healthy reproductive experience.

As practicing physicians, I believe we should be more mindful, more concerned and more involved in the problems, and particularly in the trends, in medical education. As physicians, I believe we should also be more concerned, and certainly more involved, in our country's desire to assure adequate health services for that portion of our population that we as physicians do not see and for whom we do not provide care. As obstetricians and gynecologists, I believe we have particular responsibilities in both of these areas—for the education and training of the next generation of obstetrician-gynecologists and, equally important, for the development and delivery of health services adequate to assure reproductive health and improved family life for a much larger proportion of family units in this country.

To speak of such responsibilities as being ours is not an ivory tower objective, comfortably visualized apart from the demands, the needs and the hazards of patient care. The reality has been evident throughout this country for more than two decades; adequate health services are simply not available for a very considerable proportion of the U.S. population. Accurate and commendable diagnosis, competent and adequate treatment do warrant pride and confidence in the capabilities of the American practices of medicine and surgery, but the best of care is too often not available to many, and never available to some.

The solutions are not likely to be achieved more rapidly during the next few decades if several generations of U.S. physicians are occupied only with the health needs of the patients coming to them for care. In the past two decades a number of new medical schools and greatly increased enrollments in existing U.S. Schools of Medicine will soon double the number of physicians being graduated each year in the United States. By the mid-1970's, however, it became evident that increased numbers of physicians would not be likely to provide the health services needed by the millions of Americans not economically able to pay anything or anybody for health care. Recognition of this state of affairs by consumers and politicians leaves the medical profession obligated to recognize the need for decisions that may soon, and very materially, affect the practice of medicine and surgery in the United States.

I bring these thoughts to your attention here not to predict a gloomy status for the U.S. physician, or to plead for more dedicated effort to organize improved health services for those now without health care. Rather, I would emphasize the responsibilities I believe we have as physicians to assure high quality education in medicine for the generations of medical students who will follow us. Moreover, as obstetrician-gynecologists, I believe we have far greater responsibility than we have generally recognized to assure improved health care for all U.S. women, to assure that healthy babies will be well born, that human reproduction contributes, as it should, to family health and quality of life in this country.

Everyone is talking about the need for more universally available health services. Few are doing anything about it, although the facts do not justify turning away from this major concern of our day. I believe that many physicians should be deciding that we are ready to change our patterns of practice and go into an expanded type of operation, for only if we can provide health care for the community at large, as well as care for our private patients, can the profession meet the increasing demands that are being made upon us. There seems little doubt that a governmental health corps, or some type of an expanded public health type of service, will be obliged to support a variety of trained physician-assistants to become licensed, registered, and no doubt able to assume varying responsibilities as virtually autonomous providers of various levels of health care. If we as obstetrician-gynecologists are willing to accept responsibilities not only for personally providing service but also for supervising the total OB/GYN care of the women of this country, our specialty is certain to become a major influence in the programs that will be preparing professional and nonprofessional personnel to provide the necessary health services. On the other hand, if our interests can be interpreted as those of a group interested only in the needs of those we can care for on a private patient basis, our discipline will have little influence on the development of governmentally organized programs.

I have no desire to emphasize that private practice has become a luxury that many cannot afford, but there does seem a need at this time to recognize that the profession should be feeling a broader responsibility to the society that increasingly provides the education which has enabled all of us to practice as physicians. In the day when the individual doctor could feel he had paid for his medical education, the physician could perhaps, with some reason, feel free to limit his professional responsibilities to the kind and amount of practice he preferred to undertake. Today's doctor, however, must be aware that he has been—and is continuing to be—educated at a considerable cost *to the public.* Both practicing physicians and graduating students now have reason to be increasingly aware that professional schools and hospital-based graduate studies are dependent upon considerable grant support as well as operation within tax-supported facilities and programs. Today's students and tomorrow's practitioners can hardly avoid recognition of responsibility for the many who are now without ready access to private patient care.

Before we are caught up in a whirlpool of contemporary criticisms and demands, there is increasing need to seek recognition of basic truths. Obstetricians and gynecologists need to agree on the services we believe are essential to assure women's good health; some attention must also be paid to what women who are not physicians or health workers think they need in the way of health care. We must find how these different points of view can be merged into concepts and services that will provide better health care for all women.

We continue to hear predictions, some of which sound threatening, as to what governmental intervention, perhaps really governmental control, of the practice of medicine is going to do to us. For those in an established practice, I doubt that changes will develop so rapidly as to affect the relationship they have with their patients. What I consider to be more significant than governmental influence in conditioning the character of future medical practice, are the effects of the concepts developed in preparing future generations of medical students and house officers. It is my belief that the majority of new physicians beginning practice are developing practice patterns based on the experiences they have gained during several years of the now required graduate medical education. Only 14 of the 50 U.S. states will still license a physician without completion of a program of approved graduate medical education. The years in residency programs are likely to determine the concepts and preferences, as well as the experiences and abilities, of the oncoming generations of U.S. physicians.

Patterns of future practice are being developed in the residency programs. Young physicians are looking for opportunities to enter practices that will provide them individually with the satisfaction that comes from knowing that they are doing what they *should* as well as what they *can* do.

A number of community-supported health care clinics are demonstrating ability to provide acceptable care by utilization of the services of a predominantly non-physician staff. As obstetricians and gynecologists, we are not likely to have the best of both worlds. I believe that as a specialty, we have reached a point at which we either accept responsibility for developing the health personnel who can help us provide more obstetric and gynecologic care, or we disclaim any responsibility for the care of more patients than we can personally and adequately care for on a private patient basis. Let us hope that as the supervising and responsible member of a health care unit, the physician of the future will assure adequate and acceptable health care for greatly increased numbers of patients. This, I believe, should be a major objective of the educational experiences of all physicians being prepared to cope with the problems of reproductive health.

REFERENCES

1. Mendenhall, R. C., Pearse, W. H. et al. Manpower for obstetrics and gynecology. *Am. J. Obstet. Gynec.* **130:** 927, 1978.
2. Minister of National Health and Welfare Committee on Physician Manpower (Canada): Report of the Requirements Committee. Ottawa, 1975.

2

Anatomy and Pathology of Uteroplacental Circulation

ELIZABETH M. RAMSEY, M.D.

A major development of recent decades in the field of reproductive physiology has been the recognition that the maternal-placental-fetal unit is an interlocking partnership responsible for the maintenance of pregnancy and the well-being and growth of the fetus. As a co-equal member of this triumvirate, the placenta must be accorded a new evaluation. Although it was long considered simply the mechanism for attaching the embryo to the uterine wall and for transfering nutriment from mother to fetus (in some vague and unspecified way), the organ is now known to serve the fetus as lung, kidney, liver and gastrointestinal tract and to be a veritable factory of hormones and enzymes. In addition, its role in the immunology of pregnancy is just now coming to the fore.

NORMAL UTEROPLACENTAL VASCULATURE AND CIRCULATION

Many of the functions of the placenta are intimately tied up with its vasculature and circulation. A brief review of the development of the vasculature may therefore be helpful.[9]

It will be recalled that the fertilized ovum implants on the endometrium at the time of maximal progestational growth. At this time the endometrial spiral arteries, which are prolongations of the myometrial radial arteries, extend all the way to the subepithelial capillary network and are elaborately coiled. They are promptly "tapped" by invading trophoblast from the wall of the blastocyst; continuity is established between them and the intervillous space of the placenta at an early stage. The subsequent development of the uterine arteries at the site of placental attachment (known hereafter as the uteroplacental arteries) is indicated in Figure 1. Noteworthy are the continued elongation of the vessels, their increasing coiling and back-and-forth looping, and their progressive dilatation during the first half of gestation. A salient feature is the development of terminal dilatations at the placental base.

It is generally accepted that the vis a tergo, the momentum and the velocity of maternal systemic circulation are the forces propelling maternal blood into and through the placenta. The fetal villi, suspended in the intervillous space, act as baffles, serving to lower the thrust of the incoming blood. The pressure of the afferent streams forces blood out of the intervillous space through the venous orifices in its base which connect with the uterine veins (Fig. 2). Myometrial contractions curtail or halt arterial inflow and in addition, individual uteroplacental arteries have intrinsic vasoconstrictive capacity lodged in the inner myometrial portion of their stems.

At the microscopic level, it has been demonstrated that the invading trophoblast (cytotrophoblast) not only taps the spiral arteries but also enters the lumina of the vessels progressing proximally along the inner walls.[3,10] Close to the placental base it may initially form an actual obstruction. This phase of the invasion, the intraluminal phase, lasts for some 12 weeks in man but is of shorter duration in the nonhuman primate (Fig. 3a). In the second phase the cytotrophoblast invades the walls of the arteries, replacing muscle and elastic tissue. Again the action progresses proximally and in man extends into the inner third of the myometrium, to the point where the radial artery becomes the endometrial spiral artery (Fig. 3b). The invasion has never been observed to be deeper than the myometrial-endometrial junction in nonhuman primates. In man, though not in other primates, the cytotrophoblast also penetrates the endometrial stroma as wandering giant cells (Fig. 3c). It is possible that these cells invade the arterial walls from without, providing a double challenge to their integrity. In the final stage of histological transformation, the cytotrophoblast in the arterial walls gradually disappears and is replaced by fibrous tissue mixed with fibrinoid, cellular debris and often some calcium (Fig. 3b). None of the stages of trophoblastic invasion occurs in arteries outside of the placental base, i.e., it is limited to those arteries communicating with the intervillous space and thus in direct contact with the trophoblast.

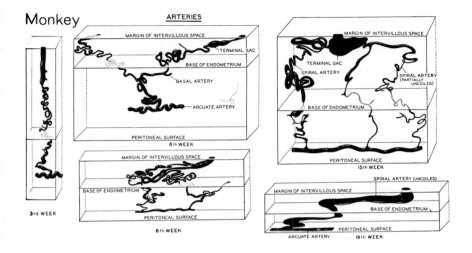

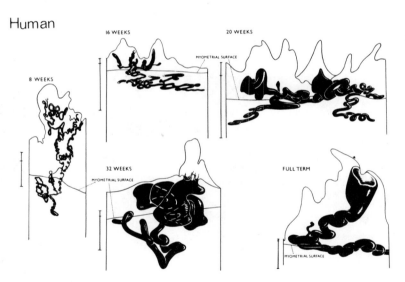

Fig. 1. Diagrammatic representations of the course and configuration of the uteroplacental arteries in the rhesus monkey and man, at comparable stages of gestation. (From: Ramsey and Harris. Contrib. Embryol. 38: 59–70, 1966. Courtesy of the Carnegie Institution of Washington.)

Correlating the gross and microscopic changes occurring in the uteroplacental arteries as pregnancy advances, it seems apparent that the replacement of muscle and elastic tissue in the vessel walls by stout but nonresilient and noncontractile elements underlies the progressive dilatation of the channels and the formation of the terminal sacs.

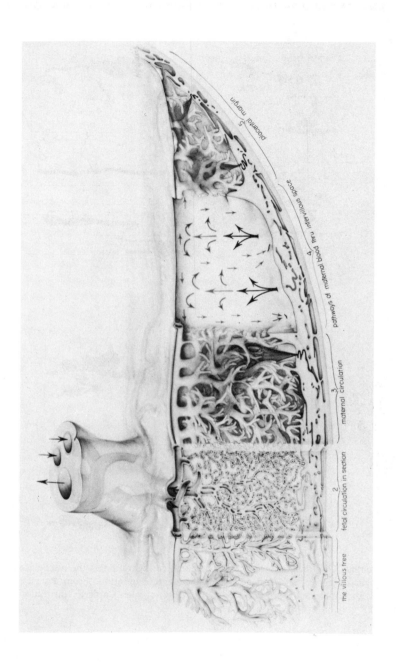

Fig. 2. Composite drawing of the primate placenta to show its structure and circulation. (Drawn by Ranice W. Crosby for Dr. E. M. Ramsey. Courtesy of the Carnegie Institution of Washington.)

Two physiologic consequences of these structural alterations are: 1) the restriction of free and effective placental circulation in the early weeks of pregnancy by the temporary clogging of arterial channels by the invading trophoblast; 2) a dramatic reduction in pressure and velocity of flow between maternal systemic values and those at the point of entry of maternal blood to the intervillous space, occasioned by the dilatation of the arteries and formation of the terminal sacs.

PATHOLOGIC UTEROPLACENTAL VASCULATURE AND CIRCULATION

Concomitant with growing appreciation of the placenta's role in normal pregnancy has come realization that its improper functioning can be a factor in pathologic conditions. Two clinical entities in particular have been widely studied in this regard: first, Small for Gestational Age Infants, so-called "placental insufficiency," and second, Preeclampsia/Eclampsia.

PLACENTAL INSUFFICIENCY

A large number of names have been applied to conditions believed to be occasioned by inadequacy of the otherwise normal placenta—Prematurity, Dysmaturity, Fetal retardation, Intrauterine growth retardation, Small for dates babies, Small for gestational age infants, etc.

Assali et al.[2] have stated that the term "placental insufficiency" has become "an umbrella used to cover our ignorance of the etiology and pathogenesis of chronic uteroplacental-fetal disturbances" and that it has also served as "a waste basket to dump a variety of disorders interfering with maternal supply of nutrients to the fetus or with fetal metabolism."

The first question, therefore, is: how close, in fact, is the association between small placentas and small babies? Statistical studies have shown that the association is not invariable. Small babies with small but otherwise normal placentas do indeed frequently occur, but small babies, on one hand, may have large placentas and, on the other, small placentas may be associated with good, big babies. One author suggests that when small babies and small placentas occur together it may be the small baby which conditions the small placenta rather than vice versa, an idea not without merit when one considers how large a part of the placenta is derived from fetal tissue. A related suggestion is that a single underlying genetic factor may be responsible for the size of both fetus and placenta. Findings in rhesus monkeys have relevance here. Some 80 percent of rhesus placentas are bidiscoid, but the single disc of the other 20 percent is no larger than the primary disc of bidiscoid placentas. It seems clear that the placenta has a

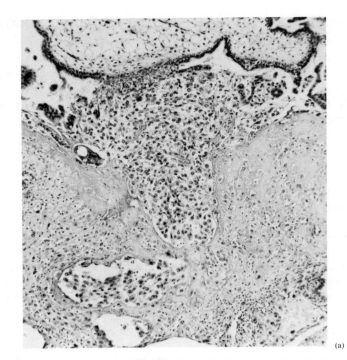

(a)

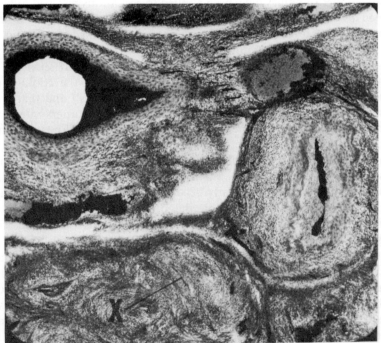

(b)

Fig. 3.

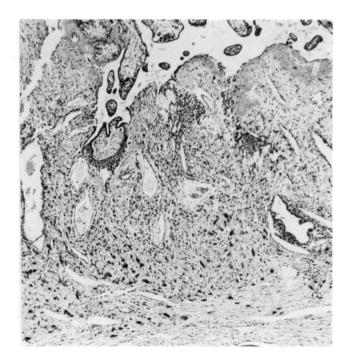

Fig. 3. Physiological changes in uteroplacental arteries. (a and c, Courtesy of the Department of Obstetrics and Gynecology, University of Virginia. b, Courtesy of the Carnegie Institution of Washington.)

a) Photomicrograph of a section made at the base of a human placenta at the 12th week of gestation. Cytotrophoblast forms a plug at the entry of a spiral artery to the intervillous space and progresses down the inner wall proximally. (U. of Va. No. 32-2)

b) Photomicrograph of a section made at the base of a monkey placenta on the 102nd day of pregnancy. In the artery on the left, above, there is replacement of the vessel wall by trophoblast; in that on the right, there is extensive fibrosis of the vessel wall. The artery at X is occluded by intrinsic vasoconstriction without wall change. (Carnegie Monkey No. 679)

c) Photomicrograph of a section of the placental base of a human pregnancy at the 17th week of gestation. There is extensive infiltration of endometrium and myometrium by trophoblastic giant cells. (U. of Va. No. 18-2)

wide margin of safety, and placental size, unless reduction is extreme, may not be the exclusive conditioning factor in production of "Small for Gestational Age" infants.

Currently, major attention is focused on other factors which may be responsible. Longo[8] has tabulated the possibilities as shown in Table 1. The author's own legend is included (italics are mine). Of special interest in the context of the present discussion are two categories: decreased area of

Table 1. **Factors that may cause small-for-gestational-age infants.** *Maternal and fetal factors are probably more common causes of this condition* than decreased transport or metabolism of trophoblast cells per se.

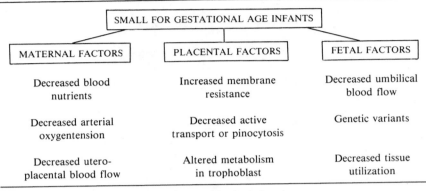

SMALL FOR GESTATIONAL AGE INFANTS		
MATERNAL FACTORS	PLACENTAL FACTORS	FETAL FACTORS
Decreased blood nutrients	Increased membrane resistance	Decreased umbilical blood flow
Decreased arterial oxygentension	Decreased active transport or pinocytosis	Genetic variants
Decreased utero-placental blood flow	Altered metabolism in trophoblast	Decreased tissue utilization

(From Longo. By courtesy of Dr. L. D. Longo and Academic Press.)

transport, and decreased uteroplacental blood flow. Three major conditions may bring about the former situation: 1) Fibrin deposition; 2) Infarction; 3) Abruption.

1. *Fibrin deposition.* In entirely normal placentas, a small amount of fibrin is deposited on the surface of a few chorionic villi. If, however, the amount is increased to the point where "disseminated intervillous fibrinosis" is the appropriate designation, it is clear that a barrier will be created mechanically preventing adequate exchange between maternal and fetal blood streams. The infant will then be adversely affected.

2. *Infarction.* Since the nutrition of the villi is derived from the maternal blood in the surrounding intervillous space, villous ischemia and necrosis will be the next stages if the foregoing process becomes aggravated, resulting in formation of placental infarcts. The infarcted areas will eventually become fibrosed if the pregnancy continues. Again, a few infarcts occur in most placentas, but a widespread area of tissue destruction will have serious consequences for the fetus. Placental infarction may also result from pathological changes in the uteroplacental arteries, as described below.

3. *Abruption.* The final morphological impairment of transfer is associated with abruptio placentae. A central separation usually entails rupture of afferent uteroplacental vessels, thus interrupting the supply of oxygenated, nutrient-rich blood to the fetus. This is particularly serious, quite apart from the maternal hemorrhage and premature delivery which may be associated. Separation at the placental margin predominantly af-

fects venous drainage channels, interrupting the flow of blood from which the fetus has already withdrawn the nutrient components. This venous blood is under less pressure than the hemorrhage from central arterial vessels and therefore dissects less widely. Thus marginal separation has less grave consequences for both mother and child.

The underlying uteroplacental pathology producing thrombosis and abruption was described by Hertig in 1945.[7] It consists of an endarteritis which may destroy the vessel walls, causing rupture, or may create occlusion of the lumen (Fig. 4). The two processes may occur simultaneously involving adjacent arteries at the placental base.

Decreased uteroplacental blood flow will of course result from the lesions described. The effect of such decreased blood flow upon placental growth has been demonstrated in animals: in sheep[5] by intraarterial injection of microspheres to create partial obstruction of the vessels; in monkeys,[15] dogs and several other nonprimate animals,[1] by controlled ligation of uterine arteries or the aorta itself. Recent studies in human patients

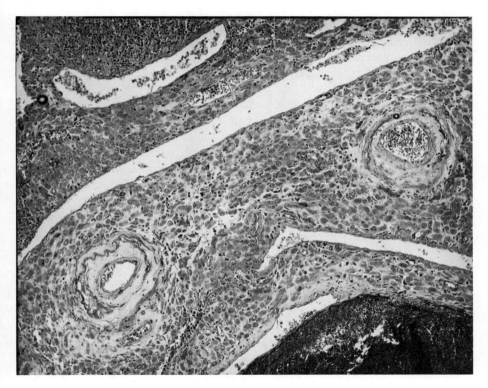

Fig. 4. Photomicrograph of human uteroplacental arteries showing marked endarteritis. (Courtesy of Dr. Arthur T. Hertig.)

extend the generalization to man,[12] the degree of fetal weight deficit reflecting the severity of the pathologic lesions.

PREECLAMPSIA/ECLAMPSIA

It has long been surmised that pathology of placental vessels forms the basis of preeclampsia/eclampsia. When Hertig reported the arterial lesions noted above, they were at once seized upon and implicated in the condition. However, although they do occur when preeclampsia complicates placental infarction or abruptio, they are not universally associated with it. In 1950 Zeek and Assali[16] demonstrated a lesion which is indeed consistently present in preeclampsia, namely, deposition of lipoid material in the smooth muscle of the arterial wall associated with infiltration of small round cells and macro-phages (Fig. 5). This lesion so closely resembles that of systemic atherosclerosis that Zeek and Assali christened it *atheroma.*

Two complicating features confuse the scene. First is the fact that hypertension is an integral part of the eclampsia syndrome and the effect of hypertension on blood vessels is well known. Hypertension without the clinical findings of eclampsia proteinuria, etc., does occur in pregnancy and the characteristic vascular changes occur,[11] actually in more acute form in uterine arteries than in systemic ones. However, in uncomplicated hypertension the lipid infiltration which is pathognomonic of preeclampsia/eclampsia is lacking.[4,12] The second confusing feature is the physiologic change in spiral arteries occurring in normal pregnancy, as described above. Before the recent establishment of this change as a normal process, the alteration in the vascular walls was understandably regarded as a pathologic development. Again the lack of lipid in muscle cells differentiates the normal process from the change exhibited by arteries in preeclampsia/eclampsia.

Robertson, Brosens and Dixon,[12] who with Sheppard and Bonnar[14] have been leaders in the study of human uteroplacental arteries in health and disease, find the distribution of the characteristic atheroma to be specific, involving arteries in which physiologic replacement of muscle and elastic tissue by trophoblast does not occur, i.e., in terminations of spiral arteries outside the placental base, in deep myometrial portions of placental bed spiral arteries, and in basal endometrial arteries. Moreover, they note that in preeclampsia/eclampsia the physiologic change extends less deeply into the placental spiral arteries than under normal conditions, penetrating only to the endometrial-myometrial junction. With muscle tissue remaining in the deeper portions of the stems, the vessels are candidates for atheroma formation, and they do in fact show this.

The effect of the atheromatous change, like that of Hertig's simple en-

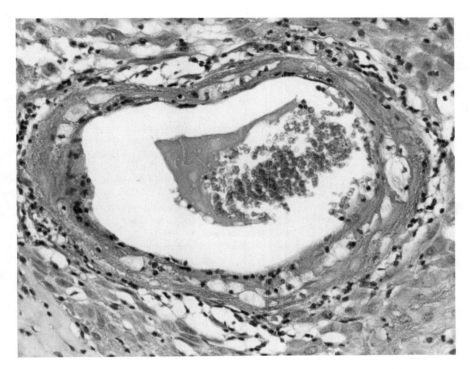

Fig. 5. 'Placental bed' biopsy; preeclampsia. Acute atherosis in a terminal segment of a spinal artery in the decidua vera. The necrotic wall contains vacuolated lipophages embedded in fibrinoid material and there are small mononuclear cells around the vessel. (From Robertson, Brosens and Dixon.[12] Courtesy of Dr. W. B. Robertson and the European Journal of Obstetrics and Gynecology and Reproductive Biology.)

darteritis, is to undermine the integrity of the vessel walls and produce varying amounts of obstruction to the lumen. Furthermore, on the basis of oxygen deprivation, tissue changes occur in the placenta itself, including degeneration of both cytotrophoblast and syncytium and of the walls of villous capillaries.[6] The usual deleterious sequelae result: decreased placental function, frequent infarction and varying degrees of fetal growth retardation.

It should be appreciated that the greater—if still seriously incomplete—knowledge of the uteroplacental vascular pathology in preeclampsia/eclampsia is not to be taken as revealing "the cause" of the syndrome, only of the mechanism by which the fetal retardation is produced. The vascular changes, like the renal lesions of eclampsia, etc., are themselves secondary to the unknown systemic factors initiating the condition.

REFERENCES

1. Abitol, M. M. Production of severe toxemia in the pregnant animal. Proc. 1st Congress of Internat. Soc. for Study of Hypertension in Pregnancy, M T Press Ltd., Lancaster, England. (In press)

2. Assali, N. S., B. Nuwayhid and C. R. Brinkman, III. Placental insuffiency, problems of etiology, diagnosis and management. *Eur. J. Obstet. Gynec. Reprod. Biol.* **5/1-2:** 87–91 and 121, 1975.

3. Brosens, I., W. B. Robertson and H. G. Dixon. The physiological response of the vessels of the placental bed to normal pregnancy. *J. Path. Bact.* **93:** 569–579, 1967.

4. Brosens, I., W. B. Robertson and H. G. Dixon. The role of the spiral arteries in the pathogenesis of preeclampsia. *Obst. Gynecol. Ann.,* pp. 177–191, 1972.

5. Creasy, R. K., C. T. Barrett et al. Experimental uterine growth retardation in the sheep. *Am. J. Obstet. Gynecol.* **112:** 566–573, 1972.

6. Fox, H. and C. J. P. Jones. Ultrastructure and ultrahistochemistry of the placenta in preeclampsia. Proc. 1st Congress of Internat. Soc. for Study of Hypertension in Pregnancy. M T Press Ltd., Lancaster, England. (In press).

7. Hertig, A. T. Vascular pathology in the hypertensive albuminuric toxemias of pregnancy. *Clin.* **4:** 602–614, 1945.

8. Longo, L. D. Disorders of placental transfer. *In*: Pathophysiology of Gestation. (N. S. Assali, Ed.) Academic Press, New York, Vol. II: 1–76, 1972.

9. Ramsey, E. M. and M. W. Donner. *Placental Vasculature and Circulation.* Georg Thieme Verlag, Stuttgart. (In press)

10. Ramsey, E. M., M. L. Houston and J. W. S. Harris. Interactions of the trophoblast and maternal tissues in three closely related primate species. *Am. J. Obstet. Gynecol.* **124:** 647–652, 1976.

11. Robertson, W. B., I. Brosens and H. G. Dixon. The pathological response of the vessels of the placental bed to hypertensive pregnancy. *J. Path. Bact.* **93:** 581–592, 1967.

12. Robertson, W. B., I. Brosens and G. Dixon. Uteroplacental vascular pathology. *Eur. J. Obstet. Gynec. Reprod. Biol.* **5/1-2:** 47–65, 1975.

13. Sheppard, B. L. and J. Bonnar. Uteroplacental arteries and hypertensive pregnancy. Proc. 1st Congress of Internat. Soc. for Study of Hypertension in Pregnancy. M T Press Ltd., Lancaster, England. (In press)

14. Sheppard, B. L. and J. Bonnar. The ultrastructure of the arterial supply of the human placenta in early and late pregnancy. *J. Obstet. Gynaecol. Brit. Commonw.* **81:** 497–511, 1974.

15. Wallenburg, H. C. S., L. A. M. Stolte and J. Janssens. Experimental infarcts in the placenta of the rhesus monkey. *Eur. J. Obstet. Gynec.* **1:** 25–33, 1971.

16. Zeek, P. M. and N. S. Assali. Vascular changes in the decidua associated with eclamptogenic toxemia of pregnancy. *Am. J. Clin. Path.* **20:** 1099–1109, 1950.

3

Cumulative Evidence Implicating Exogenous Progestogen/Estrogen In Birth Defects

JAMES J. NORA, M.D.

AND

AUDREY H. NORA, M.D.

This chapter summarizes the salient aspects of a recently completed study of five years' duration at the University of Colorado Medical Center on the possible role of progestogen/estrogen in the production of congenital malformations. In 1972, we were alerted to this potential problem by the simultaneous finding in two hospitals of two newborn infants who presented with a similar pattern of abnormalities including congenital heart disease (CHD), limb reduction and other skeletal anomalies. Maldevelopment of the gastrointestinal tract and genitourinary structures was also found. The similarity of these findings to those recognized in the thalidomide syndrome prompted us to believe that a teratogenic exposure could be responsible.

We did two preliminary case-control studies, one on patients with multiple malformations and one on patients with congenital heart disease who were already part of a long-term etiologic study.[1,2] Independently, Levy, Cohen and Fraser[3] reported a specific association between transposition

Supported by Contract NO 1–HD–4–2845 from the National Institute of Child Health and Human Development.

of the great arteries (TGA) and hormonal treatment. In the months that followed, our findings of limb reduction anomalies were confirmed by Janerich and co-workers[4] and by Hellstrom et al.[5] The pattern of multiple anomalies has been described by the acronym VACTERL (V = vertebral; A = anal; C = cardiac; T = tracheal; E = esophageal; R = renal; L = limb). Confirmation of the association of the VACTERL syndrome with first trimester exposure to progestogen/estrogen has come from several investigators, including Kaufman,[6] Balci et al.[7] and Buffoni and co-workers.[8] Oakley and associates could not detect a relationship between major malformations and maternal hormonal exposure.[9] They did not study heart defects in their preliminary investigation, but could find no increase in other single VACTERL anomalies, with the possible exception of esophageal atresia.

Subsequent reports regarding cardiovascular anomalies and maternal exposure to progestogen/estrogen in the first trimester have not been unanimous. Mulvihill et al.[10] and Yasuda and Miller[11] have been unable to confirm a specific association between transposition of the great arteries and hormonal exposure. Later reports of our ongoing studies[12,13] and those of other investigators[14] including the collaborative perinatal group[15,16] support the finding that various congenital heart defects (not limited to TGA) are associated with hormonal exposure. It should be noted here that the first clues to a cardiovascular-hormonal relationship in fetal maldevelopment may be traced to Mitchell et al.[17] who first reported "hormonal deficiency" in prospectively studied mothers who gave birth to infants with TGA. Methodologic differences and the smaller subset that TGA represents (as opposed to all congenital heart disease) may account for the failure, so far, to confirm the specific hormonal-TGA association reported by Levy et al.[3] and presaged by Mitchell and co-workers.[17]

The genitourinary system was the first in which maldevelopment was associated with maternal exposure to exogenous female hormones. Genital anomalies were reported by Wilkins[18] and subsequently by Aarskog[19] and our group.[20] Another early report of an association concerned the neural tube anomalies as described by Gal et al.[21] Laurence and co-workers could not confirm this.[22] We are not aware of any other isolated anomalies subjected to study for a maternal hormonal association, except as they may appear in two large prospective investigations, one in the United States[16] and one in France.[23] As noted earlier, the American collaborative perinatal study, involving 50,282 pregnancies, revealed a significant increase in exposure rate to exogenous female sex hormones in infants born with congenital heart lesions. No significant increase in exposure rate was found for other discrete anomalies. Patterns of anomalies were not studied. The French investigation encompassed 20,000 pregnancies (from which a subset of 7310 newborns were examined) and did not disclose an increase in hormonal exposure for any specific anomaly.

In this presentation we provide details of methodology with final results of our own investigation and relate our findings to the growing body of literature addressing this subject. We will try to answer two questions: Does maternal exposure to exogenous progestogen/estrogen during the first trimester of pregnancy represent a risk to the fetus? If there is a risk, how great is it?

SUBJECTS AND METHODS

Case Control Study 1-Multiple Anomalies. Thirty-two patients having three or more major anomalies of the VACTERL group were compared with control groups (to be described) for maternal exposure to progestogen/estrogen in the first trimester of pregnancy. For each of 16 VACTERL patients delivered before July 1, 1973,[20] two controls were chosen who were referred for evaluation of heart murmurs which were eventually demonstrated to be functional. Subjects from the two groups were matched as closely as possible for sex, date of birth, gestational age, race, socioeconomic level, area of residence, maternal age, and parity. In the VACTERL group, 11 patients were under one year of age when the history was obtained and five ranged in age from 17 months to 6 years. Eleven patients were male. The mean age for the group was 14.2 months, mean maternal age was 23.9 years, and mean parity was 2.1. Twelve patients were white, one black, and three Chicano. In the 18-month period from January 1, 1972 to June 30, 1973, twelve patients with this association were delivered in our referral area. Our control group of 32 patients consisted of 24 whites, two blacks and six Chicanos with a mean age of 14.6 months, a mean maternal age of 23.5 years and a mean parity of 2.3.

For 16 VACTERL patients (11 males) delivered from July 1, 1973 to June 30, 1977, we were unable to obtain enough controls with functional murmurs (perhaps reflecting improved diagnostic skill in the referral sector). Our two-for-one controls were most often patients with functional murmurs, but included normal subjects from the newborn nursery and well child clinic. Matching was also less exact, but an effort was made to conform to the earlier protocol. Matching for sex and approximate date of birth was the first priority. Thirteen VACTERL patients and 26 controls were white. Three from the experimental group and six controls were Chicano. The mean maternal age of the VACTERL group was 25.1 years, mean gravidity 2.06 and mean parity 1.7. In the control group the mean maternal age was 23.0 years, mean gravidity 2.25 and mean parity 1.88.

Fourteen of the 16 VACTERL patients were less than one year of age when the history was obtained.

To determine the relative importance of various anomalies in the VACTERL group as predictors of teratogenic exposures, particularly to progestogen/estrogen, other subsets of anomalies were studied. Data on thirty-nine patients with multiple anomalies and on children with discrete anomalies were collected without matching for comparison with the exposure rates in the multiple anomaly and congenital heart case-control studies.

All data were obtained by personal and detailed interviews of the mothers, conducted by trained interviewers, recorded on pre-printed forms designed for the study,[20] and analyzed using a standard chi-square 2x2 contingency format.

Case Control Studies 2 and 3—Congenital Heart Diseases.   From July 1, 1972 through June 30, 1977, 236 patients with a full variety of congenital heart lesions were studied. To reduce maternal memory bias all retrospective histories were obtained on patients less than one year of age. The first group of 60 patients was ascertained on our pediatric cardiology service and paired and matched one for one having patients with known single mutant gene and chromosomal disorders. Because the numerical limits of this genetic control group were exceeded by the numbers of patients with congenital heart lesions, a second control group was required for the remaining 176 patients. This control group consisted of infants chosen as part of our prospective cohort. Two control infants were matched with each congenital heart patient. Since these control histories were obtained prior to delivery, the possibility of interviewer bias was essentially eliminated. The physical status of the second group of control infants was assessed by chart review and personal examination.

The histories of all patients were obtained by personal interview of the mothers, following a specific protocol, recorded on pre-printed forms[12] and analyzed by the standard chi-square procedure. Matching was for sex, race, socioeconomic level, approximate date of birth, and area of residence. The limits of the period of cardiovascular development vulnerable to teratogenic influence was related to our knowledge of the completion of specific embryologic events. For example, a teratogenic event occurring after 34 days conceptional age would not be accepted as a cause of transposition of the great arteries, because trunco-conal septation is completed by that time.

Cohort Study.   From July 1, 1973 to December 31, 1976, in the antenatal care clinic of Colorado General Hospital, expectant mothers were interviewed by trained interviewers as early in their pregnancy as feasible. Additional interviews late in the pregnancy or in the immediate newborn period were accomplished in selected cases. The interviews followed a comprehensive protocol, were recorded on pre-printed forms,[20] and analyzed by the standard fourfold chi-square procedure. At the time of delivery of an infant whose mother received progestogen/estrogen in the first trimester of pregnancy, a control infant without such maternal exposure delivered during the same time period was selected. Pairing and matching for sex, race, gestational age, socioeconomic level, and area of residence was attempted within the limitations of being able to find such matches in infants born on the same day. The names of the patients were given to a participating physician to perform physical examinations without knowing which was the exposed infant and which was the control. If pairing and matching was not possible for at least sex, race and approximate gestational age, the newborn was removed from the study.

From the original prospective cohort of 143 consecutive patients with maternal exposure to hormones, 26 were eliminated for various reasons in order of frequency: failure to find a satisfactory control; lost to follow-up; physician denial; stillbirth; and inadequate or unverifiable data. The single blind requirement of the protocol (for physical examinations) did not provide enough patients for invariable matching of ethnic subgroups, socioeconomic level, maternal parity or gravidity. However, the overall characteristics of the experimental and control groups of the cohort study were similar to each other and to the groups in the three other studies from the population of our referral area. The mean maternal age in the experimental group was 24.6 years and in the control group 23.1 years.

RESULTS

Although our preliminary reports emphasized the highly tentative nature of our findings, there was a profound influence on the exposure rates in our area. Our study design for the definitive three-year segment of the investigation was based on the exposure rates being recorded in 1973. As Table 1 indicates, there was a precipitous decline in first-trimester exposure

Table 1. Prospective Maternal Hormone Exposure Rate by Year.

1973	1974	1975	1976
20/160	44/525	38/654	6/342
12.5%	8.3%	5.8%	1.75%

to female sex-hormones from 1973 through 1976. This made it impossible to achieve the number of cases we projected in our protocols, which required antenatal histories or pregnancy histories taken before the proband reached one year of age.

Case Control Study 1—Multiple Anomalies. Table 2 shows the 32 patients with VACTERL syndrome who were compared with controls (as previously defined) for maternal hormonal exposure in the first trimester. The anomalies present are signified by the letters of the acronym. For example, patient 6 had all the anomalies of the syndrome (VACTERL), whereas patient 7 had only anal, cardiac and limb anomalies (ACL). The first 16 patients were from 19 individuals ascertained before 1973. Of these, three were eliminated—the first two because they were index cases and one patient who had a chromosomal deletion (4p-). Patients 17 through 32 were ascertained over the four-year period from July 1, 1973 through June 30, 1977. The rate at which patients with this syndrome were encountered dropped from eight per year in 1972 to four per year during the subsequent years of the study.

Table 3 lists the exposures to teratogens which could be considered to be potentially significant. It is clear from these findings and from the literature that there are several potentially teratogenic agents including hydantoin, amphetamines, alcohol and Antabuse which may be found in association with the simultaneous presentation of three VACTERL anomalies. The most common agent, by far, is progestogen/estrogen. We have organized the data in several different ways: a combined group; as two separate groups, one ascertained prior to 1973 (when maternal progestogen/estrogen exposure was high in our population) and one ascertained in 1973 and after (Table 4). We also evaluated our definition of VACTERL and looked at patients with congenital heart disease plus only one other anomaly of the VACTERL group to see if this was as discriminating as three anomalies for hormone exposure. We made comparisons with congenital heart disease alone and congenital heart disease with another anomaly that was not of the VACTERL group. Finally, we made some noncontrolled comparisons with other abnormalities (Table 5).

Table 4 shows a highly significant difference (P < .001) when comparing VACTERL patients whose only known potentially teratogenic exposure was to progestogen/estrogen with unexposed controls. The estimated relative risk of acquiring VACTERL syndrome following maternal exposure to exogenous hormones is 8.41.

In Table 5, we looked at six different anomalies or patterns in relation to their predictive value for progestogen/estrogen exposure. They are displayed in descending order with the VACTERL syndrome being the

Table 2. Findings of Progestogen/Estrogen and Other
Teratogenic Exposure in VACTERL

PATIENT	DISORDER	PROGESTOGEN/ ESTROGEN OR PROGESTOGEN	OTHER POTENTIAL TERATOGENS	NO KNOWN TERATOGEN VULNERABLE PERIOD
1	VCTER	•••	+	•••
2	CERL (+)	+	•••	•••
3	ACL (+)	+	+	•••
4	ACRL	•••	•••	+
5	ACL	+	•••	•••
6	VACTERL (+)	+	•••	•••
7	ACL	+	•••	•••
8	ACR	•••	+	•••
9	VTEL (+)	+	•••	•••
10	ACL	•••	•••	+
11	VACTERL	•••	+	•••
12	VCL (+)	+	•••	•••
13	CRL	+	•••	•••
14	CTEL	+	•••	•••
15	VCTERL	+	+	•••
16	CTEL	•••	+	•••
17	VACTER (+)	+	•••	•••
18	VACR (+)	+	•••	•••
19	CTERL	+	•••	•••
20	CTERL *	+	•••	•••
21	CRL	+	•••	•••
22	CRL (+)	•••	+	•••
23	CRL (+)	•••	+	•••
24	VARL (+)	•••	+	•••
25	VCTE	•••	+	•••
26	VEL (+)	•••	•••	+
27	VTEL	•••	+	•••
28	VACR (+)	•••	+	•••
29	VCTEL(+)	•••	+	•••
30	CTERL (+)	•••	+	•••
31	VCR (+)	•••	+	•••
32	VTEL (+)	•••	•••	+

(+) = Additional anomalies.
* = 46,XX Karyotype with male phenotype.

Teratogenic exposure rate = 87.5%.
Progestogen/estrogen alone = 43%.

most discriminating. Congenital heart disease as a discrete anomaly appears to be less predictive than CHD plus one additional anomaly of the VACTERL group, but more predictive than CHD plus a non-VACTERL anomaly. One other point of interest is the neural tube defects, which will

Table 3. Frequency of Potential Teratogens in First Trimester in VACTERL Patients.

Progestogen / estrogen alone	13
Progestogen / estrogen plus other agents	2
Severe Infections alone	1
Severe Infection plus other agents	2
Hydantoin alone	1
Hydantoin plus other agents	2
Alcohol alone	1
Alcohol plus other agents	1
Antabuse alone	1
Dextroamphetamine alone	1
Thyroid alone	1
Thyroid plus other agents	1
X-ray plus other agents	2
Anesthetic gases alone	1

Table 4. Comparison of Patients with VACTERL Syndrome and Controls on the Basis of Exposure to Progestogen/ Estrogen Alone.

	PRE-1973	1973–1977	TOTAL	RELATIVE RISK (est.)
VACTERL	8/14 (57%)	5/16 (31%)	13/30 (43%)	8.41
Control	3/28 (11%)	2/32 (6%)	5/60 (8%)	
X^2	10.41	5.35	15.31	
p	< .005	.021	.001	

Table 5. Non-Controlled Comparison of Discrimination of Maternal Progestogen/Estrogen Exposure By Various Patterns and Abnormalities.

ABNORMALITY	HORMONES
VACTERL–3 anomalies (13/30)	43%
Congenital heart defects (45/236)	21%
Heart + 1 VACTERL anomaly (5/18)	28%
Heart + 1 non-VACTERL anomaly (2/21)	9%
Neural tube (5/24)	21%
Cleft lip with or without palate (1/8)	12.5%

be mentioned here as an ancillary, yet potentially interesting finding. We observed a high frequency of hormonal exposure in a small group of patients with neural tube defects (all spina bifida) who were not part of a case-control study.

Twenty-seven of the 32 patients with VACTERL syndrome had cardiovascular abnormalities—by far the most common anomaly in these infants. Fifteen of the 27 patients with heart lesions had more than one cardiac anomaly with ventricular septal defect (VSD) and atrial septal defect (ASD) being equally represented (nine patients each). Patent ductus arteriosus (PDA) was found in eight patients, dextroversion in four and total anomalous pulmonary venous return in three. No cases of transposition of the great arteries were encountered, but there were three patients with trunco-conal anomalies: one truncus arteriosus; one pseudotruncus (pulmonary atresia with ventricular septal defect); and one tetralogy of Fallot (TOF).

The reasons for hormone administration in the patients used in the case-control study were: pregnancy test in seven; threatened abortion in five; and various inadvertant administrations in three. All administrations contained synthetic progestogen or natural progesterone. Nine patients received additional estrogen. One additional patient had Clomid as the only known potential teratogen during pregnancy.

No Mendelizing disorders, such as Holt-Oram syndrome or Fanconi pancytopenia, or chromosomal anomalies were included in this group. A patient with a 4p- anomaly was one of three individuals eliminated from statistical analysis (the other two were index cases). Of the original 35 patients, 29 were karyotyped. The more common occurrence of limb reduction anomalies in males may relate to the observation that 22 of our 32 VACTERL patients were males.

Case-Control Studies 2 and 3—Congenital Heart Disease. Tables 6 and 7 summarize the findings in a study of patients under one year of age

Table 6. Case-Control Study 2.
Congenital Heart Patients Compared for Hormonal Exposure with Paired and Matched Genetic Controls.

EXPOSURE	HEART	CONTROL	X^2	p	RELATIVE RISK (EST.)
Progestogen/estrogen	14/60	3/60	8.3	.005	
Progestogen/estrogen alone	9/55	2/59	5.67	.017	5.58

Table 7.   Case-Control Study 3.
Congenital Heart Patients Compared for Hormonal Exposure
with 2 for 1 Paired and Matched Prospective Normals.

EXPOSURE	HEART	CONTROL	X^2	p	RELATIVE RISK (EST.)
Progestogen/estrogen	31/176	21/352	17.97	< .001	
Progestogen/estrogen alone	22/167	15/346	12.35	< .001	3.55

matched with controls as previously described. A total of 236 infants with congenital heart diseases were ascertained in the clinics and on the wards of Colorado General Hospital.

In the first group of 60, there were 14 whose mothers had verifiable exposure to progestogen/estrogen during early pregnancy in what was calculated to be a vulnerable period of cardiovascular development. In 3 or 60 controls with genetic diseases, there were similar histories. A p value of < .005 results from comparing these groups. In an effort to refine the study further, patients were eliminated from the heart and control groups who had known exposures to potential teratogens in addition to progestogen/estrogen. The numbers in the already small groups are further reduced, but a significant difference is still perceived (p = .021). The estimated relative risk of congenital heart disease following maternal hormonal exposure is 5.58 in this case-control study.

Larger numbers are provided in case-control study 3 in which two-for-one controls were obtained from prospective pregnancy histories. There were 31 of 176 congenital heart patients as compared with 21 of 352 controls in which there was a maternal hormonal exposure at the vulnerable period of cardiogenesis (p < .001). Eliminating cases from both the heart and control groups where there were known potential teratogens in addition to progestogen/estrogen also led to a comparison in which there was a highly significant difference (p < .001). The relative risk of congenital heart disease as estimated by the odds ratio is 3.55.

The distribution of cardiovascular anomalies in which there was maternal hormonal exposure was similar to that found on our service and in various heart registries. The most common lesions among these 45 patients were ventricular septal defect (VSD) in 14, atrial septal defect (ASD) in 10, and patent ductus arteriosus (PDA) in 9 patients. Trunco-conal malformations were slightly over-represented for transposition of the great arteries (4) and slightly under-represented for tetralogy of Fallot (3). Combinations of lesions were not as frequent as in the VACTERL group, but they were still common (15/45).

The reasons for hormone administration in these patients were as follows: pregnancy test (15); continued oral contraceptives after conception (15); threatened abortion (13); Clomid plus progestogen after conception (2). All exposures included synthetic progestogens or natural progesterone-alone (23), or in combination with estrogens or Clomid (22).

Cohort Study.   The dramatic decline in exposure rate during the definitive stage of the study permitted us to study the outcome of pregnancy in only 118 verifiable first-trimester exposures and their paired and matched controls. This provided considerably fewer patients than our protocol projected as required for tests of significance. In Table 8 are listed the major abnormalities found in the exposed and control groups. Eleven of 118 patients with histories of maternal hormonal exposure had major malformations compared to 4/118 in the control group. A total of 16 malformations were found in the 11 patients, including three malformations in one patient consistent with the definition of VACTERL. The numbers in both the treated and control groups are small and yield denominators of 0 in some cases, which prevents the projection of real numbers for relative risk. Relative risks were 6.00 for congenital heart disease and 2.75 for the occurrence of some major malformation in the offspring of a mother with an exposure to progestogen/estrogen in the vulnerable period of embryogenesis. The relative risk for congenital heart disease is comparable to that obtained by odds-ratio estimates from the retrospective study.

Although McNemar's chi-square was suitable for the paired design, the numbers were too small (at least for cardiac and other discrete malformations) to make this the preferable significance test. A standard fourfold

Table 8. 118 Prospective Hormone Exposures with Controls.

ABNORMALITY	HORMONE	CONTROL	X^2	p	RELATIVE RISK
Cardiac	6	1	3.68	.005	6.00
Neurological	4	0			
Skeletal	3	1			
Anal atresia	1	0			
Renal	1	0			
Vertebral	1	0			
Inguinal hernia	0	2			
Total abnormalities	16	4			
Total patients with abnormalities	11	4	3.49	.062	2.75

contingency table format yielded chi-squares of 3.68 (p = .055) for cardiovascular anomalies and 3.49 (p = .062) for patients with major abnormalities. The types of cardiovascular anomalies in the treated group were: one newborn with total anomalous pulmonary venous return, pulmonary stenosis and PDA. This patient died in the early postoperative period. Another newborn had a successful ligation of a PDA. One infant has a PDA which has not required surgical intervention. Three babies were diagnosed as having VSD alone (one case), or in combination with other lesions (one with PDA and one with ASD).

An excess of neurological abnormalities was evident in the treated group: one patient had hydrocephalus plus seizures; one had seizures alone; one, developmental delay with oculomotor apraxia and bilateral clonus; and one with severe developmental delay alone.

DISCUSSION

It is estimated that approximately 8.5 million women are taking contraceptive hormones in the United States. We do not know if the decline in exposure rate to hormones during pregnancy is national or more peculiar to our referral area. However, a projection based on data from 1973 would show that there is an exposure to progestogen/estrogen during the vulnerable period of embryogenesis in 300,000 pregnancies per year.

Is it possible to demonstrate with a high degree of confidence the presence or absence of teratogenic effect if the suspected agent is common, poorly recorded and produces only a small increase in malformations? This epidemiologic problem may apply to many agents in addition to progestogen/estrogen. The solution is not merely an academic exercise, but one of considerable importance if we are to make a significant impact on the reduction of the majority of common birth defects. In the past we have looked at and commented on such problems as maternal memory bias, "priming," dating exposures, verifying esposures and using records and interviews in data collection.[24] We have concluded that: mailed questionnaires are of very limited value; hospital records are frequently counterproductive; maternal memory bias greatly diminishes the validity of pregnancy histories taken when the proband is over one year of age; the way a question is asked markedly influences the answer; 40 per cent of prescriptions written for patients are not filled at all, and an additional 20 per cent are not taken at the time prescribed; and prescription medications are frequently taken by persons other than those for whom they were prescribed. We have come to agree with Doll that the "hazards of the first nine months are an epidemiologist's nightmare."[25]

Histories of exposure to oral contraceptives and hormonal pregnancy tests add further epidemiologic problems. For some reason women do not regard The Pill and oral hormonal pregnancy tests as "drugs," or as being comparable agents. Questions regarding these drugs must be very specific. Medications "to prevent miscarriage" are also seldom equated with The Pill. There is rarely a chart record of prescriptions of oral contraceptives (if there is a prescription), and the relationship of the prescription to the actual use of the drug is as poor or poorer than for other drugs. Add to these problems the difficulties in knowing when conception occurs while taking The Pill, breakthroughs, thinning endometrium, menstrual irregularities, spotting and the standard instructions to continue taking The Pill through a missed period and you have obstacles sufficient to derail the most carefully planned studies.

Unusual Patterns and Rare Anomalies.

The investigator who seeks to implicate a teratogen is greatly assisted in his task if the teratogen produces a rare anomaly or unusual pattern of anomalies. It is difficult to start with a common malformation such as patent ductus arteriosus and search for environmental triggers. If the PDA is accompanied by cataracts and deafness (as in rubella syndrome) or by phocomelia (as in the thalidomide syndrome), the search is much more likely to be successful.

This is the reason for investigating the VACTERL syndrome. Serious maldevelopment of simultaneously developing structures should point to a profound insult. Thalidomide caused a pattern of anomalies that would be consistent with our definition of VACTERL syndrome today. Certain of the more common chromosomal aberrations malform structures in the VACTERL group (but do not often produce a comparable pattern). Other uncommon chromosomal anomalies produce what could be diagnosed as VACTERL syndrome. Some Mendelizing disorders, such as Holt-Oram, Roberts, and Fanconi syndromes, may often have two features of the VACTERL syndrome, but are usually discriminated by other findings. The frequency of the VACTERL syndrome has been estimated to be about 1:3500.[26]

A teratogenic insult proved to be the most common association with the VACTERL syndrome. Histories of maternal exposure to alcohol and hydantoin are found in cases of VACTERL syndrome, but progestogen/estrogen is far more common. We have therefore concluded that the association of hormonal exposure with this unusual pattern of anomalies—a Baconian exception—provides the strongest etiologic evidence we are likely to get from retrospective studies. The statistical differences are highly significant. It might also be noteworthy that reports of this association of anomalies began to appear in the literature in the 1960's[27-30] when use of oral contraceptives and hormonal pregnancy tests became widespread. We may also see a downward trend nationally in the frequency rate of VACTERL syndrome with decreasing hormonal exposure during pregnancy, if our recent experience in Denver is an indicator.

So far, a search for rare *single* anomalies has provided equivocal results. Hormonal association with limb reduction anomalies has been supported in two series[4, 5] and discounted in two series.[9, 31] Reports of the four series did not specify whether or not their protocols called for separate analysis of limb reductions as single anomalies versus limb reductions as part of a pattern of anomalies. The difference in results may be attributable to design. Our experience is that limb reduction anomalies, as single abnormalities, do not correlate as well with hormonal exposure as they do as part of the VACTERL syndrome.

The investigation of transposition of the great arteries, as a relatively rare anomaly associated with hormonal exposure, has not been as useful as was hoped. Levy and co-workers[3] found an association which could not be confirmed by Mulvihill et al.[10] and Yasuda and Miller.[11] In our preliminary report we felt that there was an excess of cases of trunco-conal abnormalities which we have attributed, in part, to the very early exposure in embryogenesis that usually occurs with progestogen/estrogen. Our subsequent studies do not reveal a clear excess of trunco-conal anomalies. What may be relevant to later investigations of this relationship is that we have been experiencing a significant decline in TGA in our referral area during the past three years. Anecdotally, other pediatric cardiology centers are discussing similar declines. The number of cases of TGA is simply not sufficient to analyze. One would like to believe that there is a specific relationship between hormonal exposure and TGA and that the decline in cases reflects a decline in exposure rate to exogenous sex hormones. Unfortunately, we do not have data to do more than speculate about this possibility. We also do not have data to reach conclusions about the possible relationship of "hormonal deficiency"[17] to TGA.

The contribution of progestogen/estrogen taken within three months of conception was looked at in this context in our prospective cases. Two patients with major malformations were found in 120 such exposures (one PDA and one microcephaly). This does not exceed expectation.

Garden-Variety Lesions.

There is an immediate handicap when one selects common abnormalities to study teratogenesis. The possible advantage to the use of congenital heart diseases as a category is that they seem to be the most common single lesions associated with progestogen/estrogen exposure—and are the only single anomalies confirmed by the U.S. collaborative perinatal study as being associated with hormonal exposure.[16,31] Enough cases with well-matched controls were accumulated in our investigation to give us confidence in our data. The statistical results are highly significant. We do not have enough patients in other categories of malformations to answer questions about risks for other single lesions. The other singly occurring abnormality of clinical, if not statistical, concern from our data is neurologic disease. From both retrospective data (Table 3) and prospective data (Table 8), there appears to be an over-representation of neural tube and neurologic disorders—more consistent with the findings of Gal et al.,[21] than with Laurence and co-workers.[22]

Prospective Evidence.

Caution dictates that a call be made for more data. The large U.S. perinatal prospective study[16] was not designed for specific and detailed exploration of the hormonal-malformation association. It covered an intake period from 1958 to 1965, and is thus not representative of recent exposure rates or dosages of medications. These authors have also called for more data. The prospective French study,[23] which spans the years 1963 to 1969, is hard to interpret. The cohort of approximately 7200 newborns examined is relatively small and the malformation rates for the entire study are much lower than are comparable data from the United States. The overall malformation rate is 1.6 per cent (as opposed to 3 per cent) and the frequency of congenital heart disease is 0.3 per cent (as opposed to $\approx$ 1 per cent). The exposure rate to exogenous sex hormones is so low that very little case material is produced. We have also conducted a historical cohort study of 10,600 charts and found such enormous misclassification bias due to under-reporting that we could place no confidence in the findings.

Our small cohort investigation of 118 pairs is specific, controlled and recent, but we have too few cases to satisfy the study design. Our experience during the last six months of the study led us to project that it would take at least 18 months to ascertain enough patients to detect a fourfold increase in malformations at a .05 significance level, and that a twofold increase would not likely be detected in the foreseeable future. However, prudence requires that in the absence of projected numbers, we recognize the biologic significance of the data as opposed to the statistical significance. A modest conclusion which may be reached is that two of three prospective studies provide evidence consistent with an association between maternal exposure to exogenous female hormones and congenital heart disease. One prospective study does not. A twofold to fourfold range of increase in congenital heart defects may be projected by combining the two positive prospective studies.

An additional conclusion is that the weight of evidence from various types of studies, conducted by several groups, supports an association.[1-8, 12-21, 32] We feel that although our preliminary data and the preliminary data of other groups had to be offered and accepted with considerable caution, the evidence is now strong enough to pursue a more aggressive course of recommendations concerning progestogen/estrogen exposures during pregnancy. A twofold to fourfold increase in malformations resulting from exposure to an agent complicating a few hundred pregnancies per year is inconsequential in an epidemiologic sense. However, if the agent produces 300,000 exposures per year (as we projected for sex hormones from earlier data), as little as a twofold increase in risk for congenital heart disease would yield 3000 newborns per year with cardiac anomalies—more than any other precisely defined cause. During the past two decades, there has been a reported increase in incidence of congenital heart diseases from 0.3 percent to approximately 1 percent. This should not be dismissed as merely reflecting changes in ascertainment and diagnostic acumen when environmental teratogens have yet to be ruled out.

The Food and Drug Administration has taken the position that there is no justification for using progestogen/estrogen in threatened abortion or as a pregnancy test. This would eliminate most hormonal exposures in our own series. The Nader Health Research group contends that there has been no recent decline in hormone prescriptions specifically for threatened abortion.[33] From the number of communications we receive from malpractice attorneys, a frightening trend is becoming apparent. Our group and others are only beginning to arrive at confident decisions regarding the possible teratogenicity of these agents—and these decisions are fraught with pitfalls. However, our legal colleagues are prepared to follow rules of evidence that would establish teratogenesis through passionate litigation, rather than through dispassionate investigation.

The prudent physician will do well to adhere to the FDA guidelines abrogating progestogen/estrogen in threatened abortion and pregnancy testing. A next step would be an educational campaign promoting all reasonable precautions to avoid inadvertent hormonal exposures during pregnancy and for avoiding pregnancy within three months of terminating oral contraceptives. There will continue to be some unavoidable and accidental exposures at our present level of technology. However, the experience in the Denver referral area suggests that exposures may be dramatically reduced.

REFERENCES

1. Nora, J. J. and Nora, A. H. Oral contraceptives and birth defects. Preliminary evidence for a possible association. (Abstract) *Ped. Res.* **7**: 321, 1973.
2. Nora, J. J. and Nora, A. H. Birth defects and oral contraceptives. *Lancet* **1**: 941–942, 1973.
3. Levy, E. P., Cohen, A. and Fraser, F. C. Hormone treatment during pregnancy and congenital heart defects. *Lancet* **1**: 611, 1973.
4. Janerich, D. T., Piper, J. M. and Glebatis, D. M. Oral contraceptives and limb-reduction defects. *New Engl. J. Med.* **291**: 697–700, 1974.
5. Hellstrom, B., Lindsten, J. and Nilsson, K. Prenatal sex-hormone exposure and congenital limb reduction anomalies. *Lancet* **2**: 372–373, 1976.
6. Kaufman, R. L. Birth defects and oral contraceptives. *Lancet* **1**: 1396, 1973.
7. Balci, S., Say, B., et al. Birth defects and oral contraceptives. *Lancet* **2**: 1098, 1973.
8. Buffoni, L., Tarateta, A. and Pecordri, D. VACTERL. *Min. Gin.* **28**: 382–384, 1976.
9. Oakley, G. P., Flynt, J. W. and Falek, A. Hormonal pregnancy tests and congenital malformations. *Lancet* **2**: 256–257, 1973.
10. Mulvihill, J. J., Mulvihill, C. G. and Neill, C. A. Congenital heart defects and prenatal sex hormones. *Lancet* **1**: 1168, 1974.
11. Yasuda, M. and Miller, J. R. Prenatal exposure to oral contraceptives and transposition of the great vessels in man. *Teratology* **12**: 239–243, 1975.
12. Nora, J. J. and Nora, A. H. Genetic and environmental factors in the etiology of congenital heart diseases. *South. Med. J.* **69**: 919–926, 1976.
13. Nora, J. J. and Nora, A. H. Contraceptive hormones and congenital heart disease. *Teratology* **15**: 331, 1977.
14. Harlap, S., Prywes, R. and Davies, A. M. Birth defects and estrogens and progesterones in pregnancy. *Lancet* **1**: 682–683, 1975.
15. Hook, E. B., Heinonen, O. P. et al. Maternal exposure to oral contraceptives and other female sex hormones: relation to birth defects in a prospectively ascertained cohort of 50,282 pregnancies. (Abstract) *Teratology* **9**: A21, 1974.
16. Heinonen, O. P., Slone, D. et al. Cardiovascular birth defects and antenatal exposure to female sex hormones. *New Engl. J. Med.* **296**: 67–70, 1977.
17. Mitchell, S. C., Sellman, E. H. and Westphal, M. C. Etiologic correlates in a study of congenital heart disease. *Am. J. Cardiol.* **28**: 653–657, 1971.
18. Wilkins, L. Masculinization of female fetus due to use of orally given progestins. *JAMA* **172**: 1028–1031, 1960.
19. Aarskog, D. Intersex changes masquerading as simple hypospadias. Birth Defects: Original Article Series VII, No. **6**: 122–130, 1971.
20. Nora, A. H. and Nora, J. J. A syndrome of multiple congenital anomalies associated with teratogenic exposure. *Arch. Environ. Health* **30**: 17–21, 1975.
21. Gal, I., Kirman, B. and Stern, J. Hormonal pregnancy tests and congenital malformations. *Nature* **216**: 83, 1967.
22. Laurence, M., Miller, M. et al. Hormonal pregnancy tests and neural tube malformations. *Nature* **233**: 495–496, 1971.
23. Spira, N. Goujard, J., et al. Etude du role teratogene des hormone sexuelles. *C. Rev. Med. Fr.* **12**: 2683–2694, 1972.
24. Nora, J. J. and Fraser, F. C. Medical Genetics: Principles and Practice. Philadelphia, Lea & Febiger, 1974, pp. 275–286.
25. Doll, R. Hazards of the first nine months: an epidemiologist's nightmare. *J. Irish Med. Assoc.* **66**: 117–126, 1973.

26. Corcoran, R. and Entwistle, G. D. VACTERL congenital malformations and the male fetus. *Lancet* **2:** 981–982, 1975.
27. Kirkpatrick, J. A., Wagner, J. L. and Pilling, G. P. A complex of anomalies associated with tracheoesophageal fistula and esophageal atresia. *Am. J. Roentgenol.* **95:** 208–211, 1965.
28. Harris, L. C. and Osborne, W. P. Congenital absence or hypoplasia of the radius and ventricular septum. Ventriculo-radial dysplasia. *J. Pediat.* **68:** 265–272, 1966.
29. Say, B. and Gerald, P. S. A new polydactyly/imperforate anus/vertebral anomalies syndrome. *Lancet* **2:** 688, 1968.
30. Quan, L. and Smith, D. W. The VATER association. *J. Pediat.* **82:** 104–107, 1973.
31. Heinonen, O. P., Slone, D. and Shapiro, S. Birth Defects and Drugs in Pregnancy. Littleton, Mass., Publishing Sciences Group, 1977, pp. 93–108.
32. Nora, J. J. Nora, A. H. et al. Congenital abnormalities and first trimester exposure to progestogen/estrogen. *Lancet* **1:** 313–314, 1976.
33. Wolfe, S. Personal communication.

4

Antenatal Diagnosis

THEODORE KUSHNICK, M.D.

The indications for antenatal diagnosis have been expanding rapidly, as outlined in Table 1. Thus studies are performed for chromosomal abnormalities in the fetus on five bases; for metabolic diseases in increasing numbers of individually rare biochemical disorders; for neural tube defects, which are now approaching the point of being detected in most pregnancies because of increasing sensitivity of maternal serum alpha-fetoprotein tests; for the few but still existent severe erythroblastosis fetalis fetuses of Rh negative mothers; and increasingly, for those syndromes and defects which have eluded chromosomal or biochemical detection. For the latter group, there is greater sophistication in the use of ultrasonographic and x-ray techniques and fetoscopy.

At present, the most frequent indication for antenatal studies is still detection of fetal chromosome abnormality for reasons of advanced parental ages. However, antenatal diagnostic studies do include techniques and methods other than amniocentesis for cytogenetic evaluation. The other approaches to prenatal diagnosis will be discussed from the aspect of tests proceeding from the least to the most invasive method.

Table 1. Indications for Antenatal Diagnosis.

CHROMOSOMAL ABNORMALITY

1. Advanced parental age
2. Translocation chromosome carrier parent
3. Parent with mosaic cell line
4. Previous chromosomally abnormal child—any parental age
5. Previous chromosomally abnormal abortus—any parental age

METABOLIC DISEASES

1. In mother—detectable and/or treated
2. Both parents known carriers
3. Mother known or suspected carrier of X-link disease
4. Previous affected child—same parents

NEURAL TUBE DEFECTS

1. Previous affected child
2. Positive maternal serum α-fetoprotein X 2

RH ERYTHROBLASTOSIS FETALIS, SEVERE

DEFECTS WITHOUT AMNIOCENTESIS TEST MARKERS

1. Skeletal dysplasias
2. Specific syndromes

ANTENATAL DIAGNOSIS FROM MATERNAL SPECIMENS

As indicated in Table 2, much information can be derived regarding risks to the fetus from tests performed on maternal blood and urine samples. The determination of maternal Rh type and anti-Rh levels for possible erythroblastosis fetalis complications, and the maternal Rubella antibody titer for immune status has become virtually routine in most obstetric practice. The mother's blood phenylalanine levels can be a warning of ongoing damage to the fetus because of hyperphenylalaninemia or, by detecting a childhood-treated maternal phenylketonuria, who should resume her diet for pregnancy.

Maternal serum alpha-fetoprotein determinations for every pregnancy are on the verge of becoming a reality. This technique would enable the obstetrician to detect most first occurrences of neural tube defect in a family.[2] Approximately 90 percent of anencephalic fetuses and 80 percent of those with spina bifida can be detected with a "fine-tuned" maternal serum test. Although it was originally believed that 3 percent of all pregnancies would require amniocentesis for two positive maternal serum alpha-feto-

Table 2. Antenatal Diagnosis—Maternal Specimens.

Blood
Rh type, antibodies
Phenylalanine
Rubella titer
α-fetoprotein

Grandmother & mother: CPK, pyruvate kinase, $LDH_{4,5}$ ratio, (electromyography, muscle biopsy)

Grandmother & mother: AHG clotting activity/antigen ratio, procoagulant factor VIII antigen

Other serologic titers
Urine
Reducing substances
Methylmalonic acid
Estriol
Pregnanetriol

protein values, subsequent large-scale evaluation demonstrated that only 1.7 percent of the pregnancies yielded two positive tests. After ultrasonography and other evaluation, however, only 0.63 percent of the total group studied required amniocentesis, with a resultant 46 percent exhibiting neural tube defects.

Evaluations for X-linked recessive disease carrier states for progressive muscular dystrophy and hemophilia A can demonstrate, with 90 percent accuracy, whether or not the mother is a carrier. The recent development of an immunoradiometric assay for procoagulant factor VIII antigen has raised the possibility of in utero testing of male fetuses for hemophilia A.[7]

Maternal urine testing offers a simple screening technique for maternal galactosemia with its possible requirement for reduced galactose in the maternal diet to avoid fetal cataract formation. Basically, a urine which is positive for reducing substances by clinitest but specifically negative for glucose would lead to a presumptive diagnosis of galactosemia. Methylmalonic acidemia, although a rare disease, can be followed in pregnancies subsequent to the birth of an afflicted infant. Maternal urine will reflect increasing amounts of methylmalonic acid by virtue of its transfer from the fetus to the mother. Indeed, it is possible to follow the beneficial results of in utero therapy by giving the mother intramuscular vitamin B_{12} during the later months of pregnancy, producing a decrease in the amount of methylmalonic acid excreted in maternal urine.

Urine estriol and pregnanetriol determinations are of value late in pregnancy for determinations of possible anencephaly and recurrence of adrenogenital syndrome. There is no early antenatal diagnosis for the latter condition, although one amniotic fluid determination was reported to show elevated pregnanetriol by the 20th week of gestation.

ULTRASONOGRAPHY

A single session of ultrasonographic evaluation can provide extensive data concerning the fetus, as illustrated in Table 3. This procedure can also serve as a guide for subsequent amniocentesis and/or fetoscopy. Serial ultrasonographic evaluations can elicit information regarding the rate of fetal growth and be reassuring in regard to a normal pregnancy.

X-RAY EXAMINATION

Roentgenographic examination, like ultrasonography, is a safe non-invasive technique for evaluating the fetus, as long as there is a limitation on the number of x-rays taken. By the 16th to 20th week of gestation, the fetus has sufficient calcification of the skull, vertebrae, long bones and ribs to provide radiopacity. By the 20th to 23rd week, the pelvis is calcified. As outlined in Table 4, detection of syndromes involving these bones becomes feasible in the mid-trimester. However, x-ray examination is unsatisfactory for evaluating syndromes involving hands and feet, e.g., in polydactylism or absence of thumbs.

Roentgenographic examination is unsatisfactory for achondroplasia unless it is the rare form which is inherited as an autosomal recessive gene or is homozygous for a double dose of the autosomal dominant gene. The more common heterozygous autosomal dominant form does not offer sufficient long bone change so that it can be detected during mid-pregnancy. The bones that are calcified offer sufficient data to permit diagnosis of

Table 3. Ultrasonography.

Single
Twins
Gestational age
Anencephaly
Hydrocephalus
Large myelomeningocele
Polycystic kidneys
Lack of urine
Poly- and oligohydramnios
Limb motions
Guide for: amniocentesis, fetoscopy
Serial
Normal growth rates

Table 4. X-Ray Examination.

Indications at:
1. 16–20 weeks—skull, long bones, vertebrae, ribs
2. 20–23 weeks—above plus pelvis

Unsatisfactory for:
1. Hands
2. Feet
3. Polydactyly

Detects:
1. Achondroplasia—autosomal recessive and homozygous autosomal dominant only
2. Short-rib syndromes
3. Vertebral-rib dysplasias
4. Anencephaly
5. Autosomal recessive osteogenesis imperfecta fractures

Amniography:
1. Encephalocele
2. Myelomeningocele
3. ? Swallowing disorders
4. Diaphragmatic hernia
5. Some G.I. obstructions

short rib syndromes such as Saldino-Noonan[8]; vertebral and rib dysplasias such as Jarcho-Levin syndrome[4]; absence of skull as in anencephaly; and the autosomal recessive form of osteogenesis imperfecta by virtue of the fractures of the long bones. Osteogenesis imperfecta of the tarda type does not cause early fractures and thus is not amenable to antenatal diagnosis.

The instillation of lipid and water-soluble radiopaque dyes into the amniotic fluid has been used to demonstrate abnormalities reflected as body surface changes, e.g., myelomeningocele; subsequent swallowing of the material by the fetus permits the diagnosis of specific gastrointestinal diseases.

AMNIOCENTESIS

As outlined in Table 5, amniocentesis offers the possibility of detecting many conditions for which there are biochemical or cellular markers. The procedure is best performed at the 16th week of gestation in order to provide the maximum amount of cell growth on culture. For those conditions in which the sex chromosome constitution must be determined for X-linked recessive disease, amniocentesis can be performed at the 14th or 15th week of gestation (preferably the latter). The earlier timing is necessary to permit fetoscopy if fetal blood specimens are to be obtained from a male fetus.

Table 5. Amniocentesis.

Fluid
1. α-fetoprotein
2. Enzymes - unreliable
3. Chemical products—unreliable
4. Lu-ABH secretor—myotonic dystrophy linkage
5. *Late* pregnancy—erythroblastosis fetalis, pulmonary surfactant, adrenogenital syndrome

Direct Cell Exam
1. X and Y—unreliable
2. Some metabolic diseases—for glycogenosis II, electron-microscopy
3. Enzyme determination—require cultivation for certainty
4. Viral isolation

Cell Culture
1. Chromosomes
2. Sex determination
3. Abnormal cultured cell appearance = neural tube defects
4. Metabolic-enzyme tests
5. Linkage—G6PD for hemophilia A
6. α-Thalassemias—DNAs for molecular hybridization

? Breakage and Mitosis Rates
1. Radiation, chemicals, viruses, etc.

Fluid

As indicated, the amniotic fluid alpha-fetoprotein is an accurate determinant for anencephaly, a large leaking spina bifida, omphalocele, congenital nephrotic syndrome of the autosomal recessive type, scalp and other skin defects, early fetal demise and possibly, ataxia-telangiectasia. For reliability, most biochemical tests require cultivation of the cells for subsequent enzymatic analysis. In certain families at risk for myotonic dystrophy, the Lutheran or Lewis blood group ABH secretor status of the fetus is such that myotonic dystrophy can be detected by virtue of the linkage of these separate genes. Amniotic fluid examination in late pregnancy can offer assistance with regard to the severity of erythroblastosis fetalis, lung maturity of the fetus, etc.

Cells

Direct cell examination is not reliable for sex differentiation of the fetus. It can be utilized for a few biochemical disorders, e.g., the use of electron microscopy of cells for glycogenosis type II. The isolation of viruses from the cell pellet does not resolve the question of whether or not the viral infection is localized to the placenta or has spread to the fetus.

Cell Culture

As defined in Table 5, diagnostic accuracy is excellent following culture of amniotic fluid cells, regarding cytogenetic aspects, sex determination, or detection of metabolic errors. The appearance of the cells on culture, as well as their rapid adherence to the culture flask, can be an early warning signal regarding neural tube defects, if previously undetected.[3]

Attempts have been made to detect an affected male fetus with hemophilia from the hemophilia A gene's close location to the glucose-6-phosphate dehydrogenase gene on the X chromosome. Such a technique is quite valid in the black race where there is a high frequency of G6PD polymorphism which allows for differentiation of AB, A, or B type in the mother and the previously affected hemophiliac.[1] For example, in families with an affected G6PD-A hemophiliac child, G6PD typing of the fetus' cells can permit detection of subsequent G6PD-A affected fetuses, or non-affected G6PD-B fetuses, if the mother is G6PD-AB.

The recent development of DNA molecular hybridization techniques permits diagnosis of alpha thalassemia from cultured *amniotic* cells, without resorting to fetoscopy to obtain fetal *blood* specimens.[6]

Laboratory investigations are ongoing with respect to chromosomal breakage and mitosis rates after exposure of the fetus to radiation, chemicals, viruses, etc. Basically, it is necessary to establish the normal breakage and mitosis rates in order to determine if there is an increase after such environmental exposure; and to correlate pregnancy outcome with any such chromosomal changes.

FETOSCOPY

As indicated in Table 6, fetoscopy has been utilized mainly to obtain fetal blood specimens by placental venepuncture and to examine the microanatomy of the fetus. "Blind" placental blood aspirations carry the risk of causing abortions. However, placental vein aspiration for small quantities of blood permits detection of the hemoglobinopathies without such risks. Creatine phosphokinase determination done on the fetal blood specimen can detect a male with progressive muscular dystrophy. There is hope for a technique to detect hemophiliac males in the near future.[7]

Physical examination of the fetus allows those syndromes involving the digits, nails, abnormal facies, and some dermatologic syndromes to be diagnosed. Visualization of the digits may demonstrate polydactyly syndromes; conditions with absent thumbs; those with nail dysplasias; and ectrodactyly.[5] Skin biopsy for a "harlequin" fetus is feasible.

Fetoscopy has also raised the possibility of future intrauterine intravenous treatments.

Table 6. Fetoscopy.

Blood Tests
1. Hemoglobinopathies—SS, α and β Th, SC
2. CPK - Progressive muscular dystrophy $\left.\right\}$ If XY chromosome
3. ? Procoagulant factor VIII - hemophilia A
Physical Examination
1. Digits, nails, facies, skin
2. Polydactyly syndromes
3. Ectrodactyly
4. Absent thumbs, digit syndromes
5. Dermatologic syndromes—gross
Skin Biopsy
1. "Harlequin" fetus
Future
1. ? I.V. therapy

REFERENCES

1. Edgell, C-J. S., Kirkman, H. N. et al. Prenatal diagnosis by linkage: Hemophilia A and polymorphic glucose-6-phosphate dehydrogenase. *Am. J. Hum. Genet.* **30:** 80, 1978.
2. Ferguson-Smith, M. D., Rawlinson, H. A. et al. Avoidance of anencephalic and spina bifida births by maternal serum alpha-fetoprotein screening. *Lancet* **1:** 1330, 1978.
3. Gosden, C. M. and Brock, B. J. H. Morphology of rapidly adhering cells as an aid to the diagnoses of neural tube defects. *Lancet* **1:** 919, 1977.
4. Kushnick, T. and Filkins, K. Prenatal diagnosis of fetal skeletal normalcy after previous Jarcho-Levin syndrome. Abstr. 10th Natl. Found.—MOD Birth Defects Conf., San Francisco, Cal., June 12–14, 1978, p. 145.
5. Mahoney, M. J. Fetoscopy in the prenatal diagnosis of anomalies. Presented at 10th Natl. Found.—MOD Birth Defect Conf., San Francisco, Cal., June 12-14, 1978.
6. Orkin, S. H., Alter, B. P. et al. Application of endonuclease mapping to the analysis and prenatal diagnosis of thalassemias caused by globin-gene deletion. *New Engl. J. Med.* **299:** 166, 1978.
7. Peake, I. R. and Bloom, A. L. Immunoradiometric assay of procoagulant factor-VIII antigen in plasma and serum and its reduction in haemophilia. *Lancet* **1:** 473, 1978.
8. Richardson, N. M. Beaudet, A. L. et al. Prenatal diagnosis of recurrence of Saldino-Noonan dwarfism. *J. Pediatr.* **91:** 467, 1977.

RECOMMENDED READING

1. Crandall, B. F. Lebherz, T. B. et al. Neural tube defects: Maternal serum screening and prenatal diagnosis. *Ped. Clin. N. Amer.* **25 (3):** 619, 1978.
2. Miles, J. H. and Kaback, M. M. Prenatal diagnosis of hereditary disorders. *Ped. Clin. N. Amer.* **25 (3):** 593, 1978.

5

Clinical Pregnancy Test

WILLIAM J. HARTKO, M.D.

AND

JAMES R. JONES, M.D.

The search for a reliable method of confirming pregnancy extends far back into mankind's past. Four thousand years ago the Egyptians were taking advantage of the large amounts of estrogen contained in the urine of pregnant women, and of its ability to cause accelerated germination in grain seed, to verify pregnancy. Since then, many "tests" have been used, most of which possessed serious shortcomings. In the last fifty years, however, greater success has been achieved, primarily by taking advantage of the biological properties of a placental glycoprotein hormone, human chorionic gonadotropin (hCG). HCG is produced in a relatively predictable pattern in normal pregnancy, and occasionally in other conditions. Outlined in the following chapter are the techniques involved in several currently used tests, not in a manner to enable the reader to begin to perform a radioimmunoassay or radioreceptor assay at his or her hospital, or to "rate" various commercial varieties of any testing modality, but rather in an effort to define the capabilities of these tests to help care for women in their gynecological and obstetrical needs.

Tests which have receded from current clinical use will be ignored or touched on only briefly. Our emphasis will be on the newer tools available to us[1]: the radioimmunoassay and radioreceptor assay. The immunologic tests, both direct and agglutination inhibition, have been extensively compared and references are readily available.[2-7] Pregnancy testing today has reached a level of sophistication by which pregnancy can be diagnosed accurately even before the time of the first missed period, and the "quality" of a pregnancy can be investigated.

HUMAN CHORIONIC GONADOTROPIN (hCG)

Because most of the commonly used tests to detect pregnancy are based on the presence of hCG, let us first discuss this hormone.

Human chorionic gonadotropin is one of four major glycoprotein hormones in the human. The other three are: follicle-stimulating hormone (FSH), luteinizing hormone (LH), and thyroid-stimulating hormone (TSH). Each of these hormones possesses a similar quaternary structure with two dissimilar polypeptide chains which are designated as α and ß-subunits. For each of the four glycoproteins, the α chains are structurally and immunologically identical. In recombination experiments, the α chain from one hormone may be substituted into any of the other glycoproteins without obvious biologic or immunologic effect. Neither the α nor the ß-subunit is biologically active by itself, activity being a property of the combined subunits. The nature of that activity, both biologically and immunologically, is therefore determined by the specific ß-subunit. The ß-subunits, not unexpectedly, are quite dissimilar in their amino acid sequence and content. A further discussion of the activity of the other three glycoproteins is beyond the scope of this presentation.

The occurrence of hCG in nature is dependent on its production and secretion by trophoblastic cells during pregnancy. Characteristically, hCG production begins quite early in the course of a pregnancy: soon after, or perhaps at the time of, implantation of the blastocyst.[8-10] Human chorionic gonadotropin can be detected in maternal plasma about 9 to 11 days after ovulation, or 3 to 5 days before missed period. Thereafter, as is shown in Fig. 1, hCG rises rapidly, peaking between 56 and 68 days after conception and then slowly decreases, reaching its nadir at about 126 days. Afterwards, it remains stable at a low level until the termination of placental function (delivery of the placenta). This "plateau" level of hCG in the latter part of pregnancy may be less than the amount of hCG detectable by some of the agglutination inhibition pregnancy tests (slide test). The rapid rise in hCG in early pregnancy is related to the rapid increase in the number of trophoblastic cells.[11] At present there are no known classical "controls" over the secretion of hCG. It does not appear to function in either a positive or negative feedback system.

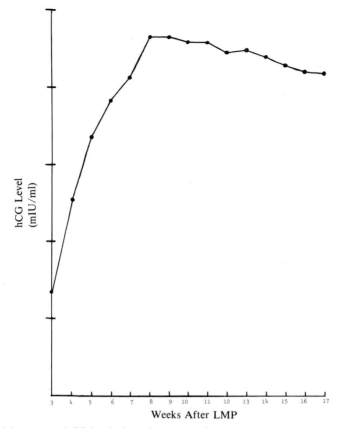

Fig. 1. Mean serum hCG levels throughout normal pregnancy.

The physiological role of hCG is incompletely understood at this time. It is believed that early secretion of hCG is necessary to maintain a functional corpus luteum, until estrogens and progestins required for the maintenance of pregnancy are produced in sufficient quantities by the fetoplacental unit.

Recent studies suggest that hCG may be involved in protecting the fetus from immunologic attack by the mother. The response of maternal lymphocytes to challenge by fetal lymphocytes in mixed lymphocyte culture is markedly reduced by the addition of hCG to the cultures. The possibility exists that the high local tissue concentrations of hCG in the placenta and uterine placental site may suppress the sensitization of maternal lymphocytes exposed to fetal antigen, thus protecting the fetus from immunologic rejection.[12]

The rapid rise in hCG in early pregnancy is probably responsible for the concomitant marked rise in circulating testosterone (and dihydrotestosterone) found in male fetuses.[13] This rise in androgens, limited to the male fetus, is responsible for internal and external virilization.

A number of investigations have detected the "inappropriate" presence of hCG in a number of benign and malignant conditions.[14] The hCG found in these circumstances may be either of the normal hCG structure or of some altered form.[15]

Concentrations of hCG are usually reported in International Units (I.U.) or milli International Units (mIU). When measured in urine the unit is usually I.U./liter; in blood, mIU/ml. Although, there is a tendency to report in metric units (nanograms, picograms, etc.) we shall, in this chapter, continue to use the International Unit system.

ASSAY PROCEDURE

Biological

The first reliable pregnancy test was developed by Asheim and Zondek in 1927.[16] Like most of the tests that followed, it took advantage of the presence of hCG in the urine or serum of pregnant patients to trigger a reaction in a test system. Their test system was the mouse, and the reaction was biological: the formation of hemorrhagic follicles in the ovaries of the immature mice. Other investigators employed other species and looked at other reactions, but the principle was the same. While the bioassays were quite precise they had several drawbacks.[17] They required large numbers of animals with storage space and personnel to care for them, technicians to purify the urine that was to be injected into the test animals, and several days of "incubation." These tests also required rather large amounts of hCG, and thus a firm diagnosis of pregnancy could not be established until 25 to 35 days after the time of ovulation. An exquisite attention to detail was required throughout the entire procedure and frequently this was not within the usual operating capacity of hospital laboratories. For these reasons, the biologic pregnancy tests have disappeared from clinical use. Because of their precision they are still used in laboratories to validate some of the newer pregnancy tests.

Immunologic

The appearance of the immunologic pregnancy tests in the early 1960's provided significant major advantages over the biologic pregnancy tests. Among these advantages was a much shorter incubation period and the ability to do away with the large stores of laboratory animals. In general, the immunologic tests have a much higher index of reproducibility and are therefore more reliable clinically. The immunologic tests are of two types: direct agglutination and the agglutination inhibition tests. Of the two tests, the latter is used more commonly. The techniques are outlined in Figs. 2 and 3. Briefly, the agglutination inhibition test (Fig. 2) begins with an antiserum to hCG (anti-hCG) being added to a sample of urine of serum. If present, hCG will bind to it an antibody-antigen combination and the anti-hCG will become unavailable for further reactions. If hCG is not present, the anti-hCG will exist unencumbered in the solution. Next, if a carrier substance (e.g., sheep RBC's or latex particles) which has been coated with hCG is added to the solution, the free anti-hCG will cause an agglutination of the hCG-coated carrier. If the patient is pregnant, however, the anti-hCG would already be bound and unable to cause agglutination. In the agglutination inhibition pregnancy tests, absence of agglutination indicates the presence of hCG and therefore a pregnancy.

In the direct agglutination tests (Fig. 3) the carrier substance is coated directly with anti-hCG. Therefore, if hCG is present in the sample, agglutination will occur. Thus in the direct agglutination test, the presence of agglutination signals pregnancy.

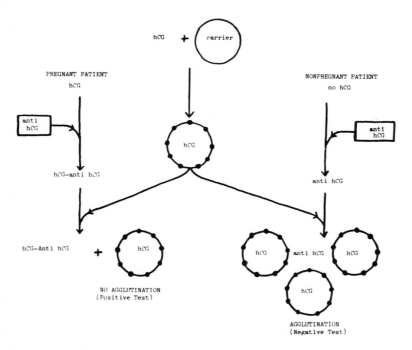

Fig. 2. Agglutination inhibition pregnancy test (see text).

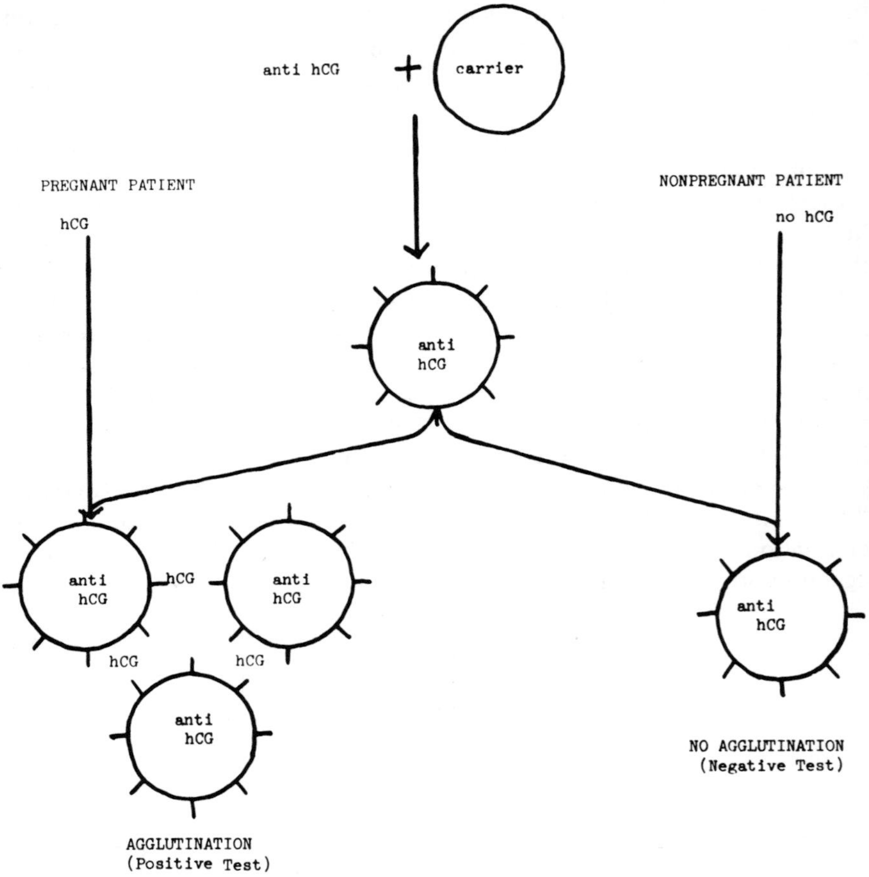

Fig. 3. Direct agglutination pregnancy test (see text).

The above-described immunologic tests are usually carried out on urine samples. They cannot distinguish between whole molecules of hCG and LH. This cross-reactivity limits the clinical usefulness of the direct agglutination and agglutination inhibition tests. In order to avoid confusion with LH, both test systems are "set" at a level of detectability (mIU/ml urine) that is beyond the level of the usual maximal LH surge.

This "high setting" renders these tests unreliable when "negative" in very early pregnancy. Another problem related to the cross-reactivity of hCG and LH is found in the "perimenopausal" patient. In this circumstance, care must be taken to distinguish between the elevated LH levels associated with ovarian failure and the hCG increases of early pregnancy.

Quantitation of the amount of detectable hCG in the immunologic tests is possible by varying the dilution of the test samples, but this is not a common practice at this time.

As a general rule, in the "slide" agglutination inhibition test the carrier consists of latex particles. The test usually requires one to three minutes to perform, and has a relatively high "threshold." This means that the test becomes positive relatively late, and that it may be negative in the 2nd and 3rd trimesters and in abnormally developing pregnancies. The direct agglutination slide test is comparable, but with a lower threshold.

The "tube" agglutination inhibition test usually has red blood cells as the carrier substance, takes about two hours to perform, and has a lower threshold (Table 1).

Radioimmunoassay

The radioimmunoassay (RIA) for hCG represents a major advance in our ability to diagnose and assess the quality of a pregnancy. Its usefulness spans almost the entire spectrum of obstetrical and gynecological practice from reproductive endocrinology to perinatology to oncology. RIA as ap-

Table 1.   Commercially Available Immunologic Pregnancy Test.

AGGLUTINATION INHIBITION	SENSITIVITY
A. Slide Test	(mIU/ml urine)
Pregnosticon Dri-Dot (Organon)	1500
Pregnosticon (Organon)	1500
Pregnosis (Roche)	1500
UCG (Wampole)	2000
Gest State (Lederle)	3000
Gravindex (Ortho)	3500
B. Tube Test	
Pregnosticon Accuspheres (Organon)	750
Pregnosticon (Organon)	750
Placentex (Roche)	1000
UCG-hypotest (Wampole)	1000
UCG-(Wampole)	1000
Gravindex Tube (Ortho)	500
DIRECT AGGLUTINATION	
Slide test	
DAP-(Wampole)	2000

plied to hCG was first reported in 1964[18] and a more refined procedure was described by Odell et al. in 1967.[19]

The technique takes advantage of the ability of an antibody to bind specifically to a given antigen, and it can be described briefly as follows: First, a highly purified form of hCG must be available. A portion of the hCG is iodinated with radioactive iodine (^{125}I or ^{131}I). Another portion of the hCG is to be used in preparing a standard (hCG). The final portion is used to produce antibody to hCG in an experimental animal. This antibody can be designated Ab•1. Using Ab•1 a second antibody, Ab•2, is then produced in a different species of experimental animal. Ab•2 is therefore directed against the Ab•1 initially produced. Thus, if Ab•1 is anti-hCG, the Ab•2 is anti (anti-hCG). With these two antibodies (Ab•1 and Ab•2), the purified (hCG) and the labled hCG (hCG*), the procedure itself can begin.

The first step in the RIA is the construction of a standard curve.

To a suitably buffered and stabilized solution, a fixed amount of labled hCG (hCG*) is added. A number of different solutions are then prepared by the addition of varying known amounts of standard hCG. To each of these various concentrations is then added a fixed amount of Ab•1. These solutions are allowed to incubate for fixed lengths of time (usually 36 to 72 hours). As a general rule, shortening the incubation period tends to decrease the sensitivity of the procedure. After incubation each solution contains a mixture of antibody-bound and unbound hCG and hCG* and no excess antibody.

The reaction can be described as:

(1) hCG+hCG*+Ab•1→hCG+hCG*+(hCG−Ab•1)+(hCG*−Ab•1)

Thus each standard solution contains hCG, hCG*, hCG − Ab•1, hCG* − Ab•1. Since both the hCG* and Ab•1 were added in known amounts, then hCG/hCG* is proportional to hCG − Ab•1/hCG* − Ab•1. At this point the second antibody is added and further incubation permitted.

This second reaction can be described as:

(2) hCG + hCG* + (hCG − Ab•1) + (hCG* − Ab − 1) + Ab•2 → hCG + hCG* + (hCG − Ab•1 − Ab•2) + (hCG* − Ab•1 − Ab•2)

These large antigen-antibody complexes (hCG − Ab•1 − Ab•2 and hCG* − Ab•1 − Ab•2) are separated from the solution by centrifugation. The radioactivity in the double antibody bound (heavier fraction) is then counted. A graph can then be constructed showing the relationship of radioactivity in the removed "large complex" portion versus the amount of radioactivity initially added to the solution. This can be described by an equation, B/Bo × 100%, where B is the number of counts found in the "large complex" portion, and Bo is the number of counts added to the solution initially (Fig. 4). Thus, as the amount of hCG in the solution increases, the amount of hCG* that can be bound into the large antibody complexes decreases. The amount of hCG in any solution is found to be inversely proportional to the amount of bound hCG*. It is then obvious that as the amount of hCG in any solution is increased, the radioactivity in the separated large antibody complex portion will decrease. The plot of (B/Bo × 100%) against the log dose of hCG standard added produces a sigmoidal curve in which the central region approaches linearity. The data thus accumulated can be manipulated in a variety of mathematical ways so that, with unknown samples, B/Bo can be determined and the amount of contained hCG can be calculated from the standard curve.

A major modification of this technique was reported by Vaitukaites and co-workers.[20] Because the α chains of both hCG and LH are indentical, and the ß chains are similar (much more so than FSH and TSH), the radioimmunoassay directed against whole molecule hCG does not adequately discriminate between hCG and LH. Thus the whole molecule hCG radioimmunoassay measures both hCG and LH. In certain circumstances

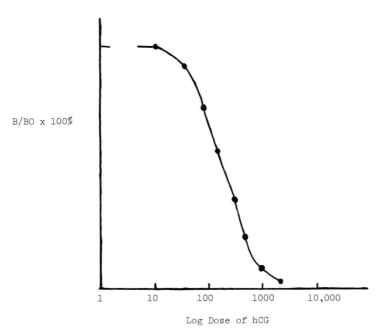

Fig. 4. Semi-logarithmic plot of B/Bo x 100% versus concentration of hCG (standard curve).

(the midcycle LH surge, in treated trophoblastic disease, etc.) this overlapping can lead to error. By extracting highly purified hCG ß-subunit, it is possible to create antisera directed specifically against the ß-subunit. Therefore the usual radioimmunoassay techniques can be performed to identify the ß-subunit which largely eliminates cross-reaction with LH. This allows greater specificity and enables the detection of very small amounts of hCG. Because of these advantages, and the comparable effort required, the ß-subunit hCG has become the test commonly performed.

Radio Receptor Assay (RRA)

The newest advance in the diagnosis of pregnancy has been the radioreceptor assay (RRA). This technique was first developed to identify estrogen and ACTH[21,22] and was soon adapted for use in the determination of human chorionic gonadotropin and luteinizing hormone.[23-25] This test is based on the presence of gonadotropin receptors within the ovaries of humans (and other species) which specifically bind hCG and LH. Like the radioimmunoassay directed against whole molecule hCG, the RRA does not differentiate between hCG and LH. Unlike the RIA, and RRA is not determined by the immunologic or structural properties of hCG, but by its *in vitro* biological activity. Conditions may exist, at least in the laboratory, where a molecule of hCG can be altered so as to yield a negative result on RRA, but still maintain enough of its structure to maintain its immunologic character and result in a positive RIA. This difference was noted as early as 1964 by Paul and Odell[18] in their pioneering work on the RIA and may have some ultimate importance in assessing changes associated with neoplastic processes.

The first step in the RRA for hCG/LH is the preparation of a standard curve. To a series of solutions that have been properly buffered and stabilized, a fixed amount of radioactive labeled hCG(hCG*) is added as well as a fixed amount of receptor membrane (typically derived from bovine corpora lutea), and various amounts of standard hCG. These solutions are allowed to incubate for a *short* period of time (15 to 30 minutes) after which each solution contains receptor membranes to which both hCG and hCG* have become bound in accordance with the principles of competitive binding. That is to say, the amount of bound hCG* and hCG is proportional to their relative concentration initially. The solution is then centrifuged and the heavier membrane fragments are collected. The radioactivity of the membrane fragments in each solution is recorded, and a graph is constructed plotting the known amount of standard hCG added against the radioactivity. To determine the hCG level of an unknown sample, the same procedure is followed and when the amount of residual radioactivity is determined, it is inserted into the standard curve and the amount of endogenous hCG is determined. The entire procedure can be completed in one hour, making the RRA equivalent to that of the immumologic pregnancy test in performance time, but with a sensitivity equal to that of the RIA. The disadvantage of the RRA is that it requires the use of a gamma counter and a technician trained in radioisotope techniques.

In both the RRA and the RIA, there is added a standard amount of plasma containing basal levels of LH and other plasma proteins. This is done to minimize the actions of the substances in the determination of hCG.

The radioreceptor assay has recently been modified and marketed as a commercial kit (Biocept-G, Wampole Labs). This kit provides an abbreviated version of the above procedure which compares an unknown sample to a standard. This allows a qualitative determination of hCG (the standard is "set" so that levels of hCG above 200 mIU/ml are detected by the test), so that a "yes or no" determination of pregnancy can be made.

The primary function of these tests is to detect the presence of pregnancy, and at the appropriate time, each of them is quite effective as can be seen in Table 2. The RIA and RRA become positive sooner and remain positive longer, but are more involved and more expensive than the immunologic tests which are quite satisfactory at the time of usual clinical interest, i.e. the weeks between the first and third missed periods.

However, both the RIA and RRA have been found useful in the screening of patients for early induced abortion. Using a modified RIA with only a 2-hour incubation period, Kosasa et al.[26] were able to identify hCG in 33 patients out of a sample of 51 at the time of menstrual extraction (mini abortion). Histological examination confirmed intrauterine pregnancy in

Table 2. Comparison of Currently Available Pregnancy Test Methods.

	SENSITIVITY (mIU/ml)	CROSS REACTION WITH LH	MINIMAL TIME FOR CLINICAL RELIABILITY (days after ovulation)
Bioassay	1,000	yes	25–35
Immunologic	500–3500	yes	25
Radioimmuno Assay hCG	1	yes	6–9
ß-subunit	1	no	6–9
Radioreceptor Assay	1	yes	6–8

Modified from: Landesman, R. and B. B. Saxena, Fert. Steril. **27**: 357, 1976.

29 of the 33 cases. Three of the remaining four patients had very early pregnancies which were not removed by menstrual extraction. The remaining patient had an ectopic pregnancy.[26] Roy and associates report almost equal success with the radioreceptor assay.[27] Thus the use of either of these procedures at a time when the immunologic pregnancy tests are still unreliable may obviate an elective surgical procedure which has risks, minor though they may be. The cost of the assay is only a small portion of the cost of an abortion procedure, and thereby constitutes an economic saving.

Another function for these tests is also apparent from the above reports. Both of these tests, especially the RRA because of its shorter incubation period, may be helpful in the diagnosis of ectopic pregnancy. The immunologic pregnancy tests are positive in only 50 to 73 percent of patients with ectopic pregnancy.[28,29] In contrast, in their extensively reported work using the radioreceptor assay, Saxena and Landesman[30,31] reached the conclusion that "two negative RRAs performed on subsequent days virtually excluded the diagnosis of ectopic pregnancy." In fact, it is a rare instance in which an ectopic pregnancy is not detected by RRA, and in those cases, the trophoblastic tissue had become fibrotic and presumably ceased to function.[32] This last statement refers to the quantitative RRA; the qualitative test with a false negative rate of 10.6 percent[33] is not as reliable as the quantitative RRA. In a patient with a compatible history and physical examination, a positive RRA may be the impetus for surgical intervention at a point prior to rupture of the fallopian tube.

Similar results have been obtained with the ß-subunit RIA.[17] Using either the ß-subunit RIA or RRA, an interesting observation has been made; in those patients with fertilized ova in whom the assay is performed prior to the first missed period, maternal hCG levels are detectable within a rather predictable range. Beyond this point patients displayed two patterns of hCG secretion; the majority showing increasing ("normal") concentrations, and a smaller subset with lower levels. The latter group tended to end in spontaneous abortions. The implication is that most pregnancies destined to abort will show deterioration, at least with respect to hCG, at some point after the implantation. When the question of the abnormal pregnancy was explored further, these tests functioned as early placental function tests. Using the RIA for hCG, Braunstein and co-workers[17] were able to predict almost 60 percent of pregnancies which would end in a first or second trimester abortion. In a smaller group, Saxena and Landesman, using the RRA were also able to predict most of the patients who would encounter difficulties. In those patients who were to abort late in pregnancy, they were able to demonstrate a change from values in the normal range to values which either decreased or plateaued in an abnormal range. Conversely, in several patients initially judged to be at risk for abortion, the hCG values were found to return to the normal range and these patients did not abort. This raises the possibility that patients at risk could be screened periodically and those at increased risk could be identified and treated.

Another area in which screening of the obstetrical population might be of significant benefit is in multiple pregnancy. When screening is carried out beyond the time of the missed menses (Fig. 5) the range of values of

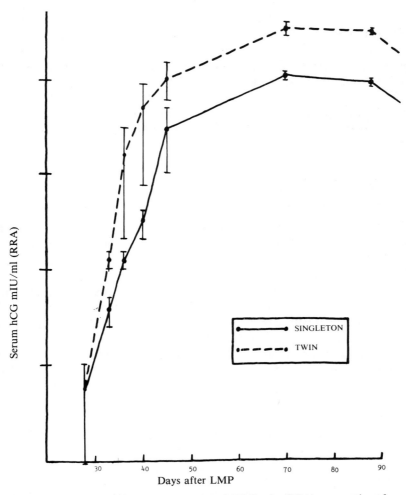

Fig. 5. Semi-logarithmic plot of mean serum hCG levels (RRA) versus time from last menstrual period (LMP) in singleton and twin pregnancies. The vertical lines indicate the observed ranges.

hCG for singleton and twin pregnancies do not overlap.[31,33] Presumably an abnormally developing twin pregnancy might not be so easily separable from a singleton pregnancy, and trophoblastic disease might mimic a multiple gestation. However, the RRA could serve to select those patients who would have the multiple gestation confirmed by ultrasonography later in the pregnancy, thereby allowing truly prospective studies of methods of reducing the morbidity of multiple gestations.

Finally, quantitation of gonadotropin hormone associated with trophoblastic neoplasms is of documented usefulness. Hammond and associates[34] have shown that patients can be separated into high and low risk groups based on a number of factors, one of which is an initial gonadotropin level greater than 100,000 IU/L of urine. Decisions regarding changes in chemotherapy often relate to the rate at which gonadotropin levels are falling on existing therapy. Boyko and Russell[35] have recently evaluated the benefits of both RIA for ß-subunit and the RRA and found them to be equivalent in most instances except at very low hCG titers. Because the RRA is easier and quicker, they have recommended this test for routine follow-up of patient with trophoblastic disease.

ON THE HORIZON

This chapter has discussed only those techniques which were of clinical importance and thus has been limited to a discussion of pregnancy tests based on the appearance of hCG. Although no test based on other pregnancy-related-substances has any clinical importance, there are several areas currently under investigation.

The most widely investigated substance is Pregnancy Specific ß, Glycoprotein (PSß,G) which can be measured by radioimmunoassay and does not cross-react with LH.[36] In their report, Grudzinskas and colleagues specifically address the question of whether PSß,G offers any value as a pregnancy test. Its time of appearance in the blood is very similar to that of hCG; however, it appears in the urine relatively late, and therefore does not seem to offer any specific advantage over the hCG-based pregnancy tests. A major possible application, suggested by the authors and by others,[37] is the development of an early pregnancy abortifacient. Unlike anti-hCG substances tested for their abortifacient properties, an anti-PSß,G presumably would not interfere with the menstrual cycle by disturbing LH levels.

Another more promising test involves a poorly described substance known as "early pregnancy factor" (EPF). This substance has been found to inhibit rosette formation by the lymphocytes.[38] This ability of the serum of pregnant women to alter lymphocytic function *in vitro* may well be an important clue to understanding why a woman immunologically tolerates the presence of the fetus. This effect has been found in mice within hours after fertilization. In very limited experience with human subjects, there seems to be a comparably rapid response. This raises the possibility that pregnancy might be diagnosed within days or even hours of fertilization. The activity of EPF appears to be independent of hCG, although hCG has a similar action on the lymphocytes. While much work remains to be done, possible applications are apparent.

Another area of investigation involves the salivary enzyme N-acetyl-ß-D-glucosaminidase. Rosado et al. have shown a characteristic pattern of activity coincident with ovulation with a secondary rise 10 to 12 days later which is absent in those patients who have become pregnant.[39] There are a number of serious problems that remain to be evaluated in this procedure and it does not have any immediate application as a clinical pregnancy test. Its value may lie in its association with ovulation as a guide to periodic abstinence to prevent pregnancy.

REFERENCES

1. Harwick, D. F. (Ed.) Early Diagnosis of Pregnancy, An Invitational Symposium. *J Reprod. Med.* **12:** 1, 1974.
2. Porres, J. M., D'Ambra, L. et al. Comparison of eight kits for the diagnosis of pregnancy. *Am. J. Clin. Path.* **64:** 452, 1975.
3. Kerber, I. J., Inclan, A. P. et al. Immunologic test for pregnancy. *Obstet. Gynecol.* **36:** 37, 1970.
4. *Medical Letter.* **17:** 6–7, Jan. 17, 1975.
5. *Medical Letter.* **7:** 31–32, 1965.
6. Lau, H. L., Linkins, S. E. and King, T. M. A capillary tube pregnancy test. *Am. J. Obstet. Gynecol.* **127:** 349, 1977.
7. Lang, L., Reiss, A. M. et al. A new more sensitive tube test for pregnancy evaluated with a selected hospital population. *Am. J. Obstet. Gynecol.* **126:** 693, 1976.
8. Hogden, G. D., Tullner, W. W. et al. Specific radioimmunoassay of chorionic gonadotropins during implantation in Rhesus monkeys. *J. Clin. Endocr. Metab.* **35:** 457, 1974.
9. Saxena, B. B., Hansen, S. H. et al. Radioreceptor assay of human chrorionic gonadotropin: Detection in early pregnancy. *Science* **184:** 793, 1974.
10. Braunstein, G. D., Rasor, J. et al. Serum human chorionic gonadotropin levels throughout normal pregnancy. *Am. J. Obstet. Gynecol.* **126:** 678, 1976.
11. Braunstein, G. D., Grodin, J. M. et al. Secretory rates of human chorionic gonadotropins by normal trophoblast. *Am. J. Obstet. Gynecol.* **115:** 447, 1973.
12. Adcock, E. W., Teasdale, T. et al. Human chorionic gonadotropin: its possible role in maternal lymphocyte suppression. *Science* **181:** 845, 1973.
13. Reyes, F. I., Winter, J. S. D. et al. Gonadotropic-gonadal interrelationship in the fetus.

In Diabetes and Other Endocrine Disorders During Pregnancy and in the Newborn. (New, M. I. and Fiser, R. H. (Eds.) New York, Alan R. Less, 1976.

14. Editorial. Ubiquitous human chorionic gonadotropins? *Lancet* **2**: 1116, 1977.

15. Vaitukates, J. L. Immunologic and physical characterization of human chorionic gonadotropin (HCG) secreted by tumors. *J. Clin. Endocr. Metab.* **37**: 505, 1973.

16. Editorial. *J. Reprod. Med.* **12**: 1, 1974.

17. Braunstein, G. D., Karow, W. G. et al. First trimester chorionic gonadotropin measurement as an aid in the diagnosis of early pregnancy. *Am. J. Obstet. Gynecol.* **131**: 25, 1978.

18. Paul, W. E. and Odell, W. D. Radiation inactivation of the immunological & biological activities of human chorionic gonadotropin. *Nature (London)* **203**: 979, 1964.

19. Odell, W. D., Ross, G. T. and Rayford, P. C. Radioimmunoassay for luteinizing hormone in human plasma or serum: Physiological studies. *J. Clin. Invest.* **46**: 248, 1967.

20. Vaitukaites, J. L., Braunstein, G. D. and Ross, G. T. A radioimmunoassay which specifically measures human chorionic gonadotropin in the presence of human luteinizing hormone. *Am. J. Obstet. Gynecol.* **113**: 751, 1976.

21. Koreman, S. G., Tulchinsky, D. and Eaton, L. W. *In* Diczfalusy, E. (Ed.) Steroid Assay by Protein Binding. Stockholm, 1970, p. 291.

22. Lefkowitz, R., Roth, J. and Pastein, I. Radioreceptor assay of adrenocorticotropic hormone: new approach to assay of polypeptide hormones in serum. *Science* **170**: 663, 1970.

23. Catt, K. J., Dufan, M. L. and Tsuruhara, T. Studies on a radioligand-receptor assay for luteinizing hormone and chorionic gonadotropin *J. Clin. Endoc. Metab.* **32**: 860, 1971.

24. Catt, K. J., Dufan, M. L. and Tsuruhara, T. Radioligand-receptor assay of luteinizing hormone and chorionic gonadotropin. *J. Clin. Endocr. Metab.* **43**: 123, 1972.

25. Lee, C. Y. and Ryan, R. J. Radioreceptor assay for human chorionic gonadotropin. *J. Clin. Endocr. Metab.* **40**: 228, 1975.

26. Kosasa, T. S., Pion, R. J. et al. Rapid hCG-specific radioimmunoassay for menstrual aspiration. *Obstet. Gynecol.* **45**: 566, 1975.

27. Roy, S., Klein, T. A. et al. Diagnosis of pregnancy with a radioreceptor assay for hCG. *Obstet. Gynecol.* **50**: 401, 1977.

28. Reid, D. E., Ryan, K. J. and Benirsche, K. Principles and Management of Human Reproduction. Philadelphia, W. B. Saunders, 1972.

29. Beling, C. G., Kemmann, E. et al. The use of radioreceptor assay of hCg in the diagnosis of ectopic pregnancy. (In preparation).

30. Saxena, B. B. and Landesman, R. The use of radioreceptor assay of human chorionic gonadotropin for the diagnosis and management of ectopic pregnancy. *Fertil. Steril.* **26**: 397, 1975.

31. Saxena, B. B. and Landesman, R. Diagnosis and management of pregnancy by the radio receptor assay of human chorionic gonadotropin. *Am. J. Obstet. Gynecol.* **131**: 97, 1978.

32. Rosal, T. R., Saxena, B. B. and Landesman, R. Application of a radioreceptor assay of human chorionic gonadotropin in the diagnosis of early abortion. *Fertil. Steril.* **26**: 1105, 1975.

33. Javanovic, L., Landesman, R. and Saxena, B. B. Screening for twin pregnancy. *Science* **198**: 738, 1977.

34. Hammond, B., Borcheret, L. G. et al. Treatment of metastatic trophoblastic disease: Good and poor prognosis. *Am. J. Obstet. Gynecol.* **115**: 451, 1973.

35. Boyko, W. L. and Russell, H. T. Application of the Radioreceptor assay for human chorionic gonadotropin in pregnancy testing and management of trophoblastic disease. *Obstet. Gynecol.* **50**: 324, 1977.

36. Grudzinskas, J. G., Gordon, Y. B. et al. Specific and sensitive determinations of pregnancy-specific-B-glycoprotein by radioimmunoassay. *Lancet* **1:** 333, 1977.
37. Editorial. New placental proteins. *Brit. Med. J.* **2:** 1044, 1977.
38. Morton, H., Rolfe, B. et al. An early pregnancy factor detected in human sera by the rosette inhibition test. *Lancet* **1:** 394, 1977.
39. Rosada, A., Delgado, N. M. et al. Cyclic changes in salivary activity of N-acetyl-B-D-glucosaminidse. *Am. J. Obstet. Gynecol.* **128:** 560, 1977.

6

Assessment and Acceleration of Fetal Lung Maturity

DAVID M. SERR, M.D., SHLOMO MASHIACH, M.D.
GAD BARKAI, M.D. AND BOLESLAV GOLDMAN, M.D.

The concept of lung maturity is of the utmost importance when considering the ability of the premature newborn to adapt to the rigors of extra-uterine life. This is particularly well shown by the evidence that a) the most common cause of neonatal asphyxia is the Respiratory Distress Syndrome (RDS); b) neonatal asphyxia is the main cause of mortality in the premature newborn; and c) neonatal asphyxia is responsible for a large proportion of neonatal morbidity, primarily cases of neurological damage, when death is prevented. The neonatal mortality rate resulting from asphyxia due to RDS reaches 10 to 15 percent of the total perinatal mortality rates and up to 20 to 35 percent of the neonatal mortality rate.[1-3] These figures do not take into account morbidity rates and their varying severity in the surviving infants.

More than 90 percent of all cases of RDS are from pregnancies of less than 35 weeks' gestational age. It is the accepted hypothesis today to regard RDS as reflecting prematurity or underdevelopment of the respiratory system.[4]

In the developmental stages[5] there is no significance to the fetal lung of the degree of oxygenation and gas exchange so long as the fetus is *in utero*.

This does not mean that the fetal lung has no function or activity during intra-uterine life. The lungs are being prepared morphologically, mechanically and metabolically for expansion and respiratory function at the moment of delivery in the face of the immediate challenges of extra-uterine breathing.

This development of the fetal lung is described as taking place in three main stages: 1) The glandular phase, 2) The canalicular phase, and 3) the alveolar phase. In the first or grandular phase which begins at about day 24 of embryonic life, there is an outpouching of the foregut, which within 2 or 3 days divides in two, forming the precursors of the major bronchi.

The development of the bronchial tree continues until the completion of the terminal bronchioles at 16 weeks' gestation. During this glandular phase, the cartilagenous elements make their appearance and the development of glands spreading along the respiratory tract begins.

The canalicular phase starts at the 16th week of gestation and continues until the 25th week. At this stage completion of the development of the terminal airways occurs and a network of blood and lymphatic pathways appears.

The alveolar stage is the third and last phase of development and begins at the 24 to 25th week of gestation, continuing until the birth process is completed. During this period the process of differentiation of the airways is continued creating the primitive alveolar saccules. These are not yet the alveoli, having neither a tubular structure nor a typical cellular lining. The true mature alveoli are formed only a few weeks prior to term.

From term on the number of alveoli per field are as follows:[6]

At term	24 million per field.		
At age of one year	120	" "	"
In the adult	296	" "	"

At the gestational age of 26 to 28 weeks the airways of the respiratory system, and the blood vessels supplying them, are sufficiently developed to potentially allow extra-uterine breathing. However, the amount of blood flow through the respiratory circulation is only 10 percent of the total cardiac output due to muscular thickness. This amount is to change to more than 50 percent after delivery as a result of the oxygenation of the blood vessels and the decrease in vascular resistance.

In all of this developmental system, one of the most interesting and important elements is the alveolar epithelium. In the adult lung there are to be found two types of epithelium. The first type consists of structurally flat cells, apparently not part of the secretory epithelium, which are known as type I cells. The second type of cells are larger, rounder, contain lamellar inclusion bodies, and are sometimes termed osmiophilic bodies (since they stain with osmic acid). These cells are capable of secretory activity and are termed pneumocytes or type II alveolar cells. In addition to these two types of cells in the adult lung, there are also mobile macrophages.[7,8]

During the early development period, the lining epithelium of the airways is columnar in type; later there is a transition to a more cuboidal type of cell accompanied by a rising content of glycogen.

There exists some uncertainty as to exactly at what gestational age in the human the differentiation into type I and type II cells occurs. There is reason to believe that this is a gradual process beginning at 20 weeks[9] and continuing until 26 to 28 weeks of pregnancy.[4,10]

It is understandable that most of the research has been carried out on the activities of the type II cells, since these cells have those exocrine characteristics and contain the substance with a lamellar structure which lines the alveoli and is known as surfactant. Inclusion bodies found in the cytoplasm of these cells represent the precursors of the alveolar surfactant layer.[11-6] These inclusion bodies increase as the respiratory system develops and at term are found in far larger quantities than the number observed in the adult lung.

The concentration of glycogen in these cells decreases and is found in an amount in inverse proportion to the degree of differentiation of the cells.[10,17-19] The number of inclusion bodies in cases of RDS is less than normal.[20-22] It can also be stated that lung maturity for extra-uterine breathing activity is dependent upon the presence of type II cells capable of excreting surfactant onto the alveolar surface. The properties of this surfactant lie in its ability to reduce surface tension and that it is essential for preventing collapse of the terminal air spaces at the end of expiration.

It would be practical, therefore, to speak from now on of lung maturity as referring mainly to maturity of the system which produces alveolar surfactant in sufficient quantities to ensure adequate extra-uterine breathing. While keeping in mind this hypothesis of the etiological cause of RDS as being due to insufficient development of the alveolar surfactant system, it would be wrong to ignore other possible causes of RDS such as inadequate development of the blood vessels and an insufficient blood-air barrier.

LUNG SURFACTANT

Surfactant supports the stability of the alveoli at the end of an expiration when their volume decreases and the tendency to collapse increases in accordance with the rule of Laplace—$P = \frac{2T}{r}$, where P is the pressure tending to collapse the interphase of curved structures such as alveoli; T = surface tension, and r = radius of the curved structure (Fig. 1).[20,23-27] Surfactant has an additional function, acting as an anti-edema factor in preventing accumulation of exudate in the lung.[28]

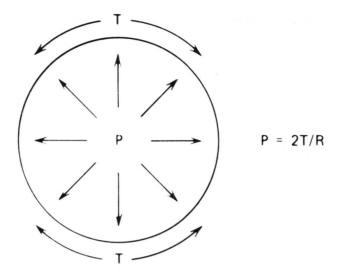

$$P = 2T/R$$

Fig. 1. The Laplace equation.

Further development of the alveoli should of itself be a cause for increase in surface tension, since the more alveoli there are, the greater the surface area of curved structures acting according to the physical rule of Laplace. It may be surmised that this would call for an increase in the amount of surfactant, but this is not the case. The need for surfactant is constant through the phases of pregnancy from 28 weeks' gestational age onward. Before 28 weeks, the airways are still in a primitive developmental stage. The reason for this apparent inconsistency lies in the presence of other factors in the lung which have bearing upon its elasticity, including the elastic fibrous tissue, the development of muscle fibres in the blood vessel walls, and the level of alpha-antitrypsin.

SURFACTANT PROFILE

Surfactant is composed of 85 to 95 percent lipids and 10 to 20 percent proteins. About 90 to 95 percent of the lipids are phospholipids and 3 to 7 percent is cholesterol.[29,30] The dominant phospholipid from the quantitative aspect is lecithin (80%),[31-34] (Table 1). The next in importance is phosphatidyl glycerol (PG) which comprises 7 to 14 percent of the total phospholipid content.[34-38] A minor component quantitatively is phosphatidyl inositol (PI).[15,32,34] Other phospholipids accounting altogether for only 6 to 12 percent of the total are sphingomyelin, phosphatidyl ethanolamine (PE), phosphatidyl serine and lysolecithin. Lecithin, PG, and PI contain a high proportion of saturated fatty acids and are therefore

Table 1. Surfactant Profile*

		PERCENT OF TOTAL Phospholipids
Lecithin		80%
Phosphatidyl glycerol (PG)		7-14%
Phosphatidyl inositol (PI)		3%
Sphingomyelin	)	
Phosphatidyl ethanolamin (PE)	)	
Phosphatidyl serin (PS)	)	6-12%
Lysolecithin	)	

* According to: Clements, J. A. (31), Gluck, L. (32), Klaus, M. (112), Body, D. R. (11), Hallman, M. (15, 36).

"surface active" in that they are able to reduce the surface tension of fluids.

BIOSYNTHESIS OF LECITHIN

There are two main pathways for lecithin synthesis (Fig. 2). The first pathway is that of the choline incorporation.[39-41] This pathway, established after 36 weeks of gestation, being more stable and less affected by factors like hypothermia, hypoxia and acidosis. The end product of this pathway is dipalmityl lecithin.

The second pathway produces lecithin by triple methylation of phosphatidyl-ethanolamine. This is the major pathway from early gestation until 35 to 36 weeks of gestation, and is more affected by the above cited factors.[40-44] The end product of this pathway is alpha-palmitic-beta-myristic lecithin.

PHOSPHATIDYL GLYCEROL (PG) AND PHOSPHATIDYL INOSITOL (PI) BIOSYNTHESIS [15,36]

These phospholipids, although produced in relatively small amounts compared to lecithin, are currently receiving more attention for the part they play in the lipid assembly with lung maturity and RDS in the newborn (Fig. 3). PI concentration peaks at about 35 weeks of gestation and then declines to low levels at term. PG appears in amniotic fluid after the 36th or 37th week and rises in concentration to term.[45] Both PG and PI are produced in the endoplastic reticulum and not in the mitochondria, even though the latter contain enzymes necessary for the production of PG. It is now thought

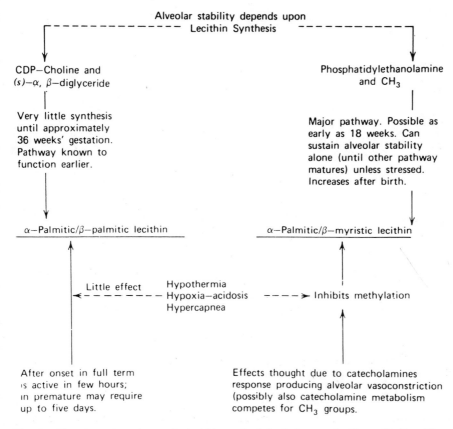

Fig. 2.   The two main pathways for lecithin synthesis in the human fetal lung. (Pediat. Clin. N. Amer., p. 371, 1973.)

that PG surfactant may be a more important factor than lecithin, and may also be more reliable for prognosis in such complications of pregnancy as diabetes.

THE REGULATION OF SURFACTANT FORMATION

The reaction leading to lecithin formation and surfactant activity is a balanced but dynamic one. The stimulus causing Type II cells to synthesize lecithin by the choline incorporation pathway just prior to term is connected to a number of regulating systems. This regulating mechanism is primarily an endocrine one, and exerts influence through DNA stimulating the synthesis of one or more enzymes. This system may be affected by exogenous pharmacological agents, e.g. steroids or aminophylin[14] which

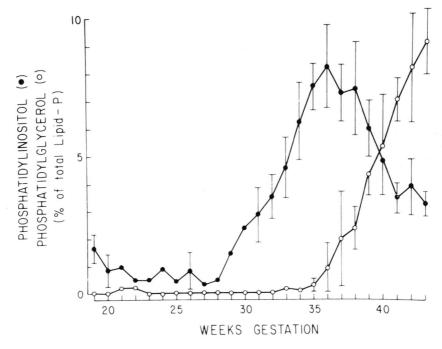

Fig. 3.   Phosphatidyl inositol (P. I.) and phosphatidyl-glycerol (P. G.) concentration in amniotic fluid as a function of gestational age. (From: Hallman et al., A. J. O. G. 125: 613, 1976.)

block the activity of the enzyme phosphodiesterase, thereby raising the level of cyclic AMP. Other such reactions include the effect of thyroid hormone upon the activation of adenylcyclase and the consequent rise in cAMP.[46]

THE SURFACTANT AMNIOTIC FLUID CONNECTION

In 1941 Potter and Bohlender[47] described a case of tracheal blockage caused by an anomaly resulting in distention of the fetal alveoli. Jost and Policard in 1948 first suggested that the fetal lung contributes secretions to the amniotic fluid,[48] when they observed that by blocking the trachea they could cause expansion of lung volume. In 1953, Reynolds showed that in fetal lambs the amount of secretion from the respiratory tract could reach 30 to 40 ml/hour.[49] In 1963, Adams et al. showed that the fluid exuding from the trachea differs in quality and constituents from amniotic fluid.[50,51] Although as mentioned before, the fetal lung is inactive regarding gaseous exhange during pregnancy, it does, however, undergo preparation for postpartum breathing by intra-uterine chest movements.[52-56] These breathing movements begin quite early in pregnancy as can be showed by the presence in the lungs of contrast media injected into the amniotic sac.[57, 58] Some authors[59, 60] have failed to confirm these observations and this may point to the irregularity of these breathing movements throughout pregnancy. The fetus begins to show chest movements in the second trimester,[60] and the amount of amniotic fluid inhaled increases in proportion to the size and advance in gestational age.[55, 56] It has been estimated that the turnover of amniotic fluid in the human fetus at term is around 200 ml/Kg per 24 hours.

It has now become feasible to follow fetal beathing movements by means of ultrasound,[62] although failure to pick up these signs by ultrasound does not necessarily mean they do not take place. Real-time ultrasonic scaning is becoming a more efficient mode for this purpose than is A-Scan. There may be factors other than gestational age and size affecting the extent of fetal chest movements and the turnover of amniotic fluid from the lungs. In fact, immature fetuses in distress have been shown to draw in less amniotic fluid to the lungs than fetuses of equivalent gestational age who are not in distress.

EVALUATION OF FETAL LUNG MATURITY

All methods for estimating fetal lung maturity are based upon examination of amniotic fluid since it bathes the fetal lung[63-65] during fetal respiratory movements.

The methods used are either chemical or physical.

BIO-CHEMICAL DETERMINATION OF LUNG MATURITY

Chemical methods estimate the qualitative or quantitative features of substances able to lower surface tension. These are as follows:

Total phospholipid concentration
Lecithin concentration
Lecithin/sphyngomyelin ratio
Palmitic acid estimation
Phosphatidyl glycerol (PG) and phosphatidyl inositol (PI) estimation.

BIOPHYSICAL METHODS OF DETERMINING LUNG MATURITY

These methods are based on the physical changes caused by the presence of surfactant in amniotic fluid. There are:

Foam stability test

Surface tension characteristics

Optical density determination

Microviscosity

Measurement of the concentration of the total phospholipid content of amniotic fluid seems a logical approach for the assessment of lung maturity since the phospholipid assembly consists mainly of lecithin.[66]

The concentration of lecithin in amniotic fluid[67-69] and the concentration of plamitic acid[69-71] are methods which have been found to be difficult to execute and which do not correlate well with the L/S ratio and clinical state. Moreover, their main disadvantage is their dependency upon the volume of amniotic fluid. This is a most important point, particularly in such high-risk pregnancies as diabetes with polyhydramnios or chronic fetal distress with oligohydramnios. Falconer has attempted to overcome these dilution problems by measuring the volume of amniotic fluid and classifying fetal lung maturity in units of volume.[72] This is not the easiest of methods, and it is also impractical in pregnancies with ruptured membranes. Lecithin measurement has the further disadvantage of being found in substances not considered part of the surfactant assembly, and thus being a possible cause of error.

The lecithin/sphyngomyelin ratio is based upon the observation that the lecithin content of amniotic fluid is low until 32 weeks and rises rapidly from 35 weeks of gestation. The association with sphyngomyelin (Fig. 4) was chosen since this substance has a different concentration curve than does lecithin, not dependent upon lung maturity and yet related to the volume of amniotic fluid. Although there are other bodies in the fluid such as membrane fragments, fetal urine, epithelial cells from several sources and other such artifacts which may contain lecithin, it should be noted that the lecithin active in lowering surface tension contains a different fatty acid composition, so these other sources of lecithin have to be eliminated by precipitation with acetone before the L/S ratio can be determined for an assessment of fetal lung maturity.[4, 73-76] Then a high clinical correlation value is found at ratios above or below L/S = 2.0 in regard to the possible development of respiratory distress syndrome. Some cases of RDS have been observed between the levels L/S = 1.50–1.99, but these were mild to moderate in degree of severity.[77]

The laboratory details of the method have been described and well established by Gluck and his associates. It is to be noted the inexactitudes in carrying out the test or failing to be precise in the acetone precipitation may cause inaccuracies leading to a high false positive rate.

All in all, in spite of its inestimable value and contribution to our knowledge of the development of fetal lung maturity, the performance of the L/S ratio remains a relatively complicated and prolonged laboratory

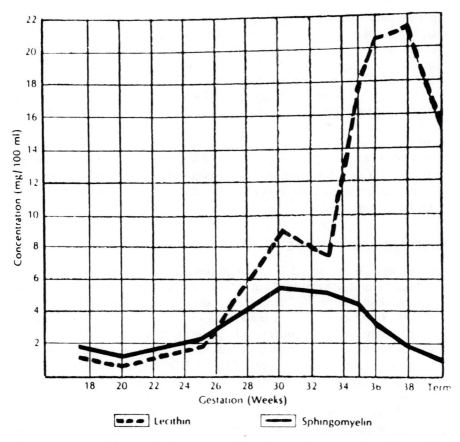

Fig. 4.   Lecithin sphingomyelin concentrations in amniotic fluid as a function of gestational age. (According to Gluck) (Brown, B. J.: Obst. Gyn. Survey, 30: 71, 1975.)

procedure requiring a high degree of skill. There are, moreover, recent reports of its possible unreliability in predicting the respiratory state of the newborn in diabetic pregnancies,[78-82] RDS having developed in some of these cases with an L/S ratio greater than 2.

The possible contamination of amniotic fluid by blood or cells containing lecithin, as well as the need for reliability in diabetic cases, has given added importance to the assessment of phosphatidyl glycerol in amniotic fluid. This compound is considered a specific pulmonary component.[34] The level of phosphatidyl inositol is measurable only when some surfactant is present in amniotic fluid. Its rise of concentration follows that of the L/S ratio, but at L/S = 3.0, there is a decrease in the level of PI. PG, however, only appears when the L/S ratio is equal to or greater than 2.0. In cases where pulmonary maturity is earlier than expected, PG will appear even before the L/S ratio reaches 2.0. On the other hand, should pulmonary maturity be delayed in the fetal lung, PG will not be found present even when the L/S ratio is above 3.0. In cases where a false positive result was given by L/S ratio determination, no PG was found.[169] In normal healthy infants, PG will appear close to the time of delivery or immediately after birth.[170]

In the tracheal effluent postnatally in cases of RDS, PI can be found while PG is absent. PI, however, is a less active surfactant functionally than is PG. L/S ratios measured in the pharynx and trachea at 6 hours of life and before, showed a ratio of less than 2.0 in cases of RDS and of more than 2.0 in controls.[19, 83-85]

BIOPHYSICAL PARAMETERS

The simplest and most widely practiced physical parameter is the foam test developed and described by Clements et al.[86] Surfactant secreted into the amniotic fluid can create bubbles or foam of high stability by shaking a test-tube. In order to exclude the effects of other components capable of creating foam such as proteins, bile pigments and free fatty acids, it is essential to prepare the amniotic fluid with ethanol. A positive test at a dilution of 1:2 excludes the possibility of RDS formation, but the test, simple as it is, lacks reliability due to the large number of false negatives.[87]

Among other physical parameters, mention should be made of surface tension balance (Wilhelmy Balance),[88, 89] and the newer optical density approach in amniotic fluid at an optical density (OD) of 650 mu. This is an optical density wavelength unaffected by pigments and bilirubin.[90] The method, however, is limited by its high rate of false negatives.

A new method based upon a different physical principle introduced for the purpose of assessing the degree of fetal lung maturity from amniotic fluid has been described recently by our team (1976) and the reliability controlled independently in the United States and in Israel.[91] This new approach for assessing lung maturity of the fetus which takes into account the whole surfactant lipid profile is independent of the volume of the amniotic fluid. The method is based on a fluorescence polarization technique where the recorded signal corresponds to the intrinsic viscosity of the lipid aggregates present in the amniotic fluid.

The physical basis of the method presented here stems from the empirical relationship between the viscosity and the surface tension of fluids. Both of these physical parameters are determined by the intermolecular forces of the fluid and are therefore interrelated. The correlation between these parameters implies that the surface tension of the pulmonary surfactant can be translated into an intrinsic viscosity parameter which, as for other lipid systems, may be expressed in terms of "microviscosity."[92, 93]

One of the most efficient techniques for determining the lipid microviscosity of all membranes and liposomes is by fluorescence depolarization of a hydrocarbon probe. It was found that 1, 6 diphenyl 1, 3, 5 hexatriene (DPH) is the most efficient probe for this purpose. This lipid microviscosity measured as the value P is directly related to the rotational motion of the probe embedded in the core of the system.

The detected degree of fluorescence polarization (P) is found to be in inverse proportion to the degree of fetal lung maturity. Estimations are carried out using the microviscosimeter (Felma)* developed for this purpose.[91] The degree of accuracy of the measured P value is estimated to be ± 0.005 by repeating measurements carried out with pool samples of amniotic fluids. The examination time is 45 minutes from the amniocentesis, and the technique is relatively simple, highly accurate, reproducible, independent or amniotic fluid volume and can be carried out by the delivery room. Figure 5 plots the P values of these samples (with their standard deviations) as related to gestational age in weeks. The downward trend in the value of P is clearly seen as pregnancy advances.

As a control study to determine the correlation between the L/S ratio and the P value, 37 samples of amniotic fluid were examined by two separate teams, and their readings correlated. A regression line shows that the coefficient was fairly good at r = 0.76 (Fig. 6).

According to the regression line, a P value of 0.307 was found to be equivalent to an L/S ratio of 2.0. This provides a working guide that laboratory-wise, P = 0.307 represents the cut-off level—lower than this RDS would not be expected to develop.

In 110 cases, P value was less than 0.312 (0.307 ± 0.005, where 0.005 represents the instrumental margin of error). None of the newborns developed RDS.

In 54 pregnancies P value was greater than 0.312. Nine of the newborn developed RDS while the rest did not. The fact that 45 of 54 cases with a P value > than 0.312 did not develop RDS gives rise to speculation about the possible existence of a "grey zone" in which the threshold could be raised for diagnosing lung maturity to above laboratory values of P = 0.312 while taking a minimal, but in some cases necessary, risk of the development of RDS.

---

* Fetal lung maturity analyzer, produced by Elscint Corp., Haifa, Israel.

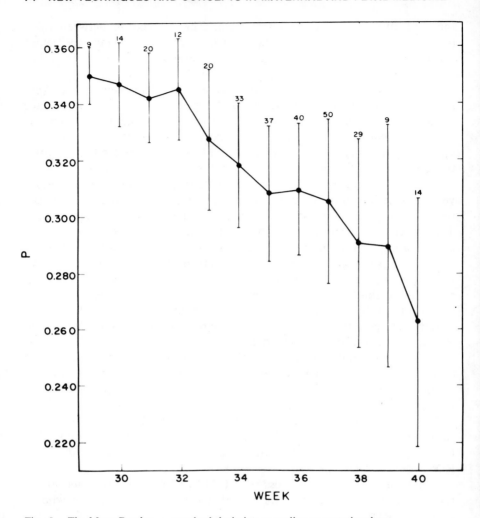

Fig. 5.   The Mean P value + standard deviation according to gestational age.

FACTORS AFFECTING THE RATE OF LUNG MATURITY

There are pathological conditions of pregnancy which may be responsible for either slowing down or accelerating the rate of development of lung maturity. Then there are pharmacological influences to be considered which may enhance pulmonary maturity either by agents of endogenous or exogenous origin.

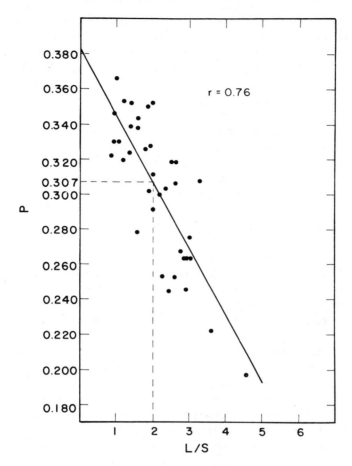

Fig. 6.   Correlation between P value and lecithin sphingomyelin ratio in 34 amniotic fluid samples.

PATHOLOGICAL CONDITIONS OF PREGNANCY[96-106]

Even though the process of pulmonary maturity follows a pattern dependent on other factors, and also upon gestational age, there often exists a chronological inconsistency in the state of the fetal lung and in the stage of pregnancy. Such inconsistencies appear mainly in pathological pregnancies and present either as a factor enhancing or delaying fetal lung maturation clinically, or according to laboratory data at birth. Enhanced maturity is usually noted in: 1) maternal hypertensive disorders or renal or cardiovascular origin, or due to severe toxemia of pregnancy; 2) hemoglobinopathies; 3) narcotic addiction (heroin, morphine); 4) diabetes mellitus (Types D, E, F, and R); 5) chorioamnionitis; 6) placental insufficiency: retroplacental bleeding, circumvallate placenta, placental infarction; 7) prolonged rupture of the membranes. In those instances where lung maturity has been hastened, there should be no danger of RDS developing despite inadequate gestational age.

Today there is evidence that prolonged premature rupture of the membranes enhances pulmonary maturity,[94-100] and that the common denominator in this enhancement in conditions involving severe diabetes (Class D, E, F, R), severe toxemia of pregnancy, placental insufficiency, hemoglobinopathies, extra-uterine infections, is stress. In all of these pathological states there is increased synthesis of endogenous glucocorticoids which speed up the activity of the enzymes essential to surfactant synthesis.

Delaying factors in lung maturation may be caused by: 1) hydrops fetalis; 2) diabetes mellitus (Types A, B, and C). In tissue culture in rabbits, Smith et al.[107] found that insulin blocks the development of lecithin, probably through stimulation and activation of the enzyme phosphodiesterase, causing a reduced level of cyclic AMP which is essential for lecithin synthesis.

Gluck et al.[108] and Epstein et al.[109] observed, however, that suppression of insulin secretion in the pancreas by a cytotoxic agent such as streptozorocin, which causes a diabetic-like state, does not result in the expected increase in L/S ratio and the accompanying increase in lecithin. Gluck therefore assumes that the developments taking place in diabetics simulate those resulting from stress in diabetes types D, E, F, and R. There are other possible factors in diabetes apart from insulin which are involved in surfactant synthesis.

Surfactant profile is a term now used to convey the assessment of fetal lung maturity; lecithin as a primary constituent constitutes only one part of this profile and has therefore reduced the specificity of the L/S ratio as a means of assessing potential RDS cases.

In most of the pathological conditions described here, the laboratory estimation of fetal lung maturity correlates well with the clinical findings. However, an important exception to this rule is in diabetic pregnancies. Several reports[79, 82 110-112] have provided data casting doubt upon the reliability of the L/S ratio in diabetes. Apparently in those cases where RDS developed in the newborn of a diabetic mother, phosphatidyl glycerol (PG) was absent. The new microviscosity method may be proven to be a reliable parameter in cases of diabetes mellitus also. In a preliminary study, fetal lung maturity was examined by this method prior to delivery in 43 cases of diabetic mothers, 16 of them insulin-dependent and 27 non-insulin dependent. In neither diabetic group was there an example of a false positive reading. Furthermore, there was no case of RDS when the P value was less than 0.312 in spite of the high cesarean section rate (50%).

PHARMACOLOGICAL AGENTS AFFECTING LUNG MATURITY

There are several substances in which enhancing fetal lung maturity causes an improved life expectancy correlating with improved results in the laboratory. Stimulation and activation of phosphodiesterase which suppresses surfactant synthesis by lowering cyclic AMP is influenced by insulin (Fig. 7). The lowering of cAMP levels inhibits the incorporation of precursors into phosphatidylcholine in isolated cells.

Intravenous administration of dibutyryl cAMP caused a significant increase in the intracellular synthesis of lamellar inclusion bodies in cells of the adult rat.[113]

Theophylline has the property of depressing phosphodiesterase, which causes an increase in cAMP and consequently an increase in production of lecithin. Theophylline is also known to increase the secretion of surfactant into the alveolar spaces.[114] In a different study on tissue culture of rabbit lung tissue, the effect of theophylline and hydrocortisone on the levels of cAMP and on the rate of incorporation of choline and methionine into phosphatidyl choline has been described. Both theophylline and hydrocortisone raise the concentration of cAMP by about 75 percent. It is surprising

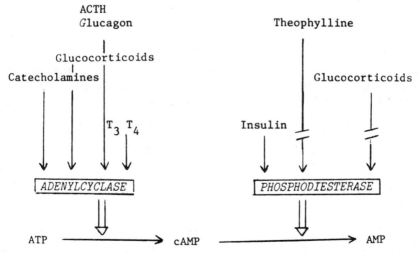

Fig. 7.   Possible site of action of certain pharmacological agents on the cyclic AMP.

that the acceleration was found to be equal for both pathways of surfactant production.[115] In this study, Barret and co-workers suggest that hydrocortisone also alters glucose metabolism by increasing the turnover of glycogen and glucose. In fact, the only hormone known to block surfactant synthesis is insulin, via its activating action on phosphodiesterase and the consequent reduction in cAMP.

PHOSTAGLANDINS

There is as yet no conclusive evidence that these lipid hormones which might function through cAMP have any direct connection on the system of surfactant synthesis.[116]

BETA-SYMPATHOMIMETIC AGENTS

The beta-sympathomimetic substances are more connected to release of surfactant from the cell to the alveolar space than they are to surfactant synthesis.[117] There are studies reporting a significant reduction in the rate of occurrence of RDS following administration of isoxsuprine.[118] However, Howie and Liggins,[119] in a now classic study, found no difference in RDS rates in pregnancies receiving a muscle relaxant such as salbutamol and/or ethanol compared to a group of pregnant women receiving other contraction-suppressing drugs. It is assumed that epinephrine acts at the intra-cellular level by activating adenylcylase and also by raising the levels of cAMP.

ESTROGENS

There is still insufficient evidence concerning the role of the estrogenic hormones in the processes of lung maturation. The effect of estrone sulphate in improving the L/S ratio has been reported. A trend towards an increased L/S ratio was noted but not to the same degree as in using steroids.[120] It has been suggested that steroids on their own are not as effective for improving lung maturity as a combination of steroids and estrogens, but this has not been substantiated.[121]

HEROIN

It would not seem reasonable that use of a narcotic such as heroin to accelerate fetal lung maturity would be acceptable without much more supporting evidence. However, note must be made of observations that the newborn of heroin addicts showed a lower rate of RDS[122] and more mature L/S ratios as a function of gestational age.[77, 123]

PHENOBARBITAL

Barbiturates prevent the release of surfactant to the alveolar spaces[114, 124] and thus delay the respiratory adjustment of premature neonates. In rabbits, the levels of intracellular surfactant developed normally following administration of phenobarbital, but the amount of surfactant secreted into the alveoli was significantly reduced. However, the incidence of RDS in mothers receiving barbiturates as treatment for convulsions has not been studied as yet. Other possible agents for accelerating lung maturity are epidermal growth factor,[125] and bromhexine.[126]

STEROIDS

The glucocorticosteroids act upon the target cell of the lung by way of receptors. In the cytoplasm of these cells there are protein structures having a close hormone affinity. These receptors are apparently to be found as early as the 9–12th week of human pregnancy.[127,128] This hormone receptor complex is connected to the cell nucleus, influences the DNA and activates the RNA messenger to effect protein synthesis.[129] It is interesting that after birth, these receptors are undetectable in both human and animal neonates.[128-130] In cases of RDS receptors are not detectable, probably because of their having been attached to endogenous steroids in large quantities. It is known that cortisol levels are particularly high following delivery.[131] There are numerous studies in monkeys, rabbits and lambs pointing to the beneficial effect of corticosteroids on the synthesis of surfactant in the third trimester of pregnancy and a consequent improvement in life expectancy.[14, 132, 133] The effect of steroid administration is on both intracellular synthesis activity and on secretion into the lung air spaces. Farrell[134] observed the accelerating effect of alpha-fluprednisone on the synthesis of lecithin in the stable pathway in rabbits by activating choline phosphotransferase. Cortisol administration, on the other hand, accelerates the synthesis of PG by activating glycerophosphatase phosphatidyl transferase.[157] An interesting study performed on tissue culture of Type II cells has shown[159] that a combination of cortisol and thyroxine enhances by a factor of × 7 the activity of cholinephosphotransferase.

The minimum time required for steroids to take effect in a tissue culture of rabbit lung is 12 hours. The optimum time for the drug to achieve its maximum effect is 24 hours. On the other hand, after 24 hours there is no further enhancing effect of the steroids.[137] However, in contrast to the effect of steroids on other body tissues, the effect on the fetal lung lasts for 5 days from the time of a single administration. There is therefore no doubt about the important role played by steroids in adequate development of the surfactant system of the lung.

There are several observations which indicate the essential role played by these hormones in the normal physiological development of lung maturity. By giving rabbits metyrapone, a blocking agent of adrenal steroids, a delay in the normal lowering of surface tension in the lung was produced.[138] Further administration of ACTH has the same effect of accelerating lung maturity as does the administration of exogenous steroids.[139, 140] Before birth, there is a significant increase in the levels of cortisol[26] in amniotic fluid[14] as well as in cord blood.[126] Acceleration of fetal lung maturity accompanies conditions of stress typical of raised steroid levels.[77, 144] In contrast, in cases of RDS the level of cortisol in the cord blood is often low.[142]

The level of cortisol in the cord blood of neonates born at vaginal delivery is far higher than the level in the cord blood of those born at elective cesarean section.[143, 145] However, there is no difference in cord cortisol levels between vaginal deliveries and cesarean sections performed abruptly during labor. This correlates well with clinical observations on the rates of RDS in vaginal deliveries and elective cesarean sections.[146]

High levels of endogenous cortisol appear with lung maturity. However, it has been observed that in cases of anencephalus or in deficient enzymatic adrenal development a delay may occur in the development of lung surfactant.[147] The most comprehensive and controlled studies on steroid effect upon acceleration of lung maturity have been carried out by Howie and Liggins[119] who gave betamethasone in a dose of 12mg/24 hours I.M. twice in the course of 48 hours, in comparison to a control group receiving 6 mg of hydrocortisone.

In the group treated by betamethasone there was an incidence of RDS of 9.0 percent significantly lower than that in the control group of 25.8 percent.[119] When correlated to gestational age, the greatest difference between the betamethasone-treated and control groups was between 30 to 32 weeks. Before 30 weeks, there was little difference, and between 32 to 34 weeks there was also a less significant difference, although the latter group showed some enhancement effect.[148] However, at more than 34 weeks' gestational age there was no significant difference between the RDS rates in the two groups. The duration of the medication is also significant. Treatment of less than 24 hours or more than 7 days reduces the beneficial effect of betamethasone administration.[148,149] It may be stated from these studies that treatment with betamethasone has increased the life expectancy of premature neonates and has significantly reduced perinatal mortality.[148]

Since many of the pregnancies in these series present as premature labors and receive ethanol or beta-adrenergic agents, Liggins and Howie attempted to isolate this factor and observed that administration of salbutamol alone does not alter the rate of RDS when compared to a control group.[119,148]

In studying the effect of premature rupture of the membranes, it was noted that this complication has no effect upon the rate of RDS when it occurs less than 72 hours from delivery. However, in a group of PRM treated up to 7 days with steroids, there is a lower rate of RDS.[148]

Other studies have examined the effect of glucocorticosteroids on the L/S ratio in amniotic fluid. In general it was reported that the effect upon lecithin production resulted in an increased L/S ratio when compared to control groups.[119,150]

It has not yet been determined which glucocorticoid is the most active in regard to pulmonary maturation processing.[119] With respect to dosage, it seems clear that doubling the dose of betamethasone does not reduce the rate of RDS and does not minimize the severity of the disease.[119]

It is possible that the take-over of all receptors explains the lack of response to corticosteroid treatment in cases developing RDS.[131] Another factor in this lack of response after delivery is the observation that apparently a period of 24 hours is required for drug activity to become effective, and within this period RDS develops.[137,148,149]

The glucocorticosteroids act upon many target organs. This activity is not always positive apart from the viewpoint of pulmonary maturity. Side effects such as increased enzymatic activity in the liver, liberation of fatty acids and reduction of glucose transfer in fat and muscle tissues, and interference with the differentiation of cells of the central nervous system can be potentially harmful.[151]

Most studies demonstrating the negative influences of steroid treatment on lung maturity have been carried out in experimental animals. However, if evidence was shown of some delay in lung and brain volume due to an apparent slowing down of mitotic development in the dendrites, the level of cholesterol in the central nervous system and in locomotor activity, there was also shown a "catch-up" growth after birth.[152] However, we should note that steroid administration after birth in the early neonatal period has been followed by neurological disorders including disturbed electroencephalograms and motor activity.[153] A study of rhesus monkeys using dexamethasone compared the amount of lung and brain tissue and DNA content in treated and non-treated animals and showed the treated group to contain less than the control group. The DNA content was significantly lower in the dexamethasone-treated group. Even at 6 months after birth, significant differences could still be detected.[154]

In contrast to these observations, more encouraging data have been reported concerning the enhancement of fetal lung maturity in cases of chronic fetal distress being accompanied by advanced neurological activity. In these cases the levels of endogenous steroids are high.[155]

Studies in experimental animals have demonstrated decreased immunological responsiveness[156] after treatment with glucocorticosteroids, a factor which may be of importance in cases of perinatal infections. There is, however, no conclusive evidence of this in the human.[148,153,157]

Liggins and Howie have described a generally low perinatal mortality[148] apart from cases of pre-eclamptic toxemia with proteinuria. Furthermore, the suspicion that mothers receiving steroids during pregnancy may give birth to newborns with affected adrenal development has been shown to be unfounded.[158] More research is required in this field for both short and long-term assessment of the pharmacological effects of drugs in the enhancement of fetal lung maturity.

THYROXINE AND LUNG MATURITY

Like steroid activity, thyroid hormone has intracellular receptors which affect gene expression.[46] Also similar to the steroid pattern immediately following birth, there is a sharp rise in the levels of T_3 and T_4.[159]

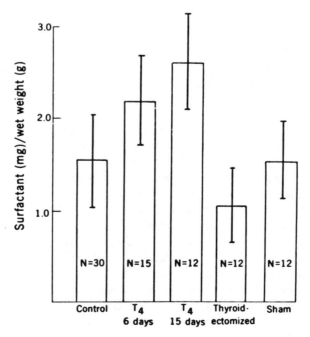

Fig. 8. The quantity of purified surfactant harvested from lung washings is expressed comparing T_4-treated with control and sham thyroidectomized rats. Brackets indicate 1 standard deviation. (From: Redding et al., Science 175: 995, 1972.)

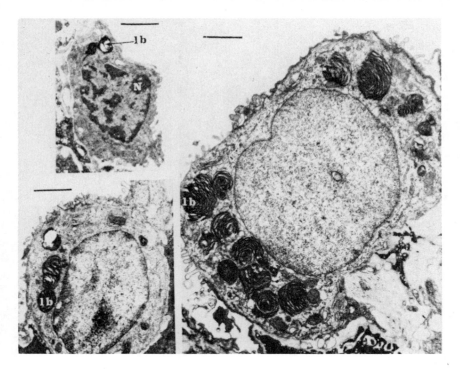

Fig. 8a.   Type II alveolar cells from thyroidectomized (upper left) euthyroid (lower left) and thyroxine-treated rats (right). A cell obtained from a thyroidectomized rat is smaller in size. The nuclear chromatin (N) is clumped and there are fewer and smaller lamellar bodies (l. b.). (From: Redding et al., *Science* 175: 994, 1972.)

Animal studies have shown that thyroxine injected into fetal rabbits or into the amniotic fluid enhance fetal lung maturity significantly.[160] In other observations it has been shown that thyroidectomy is followed by a decreased pneumocyte cell development. Thyroxine administration brought about hypertrophy of the cells and release of large amounts of surfactant from the inclusion bodies[161] (Fig. 8—see Fig. 8a). Further evidence concerning the importance of thyroid activity on human fetal lung maturation was noted in the relatively large numbers of cases of RDS found in neonates suffering from hypothyroidism.[161-163] Thyroxine does not pass over the placental barrier in significant amounts.[164] It cannot therefore be given to the mother as can steroid therapy for the purpose of enhancing fetal lung maturity.

In sheep it was demonstrated that T_4 injections into the amniotic fluid were as effective as intramuscular injections.[165] It was also shown that in humans, an intra-amniotic injection of thyroid prenatally had no deleterious effects that could be detected in the perinatal period.[166]

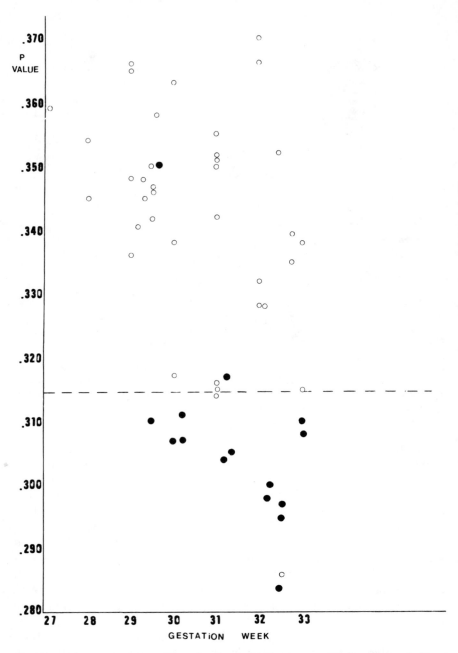

Fig. 9. P value as a function of gestational age after T_4 treatment (black points) and without such treatment (open circles). The dotted line represents the threshold of lung maturity. (Mashiach, S., et al. *J. Perinatal Medicine*. [In press])

However, it is important to note when considering the use of intra-amniotic T_4 for enhancement of lung maturity, any possible effect upon the development of the central nervous system. Experiments in newborn mice which showed effects upon the myelinization process, however, used particularly large doses of thyroxine.[167] The preliminary results of our experience with this drug have been published recently[168]: 200–500 mcg of sodium levothyroxine (T_4) was injected directly into the amniotic sac of 15 pathologic pregnancies in which premature delivery was inevitable or highly indicated between 30 to 33 weeks of gestation. Fetal lung maturity was determined by the evaluation of microviscosity "P" value as previously described. A "P" value of 0.312 was defined as the value below which development of RDS is highly improbable.

Figure 9 plots the "P" value of 50 amniotic fluids drawn from pregnan-

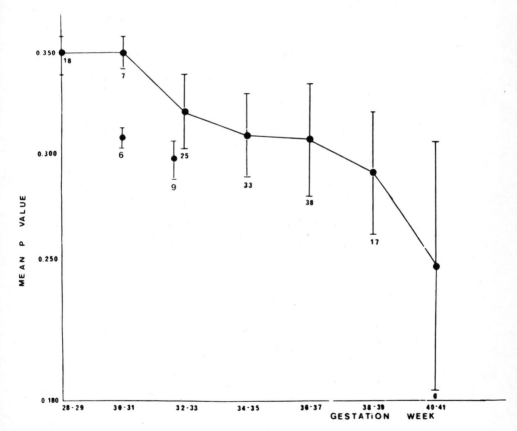

Fig. 10.   P values of two T_4-treated groups according to gestational age in comparison to the control. Black dots-mean value. Brackets-1 standard deviation. (By courtey of Dr. S. Mashiach and the Walter D. E. Gruyter Co., Berlin.)

cies of from 28 to 33 weeks. In only 15 samples, the P value was less than 0.312; 13 of these 15 samples were from pregnancies in which T_4 had previously been injected. The mean P value after thyroxine administration was compared to the mean P values in a control group where P values of amniotic fluid samples were determined but T_4 was not given (Fig. 10). There was a statistically significant difference in the rate of pulmonary ripening between the treated and the control groups of the same gestational age (30–31 weeks—$P < 0.001$; 32–33 weeks—$P < 0.005$).

The effect of intra-amniotic injection of T_4 on the outcome in newborns is shown in Figure 11. There were 12 cases of RDS among 50 cases of preterm infants born between 28 to 33 weeks of pregnancy (24%), whereas just one case of RDS among 25 preterm infants to whom T_4 treatment was given before birth (4%). This difference is statistically significant ($P < 0.007$). In preterm infants delivered between 34 to 36 weeks of gesta-

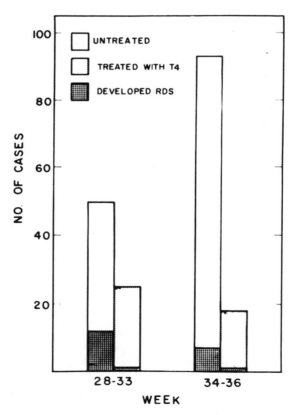

Fig. 11.   Effect of T_4 Treatment on clinical outcome (respiratory distress syndrome rate), in comparison to the control groups according to gestational age.

tion the rate of RDS was 7.5 percent (7 cases out of 93) in the non-treated group, and 5.5 percent in the T_4 treated group (1 case out of 18)—a difference not significant statistically.

These results are very similar to those of Liggins and Howie who succeeded in reducing the incidence of RDS by betamethasone therapy most markedly in infants born between 30 and 32 weeks. In infants delivered at more than 34 weeks, betamethasone therapy as well as the intra-amniotic injection of T_4 did not influence the outcome significantly.

REFERENCES

1. McKay, R. J., M. Valdes-Dapena and Arey, J. B. The fetus and the newborn infant. *In* Textbook of Pediatrics (Nelson, W. E., Vaughan, V. C. and McKay, R. J., Eds.) Philadelphia, W. B. Saunders, 1969, p. 346.
2. Pryse-Davies, J. The pathology of the lung. *Proc. Roy. Soc. Med.* **65**: 823, 1972.
3. Brown, B. J., Gabert, H. A. and Stenchever, M. A. *Obstetrical and Gynecological Survey* **30**: 71, 1975.
4. Gluck, L. M., V. Kulovich et al. Diagnosis of the respiratory distress syndrome by amniocentesis. *Am. J. Obstet. Gynecol.* **109**: 440, 1971.
5. Avery, M. E. and Fletcher, B. D. The lung and its disorders in the newborn infant. Philadelphia, W. B. Saunders, 1974.
6. Dunhill, M. S. Postnatal growth of the lung. *Thorax* **17**: 329, 1962.
7. Thurbleck, W. M. Postnatal growth and development of the lung. *Am. Rev. Resp. Dis.* **111**: 159, 1975.
8. Mason, R. J., T. P. Stossel and Vaughan, M. Lipids of alveolar macrophages, polymorphonuclear leukocytes and their phagocytic vesicles. *J. Clin. Invest.* **51**: 2399, 1972.
9. Lauweryns, J. M. Hyaline membrane disease in newborn infants. Macroscopic radiographic, and light and electron microscopic studies. *Human Path.* **11**: 175, 1970.
10. Campiche, M. A., Gautier, A., Hernandez, E. I. and Reymond, A. An electrone microscope study of the fetal development of human lung. *Pediatrics* **32**: 976, 1963.
11. Askin, F. B. and Kuhn, C. The cellular origin of pulmonary surfactant. *Lab. Invest.* **25**: 260, 1971.
12. Chevalier, G. and Collet, A. J. In vivo incorporation of choline 3–H, leucine –3H and galactose –3H in alveolar Type II pneumocytes in relation to surfactant synthesis. A quantitative radioautographic study in the mouse by electron microscopy. Anat. Res. **174**: 289, 1972.
13. Frosolone, M. F., R. Pawlowski, Charms, B. L. Relationship between intra- and extracellular surface action fractions from rat lungs. *Chest* **67**: 165, 1975.
14. Gil, J. O. and Reiss, K. Isolation and characterization of lamellar bodies and tubular myelin from rat lung homogenates. *J. Cell Biol.* **58**: 152, 1973.
15. Hallman, M. and Gluck, L. Phosphatidylglycerol in lung surfactant. II. Subcellular distribution and mechanism of biosynthesis in vitro. *Biochem. Biophys. Acta* **409**: 172, 1975.
16. Sorokin, S. P. A morphologic and cytochemical study on the great alveolar cell. *J. Histochem. Cytochem.* **14**: 884, 1966.
17. Bernard, C. L. De la matiere glycogene cosideree comme condition de development de certains tissues chez le foetus avant l'apparition de la function glycogenique du fore. *J. Physiol. (Paris)* **2**: 326, 1959.

18. Kikkawa, Y., E. K. Motoyama and Gluck, L. Study of the lungs of fetal and newborn rabbits. Morphologic, biochemical and surface physical development. *Am. J. Path.* **52:** 177, 1968.

19. Gluck, L., R. A. Landowne, Kulovich, M. V. Biochemical development of surface activity in mammalian lung. III. Structural changes in lung lecithin during development of the rabbit fetus and newborn. *Paediatr. Res.* **4:** 352, 1970.

20. Avery, M. E. and Mead, J. Surface properties in relation to atelectasis and hyaline membrane disease. *Am. J. Dis. Child* **97:** 517, 1959.

21. Kikkawa, Y., E. K. Motoyama, and Cook, C. D. The ultrastructure of the lungs of lambs. The relation of eosinophilic inclusions and alveolar lining layer of fetal maturation and experimentally produced respiratory distress. *Am. J. Pathol.* **47:** 877, 1965.

22. Schaefer, K. E., Avery, M. E. and Bensch, K. Time course of changes in surface tension and morphology of alveolar epithelial cells in CO^o induced hyaline membrane disease. *J. Clin. Invest.* **43:** 2080, 1964.

23. Macklin, C. C. The pulmonary alveolar mucoid film and the pneumocytes. *Lancet* **1:** 1099, 1954.

24. Pattle, R. E. Properties, function and origin of alveolar lining layer. *Nature* **175:** 1125, 1955.

25. Clements, J. A. and Tierney, D. F. Alveolar instability associated with altered surface tension. *In* Handbook of Physiology, Respiration. Washington D. C. *Am. J. Physiol. Soc.* **2:** 1565, 1964.

26. Clements, J. A., R. F. Hustead, R. P., Johnson, Gribetz, J. Pulmonary surface tension and alveolar stability. *J. Appl. Physiol.* **16:** 444, 1961.

27. Mead, J. Mechanical properties of lung. *Physiol. Rev.* **41:** 281, 1961.

28. Morgan, T. E.: Pulmonary surfactant. *New Eng. J. Med.* **284:** 1185, 1971.

29. Hallman, M. L. and Gluck, L. Phosphatidyl glycerol in lung surfactant. III. Possible modifier of surfactant function. *J. Lipid Res.* **17:** 257, 1976.

30. King. R. J. The surfactant system of the lung. *Fed. Proc.* **33:** 2238, 1974.

31. Clements, J. A., J. Nellenbogen and Trahan, H. J. Pulmonary surfactant and evolution of lungs. *Science* **169:** 603, 1970.

32. Gluck, L., E. K. Motoyama, H. L. Smits, Kulovich, M. V. The biochemical development of surface activity in mammalian lung. I. The surface active phospholipids; the separation and distribution of surface active lecithin in the lung of the developing rabbit fetus. *Pediat. Res.* **1:** 237, 1967.

33. Klaus, M. J., A. Clements, Havel, R. J. Composition of surface active material isolated from beef lung. *Proc. Natl. Acad. Sci., U.S.* **47:** 1858, 1961.

34. Hallman, M., M. V. Kulovich, E. Krik-Patrick, R. G. Sugarman, Gluck, L. Phosphatidylinositol (PI) and phosphatidylglycerol (PG) in amniotic fluid: indices of lung maturity. *Am. J. Obstet. Gynecol.* **125:** 613, 1976.

35. Body, D. R. The phospholipid composition of pig lung surfactant. *Lipids* **6:** 625, 1971.

36. Hallman, M., Gluck, L. Phosphatidylglycerol in lung surfactant. I. Synthesis in rat lung microsomes. *Biochem. Biophys. Res. Commun.* **60:** 1, 1974.

37. Peleger, R. C., Thomas, H. C. Beagle dog pulmonary surfactant lipids. *Arch. Int. Med.* **127:** 863, 1971.

38. Rooney, S. A., P. M. Canavan, Motoyama, E. K. The indentification of phosphatidyl glycerol in the rat, rabbit, monkey and human lung. *Biochim. Biophys. Acta* **360:** 56, 1974.

39. Weinhold, R. Biosynthesis of phosphatidyl choline during prenatal development of the rat lung. *J. Lipid Res.* **9:** 262, 1968.

40. Epstein, M. F., Farrell, P. M. The choline incorporation pathway: Primary mechanism for de novo lecithin synthesis in fetal primate lung. *Pediatr. Res.* **9:** 658, 1975.

41. Hallman, M., Raivio, K. Formation of disaturated lecithin through the lysolecithin pathway in the lung of the developing rabbit. *Biol. Neonate* **27:** 329, 1975.
42. Gluck, L., M. Sribney, Kulovich, M. V. The biochemical development of surface activity in mammalian lung. II. The biosynthesis of phospholipids in the lung of the developing rabbit fetus and newborn. *Pediat. Res.* **1:** 247, 1967.
43. Spitzer, H. L., K. Morrison, Norman, J. R. The incorporation of L-(me-14C) Methionine and (Me³H)-choline into lung phosphatides. *Biochim. Biophys. Acta* **152:** 552, 1968.
44. Gluck, L., M. V. Kulovich, A. J. Eidelman, L. Cordero, Khazin, A. F. Biochemical development of surface activity in mammalian lung. IV. Pulmonary lecithin synthesis in human fetus and newborn and etiology of the respiratory distress syndrome. *Pediatr. Res.* **6:** 81, 1972.
45. Hallman, M., Gluck, L. The biosynthesis of phosphatidylglycerol in the lung of the developing rabbit. *Fed. Prod.* **34:** 274, 1975.
46. Degroot, L. J., S. Refetoff et al. Nuclear triodothyronine binding protein: partial characterization and binding to chromatin. *Proc. Acad. Sci. (Wash.)* **71:** 4042, 1974.
47. Potter, E. L. and Bohlender. Intra-uterine respiration in relation to development of the fetal lung. *Amer. J. Obstet. Gynecol.* **42:** 14, 1941.
48. Jost, A. and Policard, A. Contribution experimentale a l'etude du development du poumon chez le lapin. *Arch. Anat. Microsc.* **37:** 323, 1948.
49. Reynolds, S. R. M. A source of amniotic fluid in the lamb. The naso-pharyngeal and buccal cavities. *Nature* **172:** 307, 1953.
50. Adams, F. H. and Gujiwara, T. Surfactant in fetal lamb tracheal fluid. *J. Pediatr.* **63:** 537, 1963.
51. Adams, F. H., Fujiwara, T. and Rowshan, G. The nature and origin of the fluid in the fetal lamb lung. *J. Pediatr.* **63:** 881, 1963.
52. Snyder, F. F. and Rosenfeld, M. Direct observation of intra-uterine respiratory movements of the fetus and the role of carbon dioxide and oxygen in their regulation. *Am. J. Physiol.* **119:** 153, 1937.
53. Barcroft, J. and Karnoven, M. J. The action of carbon dioxide and cyanide on fetal respiratory movements. The development of chemoreflex function in sheep. *J. Physiol.* **107:** 153, 1948.
54. Bonar, B. E., Blumemfeld, C. M. and Fenning, C. Studies of fetal respiratory movements. *Am. J. Dis. Child.* **55:** 1, 1938.
55. Duenhoelter, J. H. and Pritchard, J. A. Human fetal respiration. *Obstet. Gynecol.* **42:** 746, 1973.
56. Duenholter, J. H. and Pritchard, J. A. Human fetal respiration. II. Fate of intra-amniotic hypaque and ⁵¹Cr-labelled red cells. *Obstet. Gynec.* **43:** 878, 1974.
57. Reifferscheid, W. and Schmiemann, R. Roentgenographischer nachweis der intra-uterinen Atmenhewegung des Fetus. *Zentralbl. Gynaek.* **63:** 146, 1939.
58. Davis, L. A. and Potter, E. L. Intrauterine respiration of the human fetus. *J. A. M. A.* **131:** 1194, 1946.
59. Windle, W. F., Becker, R. F., Barth, E. E. and Schulz, M. D. Aspiration of amniotic fluid by fetus (an experimental roentgenological study in the guinea pig). *Surg. Gynec. Obstet.* **69:** 705, 1939.
60. McLain, C. R. Amniography. A versatile diagnostic procedure in obstetrics. *Obstet. Gynec.* **23:** 45, 1964.
61. Duenholter, J. H. and Pritchard, J. A. Fetal respiration: Quantitative measurements of amniotic fluid inspired near term by human and rhesus fetuses. *Amer. J. Obstet. Gynecol.* **125:** 306, 1976.

62. Boddy, K. and Robinson, J. S. External method for detection of fetal breathing in utero. *Lancet,* **2:** 1231, 1971.
63. Gluck, L. and Kulovich, M. V. Evaluation of fetal functional maturity. *In* Modern Perinat. Medicine. (Gluck, L., Ed.) Chicago Year Book Medical Publishers, 1974, p. 195.
64. Ross, B. B. Comparison of fetal pulmonary fluid with foetal plasma and amniotic fluid. *Nature* **199:** 1100, 1963.
65. Setnikar, I., E. Agostoni, Taglietti, A. The fetal lung, a source of amniotic fluid. *Proc. Soc. Exper. Biol. Med.* **101:** 842, 1959.
66. Schreyer, P., J. Tamir et al. Amniotic fluid total phospholipids versus lecithin-sphingomyelin ratio in the evaluation of fetal lung maturity. *Am. J. Obstet. Gynecol.* **120:** 909, 1974.
67. Laatikainen, T., T. Hokkanen, Hahti, E. Determination of amniotic fluid lecithin with a gas phase thin-layer chromatographic detector. *Scand. J. Clin. Lab. Invest.* **31:** 347, 1973.
68. Nelson, G. H. Relationship between amniotic fluid lecithin concentration and respiratory distress syndrome. Am. J. Obstet. Gynecol. **112:** 827, 1972.
69. Moore, R. A., K. T. O'Neil et al. Palmitic acid and lecithin measurements in amniotic fluid. *Brit. J. Obstet. Gynaecol.* **82:** 194, 1975.
70. Thom, H., R. Dinwiddie et al. Palmitic acid concentrations and lecithin/sphingomyelin ratios in amniotic fluid. *Clin. Chim. Acta* **62:** 143, 1975.
71. Warren, C., J. B. Holton, Allen, J. T. Assessment of fetal lung maturity by estimation of amniotic fluid palmitic acid. *Brit. Med. J.* **1:** 94, 1974.
72. Falconer, G. F., J. S. Hodge and Gadd, R. L. Influence of amniotic fluid volume on lecithin estimation in prediction of respiratory distress. *Brit. Med. J.* **2:** 689, 1973.
73. Roux, J. F., J. Nakamura, Frosolono, M. Fatty acid composition and concentration of lecithin in the acetone fraction of amniotic fluid phospholipids. *Am. J. Obstet. Gynecol.* **119:** 838, 1974.
74. Russell, P. T., W. J. Miller and McLain, C. R. Palmitic acid content of amniotic fluid lecithin as an index to fetal lung maturity. *Clin. Chem.* **20:** 1431, 1974.
75. Schirar, A., J. P. Vielh et al. Amniotic fluid phospholipids and fatty acids in normal pregnancies. Relation to gestational age and neonatal condition. *Am. J. Obstet. Gynecol.* **121:** 653, 1975.
76. Gluck, L., M. V. Kulovich and R. C. Borer: Estimates of fetal maturity. *Clin. Perinatol.* **1:** 125, 1974.
77. Gluck, L. and Kulovich, M. V. Lecithin/sphingomyelin ratio in amniotic fluid in normal and abnormal pregnancy. *Am. J. Obstet. Gynecol.* **115:** 539, 1973.
78. White, P. Pregnancy and diabetes, medical aspects. *Med. Clin. North Am.* **49:** 1015, 1965.
79. Cruz, A. C., Buti, W. C., Birk, S. A. and Spellacy, W. N. Respiratory distress syndrome with mature lecithin/sphingomyelin ratio Diabetes mellitus and low Apgar scores. *Amer. J. Obstet. Gynecol.* **126:** 78, 1976.
80. Farrell, P. M. Indices of fetal maturation in diabetic pregnancy. *Lancet* **1:** 596, 1976.
81. Harvey, D., Parkinson, C. E. and Campbell, S. Risk of respiratory distress syndrome. *Lancet* **7897:** 42, 1975.
82. Mueller-Heubach, E., Caritis, S. N. et al. L/S ratio in amniotic fluid and its value for the prediction of neonatal RDS in pregnant diabetic women. *Amer. J. Obstet. Gynecol.* **130:** 28, 1978.
83. Kanto, W. P., R. C. Borer, Roloff, D. W. Postnatal changes in the L/S ratio of tracheal aspirates from infants with severe respiratory distress syndrome. *J. Pediatr.* **84:** 921, 1974.

84. Obladen, M., T. A. Merritt, Gluck, L. Alterations in tracheal phospholipid composition during RDS. *Pediatr. Res.* **10:** 465, 1976.
85. Weller, P. H., J. Gupta et al. Pharyngeal lecithin/sphingomyelin ratio in newborn infants. *Lancet* **1:** 12, 1976.
86. Clements, J., Platzker, A. C. G. et al. Assessment of the risk of the respiratory distress syndrome by a rapid test for surfactant in amniotic fluid. *New Engl. J. Med.* 1077, 1972.
87. Caspi, E., Schreyer, P., Tamir, L. The amniotic fluid foam test, L/S ratio and total phospholipids in the evaluation of fetal lung maturity. *Am. J. Obstet. Gynec.* **122:** 323, 1975.
88. Muller-Tyl, E., Lempert, J.: The prediction of fetal lung maturity from the surface tension characteristics of amniotic fluid. *J. Perinat. Med.* **3:** 47, 1975.
89. Muller-Tyl, E., Lempert, J., Steinbereithner, K., Benzer, H. Surface properties of the amniotic fluid in normal pregnancy. *Am. J. Obstet. Gynecol.* **122:** 295, 1975.
90. Copeland, W., Stempel, L. et al. Assessment of a rapid test on amniotic fluid for estimating fetal lung maturity. *Am. J. Obstet. Gynecol.* **130:** 225, 1978.
91. Shinitzky, M., Goldfisher, A. et al. A new method for assessment of fetal lung maturity. *Brit. J. Obstet. Gynaecol.* **83:** 838, 1976.
92. Shinitzky, M., Dianoux, A. C. et al. *Biochemistry* **10:** 2106, 1971.
93. Cogan, U., Shinitzky, M., Weher, G., Nishida, T. *Biochemistry* **12:** 521, 1973.
94. Freeman, R. K., B. G. Bateman et al. Clinical experience with the amniotic fluid lecithin/sphingomyelin ratio. *Am. J. Obstet. Gynecol.* **119:** 239, 1974.
95. Richardson, C. J., J. J. Pomerance et al. Acceleration of fetal lung maturation following prolonged rupture of the membranes. *Am. J. Obstet. Gynecol.* **118:** 1115, 1974.
96. Berkovitz, R. L., Bonta, B. W., Warshaw, J. E. The relationship between premature rupture of the membranes and the respiratory distress syndrome. *Am. J. Obstet. Gynecol.* **124:** 712, 1976.
97. Bauer, C. R., Stern, L., Colle, E. Prolonged rupture of membranes associated with a decreased incidence of RDS. *Pediatrics* **53:** 7, 1974.
98. Alden, E. R., Mandelkorn, T. et al. Morbidity and mortality in infants weighing less than 1000 grams in an intensive care nursery. *Pediatrics* **50:** 40, 1972.
99. Yoon, J. J., Harper, R. G. Observations on the relationship between duration of rupture of the membranes and the development of idiopathic respiratory distress syndrome. *Pediatrics* **52:** 161, 1973.
100. Chiswick, M. L., Bernard, E. Respiratory Distress Syndrome. *Lancet* **1:** 1060, 1973.
101. Gluck, L., M. V. Kulovich, R. C. Borer, W. N. Keidel: The interpretation and significance of the lecithin/sphingomyelin ratio in amniotic fluid. *Am. J. Obstet. Gynaecol.* **120:** 142, 1974.
102. Singh, E. J., A. Mejia, Zuspan, F. P. Studies of human amniotic fluid phospholipids in normal, diabetes and drug-abuse pregnancy. *Am. J. Obstet. Gynecol.* **119:** 623, 1974.
103. Whitfield, C. R., W. B. Sproule, Brudenell, M. The amniotic fluid lecithin sphingomyelin area ratio (LSAR) in pregnancies complicated by diabetes. *J. Obstet. Gynaecol. Brit. Commonw.* **80:** 918, 1973.
104. Bustos, R., M. V. Kulovich et al. Significance of phosphatidylglycerol in amniotic fluid in complicated pregnancies. (Submitted for publication)
105. Jones, Burd, L. Z., Bowes, W. A. et al. Failure of association of premature rupture of membranes with respiratory distress syndrome. *New Engl. J. Med.* **292:** 1253, 1975.
106. Robert, M. F., Neff, R. K. et al. The association between maternal diabetes and the respiratory distress syndrome. *Pediat. Res.* **9:** 370, 1975.
107. Smith, B. T., C. J. P. Giroud, M. Robert, Avery, M. E. Insulin antagonism of cortisol action on lecithin synthesis by cultured fetal lung cells. *J. Pediat.* **87:** 953, 1975.
108. Gluck, L., Chez, R. A. et al. Comparison of phospholipid indicators of fetal lung matur-

ity in amniotic fluid of monkey (Macaca mulatta) and baboon (Papio papio). *Am. J. Obstet. Gynecol.* **230**: 524, 1974.

109. Epstein, M. F., Farrell, P. M. Primate fetal lung in gestations complicated by maternal glucose intolerance. *Pediatr. Res.* **9**: 395, 1975.

110. Liggins, G. C. Premature delivery of fetal lambs injected with glucocorticoids. *J. Endocrinol.* **45**: 515, 1969.

111. Duhring, J. L. and Thompson, S. A. Amniotic fluid phospholipid analysis in normal and complicated pregnancies. *Amer. J. Obstet. Gynecol.* **121**: 218, 1975.

112. Dunn, L. J., C. Bush, S. E. Davis, and Bhatnager, A. S. Use of laboratory and clinical factors in the management of pregnancies complicated by maternal disease. *Am. J. Obstet. Gynecol.* **120**: 622, 1974.

113. Stahlman, M. T., Gray, M. E. et al. The role of cyclic AMP in lamellar body synthesis and secretion. *Pediatr. Res.* **8**: 196, 1974.

114. Karotkin, E. H., Cashore, W. J. et al. Pharmacological induction and inhibition of lung maturation in fetal rabbits. *Pediat. Res.* **9**: 397, 1975.

115. Barret, C. T., A. Sevanian, Kaplan, S. A. Cyclic AMP and surfactant production: new means for enhancing lung maturation in the fetus. *Ped. Res.* **9**: 394, 1975.

116. Shaw, J. O. and Moser, K. M. Current status of prostaglandins and lungs. *Chest* **68**: 75, 1975.

117. Wyszogrodiski, J., H. W. Taeusch, Avery, M. E. Isoxsuprine induced alterations of pulmonary pressure-volume relationships in premature rabbits. *Am. J. Obstet. Gynecol.* **119**: 1107, 1974.

118. Kero, P., T. Hirvonen, Valimaki, I. Prenatal and postnatal isoxsuprine and respiratory distress syndrome. *Lancet* **2**: 198, 1973.

119. Howie, R. N., Liggins, G. C. Prevention of respiratory distress syndrome in premature infants by antepartum glucocorticoid treatment. *In* Respiratory Distress Syndrome. (Vilee, D. B. and Zuckerman, J., eds.) New York, Academic Press, p. 369, 1973.

120. Spellacy, W. N., Buhi, W. C. et al. Human amniotic fluid lecithin/sphingomyelin ratio changes with estrogen and glucocorticoid treatment. *Am. J. Obstet. Gynecol.* **115**: 216, 1973.

121. Charles, D., Chattoraj, S. D. Possible role of estradiol −17 beta and cortisol in the prevention of RDS. *In* Respiratory Distress Syndrome (Eds. Villee, C. A. and Ville, D. B., Zuckerman, J.) New York, Academic Press, p. 381, 1973.

122. Glass, L., B. K. Rajegowda, Evans, H. E. Absence of respiratory distress syndrome in premature infants of heroin addicted mothers. *Lancet* **2**. 685, 1971.

123. Taeusch, H. W., S. H. Carson et al. Heroin induction of lung maturation and growth retardation in fetal rabbits. *J. Ped.* **82**: 869, 1973.

124. OH, W. Surfactant formation: pharmacologic consideration. Lung maturation and the prevention of HMD. Report of the Seventh Ross Conference on Pediatric Research, 1976, p. 47.

125. Sundell, H., F. S. Serenius et al. The effect of EGF on fetal lamb lung maturation. *Pediatr. Res.* **9**: 371, 1975.

126. Lorenz, V., H. Ruttgers et al. Fetal pulmonary surfactant induction by bromhexine metabolite. VIII. *Am. J. Obstet. Gynecol.* **119**: 126, 1974.

127. Ballard, P. L., Ballard, R. A. Cytoplasmic receptor for glucocorticoids in lung of the human fetus and neonate. *J. Clin. Invest.* **53**: 477, 1974.

128. Gianopolos, G. Early events in the action of glucocorticoids in developing tissues. *J. Steroid Biochem.* **6**: 623, 1975.

129. Thompson, E. B., Lippman, M. E. Mechanism of action of glucocorticoids. *Metabolism* **23**: 159, 1974.

130. Gianpoulos, G. Variations in the levels of cytoplasmic glucocorticoid receptors in lungs of various species at different developmental stages. *Endocrine* **94:** 450, 1974.
131. Baden, M., C. B. Bauer et al. A controlled trial of hydrocortisone therapy in infants with respiratory distress syndrome. *Pediat.* **50:** 526, 1972.
132. Avery, M. E. Pharmacological approaches on the acceleration of fetal lung maturation. *Brit. Med. Bull.* **31:** 13, 1975.
133. Taeusch, H. W., M. Heiner, Avery, M. E. Accelerated lung maturation and increased survival in premature rabbits treated with hydrocortisone. *Am. Rev. Resp. Dis.* **105:** 971, 1972.
134. Farrell, P. M. and Zachman, R. D. Induction of choline phosphotransferase and lecithin synthesis in the fetal lung by corticosteroids. *Science* **179:** 297, 1973.
135. Rooney, S. A., I. Gross et al. Stimulation of glycerol phosphate phosphatidyltransferase activity in fetal rabbit lung. *Biochim. Biophys. Acta,* **398:** 433, 1975.
136. Farrell, P. M., D. W. Dundgre and Douglas, W. H. J. Enzymatic synthesis of phosphatidyl choline in homogenous cultures of apparent type II pneumocytes. *Pediatric Res.* **9:** 276, 1975.
137. Smith, B. T. Lung maturation and the prevention of H. M. D. Report of the 17th Ross Conference on Pediatric Research. Ross Laboratories, Columbus, Ohio.
138. Chernick, V. Glucocorticoid inhibition; Delayed lung maturation. 17th Conference on Ped. Res., p. 67.
139. Robert, M. F., A. T. Bator, Taeusch, H. W. Pulmonary pressure volume relationship after corticotropin and saline injections in fetal rabbits. *Pediat. Res.* **9:** 760, 1975.
140. Sundell, H., A. Triantos et al. Prevention of hyaline membrane disease with ACTH infusion in fetal lambs. *Pediat. Res.* **7:** 407, 1973.
141. Fencl, M., De M., Tulcinsky, D. Total cortisol in amniotic fluid and fetal lung maturation. *New Engl. J. Med.* **292:** 133, 1975.
142. Murphy, B. E. P. Cortisol and cortisone levels in the cord blood at delivery of infants with and without the respiratory distress syndrome. *Am. J. Obstet. Gynecol.* **119:** 1112, 1974.
143. Murphy, B. E. P. Does the human fetal adrenal play role in parturition. *Am. J. Obstet. Gynec.,* **115:** 52, 1973.
144. Hillman, D. A. Urinary 17-hydroxycorticosteroid excretion in newborn infants with respiratory distress syndrome. *Am. J. Dis. Child,* **102:** 569, 1961.
145. Migeon, C. J., H. Prystowsky et al. Placental passage of 17-hydroxy corticosteroids: Comparison of the levels in maternal and fetal plasma and effect of ACTH and hydrocortisone administration. *J. Clin. Invest.* **35:** 488, 1956.
146. Frederick, J. and Butler, N. R. Hyaline membrane disease. *Lancet* **2:** 768, 1972.
147. Kenny, F., R. Depp et al. Glucocorticoid, mineralcorticoid and estrogen metabolism in a neonate with familial congenital absence of adrenals. *Pediat. Res.* **7:** 329, 1973.
148. Liggins, G. C. Prenatal Glucocorticoid treatment; prevention of respiratory distress syndrome. 17th Conference on Ped. Res., p. 97.
149. Liggins, G. C. and Howie, R. N. A controlled trial of antepartum glucocorticoid treatment for prevention of the respiratory distress syndrome premature infants. *Pediatrics* **50:** 515, 1972.
150. Caspi, E., P. Schreyer et al. Changes in amniotic fluid lecithin-sphingomyelin ratio following maternal beta-methasone administration. *Am. J. Obstet. Gynecol.* **122:** 327, 1975.
151. Conney, A. H. Enzyme induction: Thoughts on clinical applications. 17th Conference on Ped. Res., p. 21.

152. Kotas, R., L. Mims, Hart, L. Reversible inhibition of lungs cell number after glucocorticoid injection. *Pediatrics* **53**: 358, 1974.
153. Fitzhardinge, P., Eisen, A. et al. Sequelae of early steroid administration to the newborn infant. *Pediatrics* **53**: 877, 1974.
154. DeLemos, R. A. Glucocorticoid effect: organ development in monkeys. 17th Conference on Ped. Res., p. 77.
155. Gould, J. B., L. Gluck, Kulovich, M. V. The acceleration of neurological maturation in high stress pregnancy and its relation to fetal lung maturity. *Pediat. Res.* **6**: 335, 1972.
156. Taeusch, H. W. Glucocorticoid prohylaxis for respiratory distress syndrome. A review of potential toxicity. *J. Pediat.* **87**: 617, 1975.
157. Killam. Prenatal glucocorticoid treatment: effect on surviving infants. 17th Conference on Ped. Res., p. 110.
158. Klevit, H. Corticosteroid therapy in the neonatal period. *Ped. Clin. N. Am.* **17**: 1003, 1970.
159. Erenberg, A., D. L. Phelps et al. Total and free thyroid hormone concentrations in the neonatal period. *Pediatrics* **53**: 211, 1974.
160. Wu, B., Kikkawa, Y. et al. Accelerated maturation of fetal rabbit lung by thyroxine. *Physiologist* **14**: 253, 1971.
161. Cuestas, R. A., A. Lindall, Engel R. R. Abnormal cord thyroid hormone levels in neonatal respiratory distress syndrome. *Ped. Res.* **10**: 337, 1976.
162. Friedman, W. F., Hirschkliu, N. G. et al. Pharmacologic closure of patent ductus arteriosus in the premature infant. *New Engl. J. Med.* **295**: 526, 1976.
163. Cuestas, R. A., Lindall, A., Engell, R. R. Thyroid hormone and respiratory distress syndrome of the newborn. *New Engl. J. Med.* **295**: 297, 1976.
164. Grumbach, M. M. and Werner, S. C. Transfer of thyroid hormone across the human placenta at term. *J. Clin. Endocrinol. Metab.* **16**: 1392, 1956.
165. Sack, J., Delbert, A. et al. Thyroid hormone metabolism in amniotic and allantoic fluids of the sheep. *Pediatr. Res.* **9**: 837, 1975.
166. Fisher, D. A., Dussault, J. et al. Ontogenesis of hypothalamic pituitary thyroid function and metabolism in man, sheep and rat. (Roy and Green, Ed.) Recent Progress in Hormone Research, Vol. 33. New York, Academic Press, 1977, p. 59.
167. Phelps, C. P. and Leathem, J. H. Effects of postnatal thyroxine administration on brain development. Response to postnatal androgen and thyroid regulation in female rats. *J. Endocrinol.* **69**: 175, 1976.
168. Mashiach, S., Barkai, G., Sack, J., Stern, E., Goldman, B., Brish, M., Serr, D. M. Enhancement of fetal lung maturity by intra-amniotic administration of thyroid hormone. *Am. J. Obstet. Gynecol.* **130**: 289, 1978.
169. Cunningham, M.D., Greine, J. M., Thompson, S. A., Desai, N. S.: Antenatal reduction of surfactant phosphatidylglycerol in infants of diabetic mothers with respiratory distress. *Paediat. Res.* **10** (1976) 460.
170. Hallman, M., Feldman, B. H., Gluck, L. RDS: The absence of phosphatidyl glycerol in surfactant. *Paediat. Res.* **9** (1975) 369.

7

The Significance of Fetal Size

RAJA W. ABDUL-KARIM, M.D.
AND
SHIRAZALI G. SUNDERJI, M.B., CH.B.

The great interest in fetal growth retardation is largely due to the fact that growth retarded fetuses and newborns are subject to a high incidence of complications. These are summarized in Table 1. A sound approach to the diagnosis and management of intrauterine growth retardation entails a thorough understanding of the physiologic and pathophysiologic factors regulating fetal growth. Unfortunately, our knowledge in this area is fragmentary.

The current definition of intrauterine growth retardation (IUGR) is based largely on statistical rather than biological criteria. The most commonly used index is birthweight as it relates to gestational age. Babies whose birthweights are below the normal limits are considered growth retarded. This presupposes that the limits for normalcy are well defined; in fact they are not.

The absence of a clear biologic definition of what constitutes a growth retarded baby has resulted in the lack of a universally accepted standard. Authors have employed various criteria, e.g., below the 3rd, 5th or 10th percentile. The population thus defined is not only heterogeneous, but differs with the set limits (Fig. 1).

Table 1.   Fetal and Neonatal Complications of Intrauterine Growth Retardation.[1,2,4]

1. Increase in perinatal morbidity and mortality	7. Hypocalcemia
2. High incidence of congenital (morphologic/chromosomal) anomalies	8. Hypothermia
3. Intrapartum asphyxia	9. Hyperviscosity (polycythemia)
4. Pulmonary hemorrhage	10. Poor postnatal physical growth
5. Meconium aspiration	11. Educational difficulties
6. Hypoglycemia	

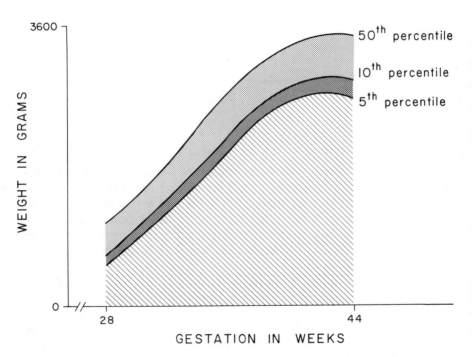

Fig. 1.   Empirical human fetal growth curve based on birthweight for gestational age to demonstrate that the population of newborn considered growth retarded differs, whether the 10th or 5th percentile limits are used. The 3rd percentile (not shown) select still another group. It should be noted that in terms of *numbers*, there are more babies who fall within the 3rd and 10th percentile than below the 3rd percentile.

The complexity of defining IUGR is further illustrated by Figure 2. Here the 5th and 95th percentiles of birthweight for gestation are superimposed upon perinatal mortality rates based on birthweight and gestational age. It is apparent that there can be up to a fourfold variation in perinatal mortality in "normal" sized babies (i.e., between the 5th and 95th percentile) born at term. It may also be argued (using perinatal mortality as the index) that all babies born between 39–41 weeks whose birthweights fall below the 50 contour may have a disturbance in their growth since they deviate from an "optimal" perinatal mortality. This obviously is unrealistic, but serves to underscore the current dilemma.

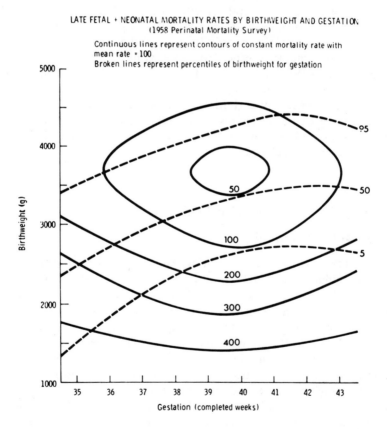

Fig. 2. Reproduced by permission from: Goldstein, H., Peckham, C. In: Roberts, D. F., Thomson, A. M. (eds). The Biology of Human Fetal Growth, Taylor and Francis Ltd., London 1976. p. 81. © 1976 Taylor and Francis Ltd.

It is therefore clear that IUGR babies represent a statistical selection which does not necessarily define all babies whose birthweights have not reached the *optimal limit. Nor does it mean that babies of similar birthweights share a common prognosis.* Furthermore, fetal length can vary independently of weight. It behooves us to define the optimal limits of fetal size not only with respect to perinatal mortality but to other indices of prenatal and postnatal development. It is to this end that research into the factors controlling fetal size can be quite rewarding.

The criterion of using birthweight as an index of growth retardation has an additional disadvantage; it is a retrospective diagnosis. Sonography constitutes a fairly reliable method for the *prenatal diagnosis* of growth retardation. It is also a method whereby the *rate of growth* can be measured and indices of fetal growth other than weight can be assessed.

Fetal size however viewed, is a significant prognosticator of prenatal and postnatal outcome. Indeed, it appears that birthweight is the more significant variable with respect to perinatal morbidity and mortality than at least some of the other indices of postnatal growth.[21,43] The significance of birthweight as an index of outcome is not limited to those fetuses or newborns designated by definition as growth retarded. Hence a thorough understanding of the mechanisms regulating fetal size is essential for the identification and possible treatment of those fetuses which have not achieved their optimal size.

PHYSIOLOGIC REGULATORS OF FETAL SIZE

Maternal Environment

The classic experiment demonstrating the key role of the *maternal environment* in regulating fetal size was done by Walton and Hammond in the late 1930's.[47] These investigators bred shire horses with Shetland ponies and found that the birthweight of the offspring was related to the size of the mother. This observation has subsequently been confirmed in other animals. Smidt et al. showed that zygotes from normal-sized pigs transferred into drarf sows developed into piglets whose birthweight was nearly halved, whereas the zygotes of dwarf pigs grown in normal sized sows resulted in piglets whose birthweight was almost doubled.[40]

In the human the evidence is of a less direct nature. A higher correlation in birthweight exists among half-sibs from a common mother than in those from a common father.[30] Furthermore, there is a correlation between the birthweight of an infant and that of its mother.[33]

Maternal Endocrine System

The normal *maternal endocrine system* has little direct influence on fetal size.[26] Maternal hormones either do not cross the placenta (e.g., the peptide and protein hormones) or do so very poorly (e.g., T4, T3 and cortisol. Cortisol is converted by the placenta to cortisone). These barriers to the transfer of maternal hormones seem advantageous to the fetus as it develops its own endocrine system free of outside control. This protective barrier, however, does not extend to maternal diseased states. The altered fetal growth in response to maternal endocrinopathies may be due to mechanisms other than the direct transfer of maternal hormones.[26] In maternal thyrotoxicosis the fetal affliction may be secondary to the transfer of immunoglobulins, e.g., LATS. The fetal macrosomia associated with maternal diabetes and sometimes seen in acromegaly may be due respectively to hyperglycemia or to somatomedin action. The fetal hyperparathyroidism associated with maternal hypoparathyroidism is probably initiated by the lowering of the maternal plasma calcium.

Maternal Nutrition

The earlier concept that the fetus is a true parasite has now been modified, and it is clear that maternal nutrition during pregnancy can influence fetal weight as well as other aspects of its development. Birthweight correlates directly with the mother's prepregnancy weight, and her weight gain during pregnancy. This subject has recently been reviewed.[3] It should be mentioned, however that severity of the fetal effect of undernutrition varies among species and that in some aspects, the primate fetus seems to be more resilient to the effect of maternal dietary restrictions than the rodent.[2,4]

Fetal Endocrine System

Based on the available evidence, *insulin* appears to be the most important hormone influencing fetal size in the human. The evidence principally comes from the association of fetal hyperinsulinemia (e.g., secondary to maternal diabetes mellitus) with fetal macrosomia, and that of congenital hypoinsulinemia with low birthweight.[25,39] In maternal diabetes mellitus, the fetal mascrosomia is inversely related to the adequacy of maternal blood sugar control. This in turn correlates with the degree of fetal hyperinsulinism. Direct support for the growth-promoting effect of insulin is found in animal studies.[23] For example, exogenous insulin injected into rat fetuses causes an increase in birthweight.[34]

Apart from insulin there is little evidence in the human that other fetal hormones significantly affect fetal weight. This is not true for other species, hence the findings in laboratory animals may not apply to the human. Although the *glucocortisides* are important in various maturational processes, they exert no major influence on fetal size in the human. Similarly, *thyroid hormones* while important in skeletal and brain maturation, seem to have little effect on fetal weight. Hypothyroid human fetuses can be of normal birthweight although their length may be shortened. This is not true in the sheep, where fetal hypothyroidism has a significant effect on its weight.[24] The difference among species may at least partly be the result of the varying amount of transferred maternal thyroid hormones.[45]

Growth hormone (GH) is another example where the role in the human fetus seems to differ from that in other species. This subject has been reviewed recently by Liggins[25] and by others.[3] In sheep, GH deficiency leads to undersized fetuses. In the human, available evidence comes from the study of three congenital anomalies[3,25]: anencephalics, fetuses spontaneously decapitated in utero, and newborns with familial HGH deficiency. While conflicting views have been expressed regarding inferences made from the study of such newborns, a critical analysis of the findings does not exclude the possibility that "normal" birthweight can be reached in the absence or deficiency of HGH. This is somewhat surprising since GH reaches high levels in fetal cord blood.

There is increasing interest in the role *somatomedin* may have in influencing fetal size. Somatomedin is a polypeptide which is stimulated by and has a negative feedback on HGH. Not much is known about its role in fetal growth. Somatomedin is decreased in maternal plasma and is found in low concentration in cord blood. The level in cord blood seems higher in large fetuses and low in IUGR. Estrogens are possible inhibitors of somatomedin.[31,41,42]

The role that *estrogens* play in modulating fetal size in the human is not known. In rabbits, estrogens exert a significant effect on both fetal and placental weights.[6,7,9] Estrogen deficiency increases both fetal and placental weights, whereas estrogen replacement constrains their growth (Fig. 3). The reduction in fetal size is directly related to the amount of estrogen; increasing the dose further leads to fetal demise. The increase in fetal and placental weights under estrogen deficiency is due to cellular hyperplasia without a change in cell size.[5,7,9]

The studies in rabbits on the role of estrogens in regulating fetal and placental weights have added another dimension to understanding the interrelationships between nutritional influences and the endocrine milieu. Nutritional deficiency in rabbits leads to weight loss in the mother, an in-

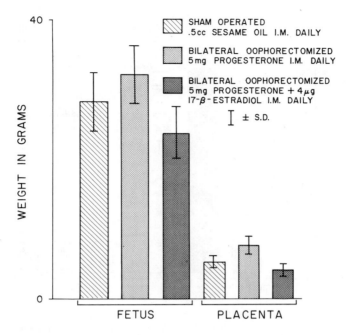

Fig. 3.   The influence of estrogen deficiency (produced by bilateral oophorectomy) on fetal and placental weight in 27-day pregnant rabbits. Estrogen deficiency induced a significant increase in both fetal and placental weight. Exogenously administered 17-B-estradiol prevented fetal and placental macrosomia in bilaterally oophorectomized rabbits.

creased rate of stillbirths and intrauterine growth retardation. The administration of progesterone reduces the rate of stillbirths but has no influence on fetal weight. Nutritionally deficient pregnant rabbits rendered estrogen deficient (by bilateral oophorectomy with progesterone supplementation) lose *more* weight but have fetuses and placentas of *normal weight.*[5] The decrease in fetal size incidental to maternal undernutrition was corrected by the increased rate of cell multiplication incidental to the estrogen deficiency (Fig. 4).

The Fetal Kidneys

The mechanism by which the kidneys influence fetal size is not clear. However, the association of renal agenesis with growth retardation in the human has been made. In sheep, fetal nephrectomy leads to growth retardation.[44,46]

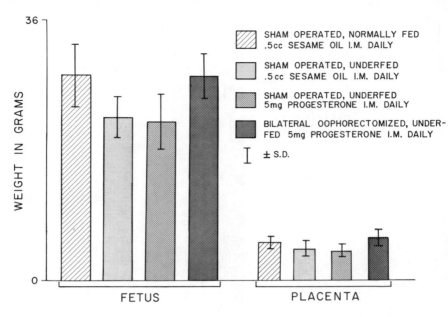

Fig. 4. Prevention of nutritionally induced fetal and placental growth retardation by estrogen deficiency in 27-day pregnant rabbits. Undernutrition significantly decreased fetal and placental weights in intact and intact progesterone-supplemented rabbits. In equally undernourished rabbits rendered estrogen-deficient (by bilateral oophorectomy) fetal and placental weights were similar to normally fed controls.

Genetic Makeup of the Fetus

This accounts for 15–20 percent of variations in birthweight. Male newborns as a rule are heavier than females. This may be related to the presence of the Y chromosome which enhances the antigenic dissimilarity between the mother and fetus and/or the action of testicular hormones. Precise number and orderly cell division are needed to insure a normally proportioned growth. The number of cells in a fetus at term is the sum total of 42 successive cell divisions of the zygote.

Nutrients

Fetal size is influenced by the amount and nature of nutrients reaching it and by its ability to utilize those nutrients. The fetal nutrient supply is dependent on maternal intake, the availability of the nutrients in the maternal blood, the adequacy of the maternal placental circulation, and the adequacy of placental transfer.

PATHOLOGIC INFLUENCES ON FETAL GROWTH

The size a fetus attains is influenced not only by physiologic regulators but also by the presence or absence of certain pathologic states. The majority of the latter are associated with fetal growth retardation. Table 2 provides a summary.

Diagnosis of IUGR

Suspected IUGR must be sharply differentiated from an error in gestational age. Clinically, IUGR must be considered in any pregnancy associated with a complication known to retard fetal growth, as well as in those women with a previous growth retarded newborn. Clinical suspicion, abdominal palpation and fundal height measurements are useful but more precise documentation is needed. Of the hormonal tests available, 24-hour maternal urinary estrogen levels correlate best with fetal weight.[4] A most helpful tool in the diagnosis and followup of IUGR is serial ultrasonography. This should not supersede but should be used in conjunction

Table 2.   Pathologic Influences Associated with Intrauterine Growth Retardation. (Compiled from[1,2,4])

I. Fetal Afflictions
    1. Congenital Anomalies
    2. Infections
    3. Drugs
    4. Radiation
    5. Immunologic factors
II. Placental Abnormalities
    1. Extensive infarcts
    2. Hemangiomas
    3. Single umbilical artery
III. Maternal Illness and/or Deficiency in Nutrient Support
    A. Vascular Insufficiency
        1. Essential hypertension
        2. Chronic renal disease
        3. Severe diabetes mellitus
        4. Preeclampsia
    B. Chronic abruption with recurrent bleeding
    C. Multiple gestation
    D. Undernutrition
    E. Hypoxemia
        1. Altitude
        2. Smoking
        3. Cyanotic Heart Disease

with clinical judgment; ultrasonography has added significantly to precision in diagnosing IUGR. An indepth discussion of ultrasonography is outside the scope of this chapter. A summary of the ways ultrasonography can be employed in the diagnosis and management of IUGR is presented in Table 3.

Serial fetal biparietal diameter (BPD) measurements have identified two forms of IUGR that differ in etiology and prognosis[10-12] (Table 4.)

1. *Low profile growth:* The fetal BPD continues to grow, although the measurements fall below normal.

2. *Late flattening growth:* A cessation or slowing in the growth of the BPD occurs in a previously normally growing fetus.

Fancourt and Campbell[15] have provided data on the 4-year follow-up of

Table 3. Summary of Ultrasonographic Methods to Assess Fetal Growth.[11,20]

A. Biparietal Diameter
  1. Normal rate of growth
    14–30 weeks 3.3 mm/wk (average)
    30–36 weeks 2.0 mm/wk   ''
    36–40 weeks 1.2 mm/wk   ''
  2. Accuracy: Nearly 20% either false
    Positive or false negative
B. Head Circumference

Weeks	Rate of Growth
14–30	11.5 mm/wk Average
30–36	7.2 mm/wk Average
36–40	1.8 mm/wk Average

C. Abdominal Circumference
  1. Predictive accuracy of a single measurement

Week Performed	% of Babies Below 5th Centile Detected
32	87
36	75

  2. Rate of growth

Week	Rate
14–36	11.6 mm/wk Average
after 36	7.4 mm/wk Average

D. Abdominal to Head Circumference Ratio

Week	Ratio
< 36	< 1
36	1
> 36	> 1

E. Total Intrauterine Volume (TIUV),
  Longitudinal (L), Transverse (T),
  and Antero-Posterior (AP) Diameter
  of Uterus are Measured TIUV = L X T X AP X 0.5233

Table 4. Patterns and Characteristics of Intrauterine Growth Retardation Based on Fetal Biparietal Diameter Measurement[10-12]

1. *Low Profile Growth*
    A. Infant symmetrically small
    B. Rarely asphyxic at birth-apgars usually normal
    C. Associated with congenital anomalies
    D. Rarely associated with maternal disease
    E. Urinary estrogens, oxytocin challenge test—usually normal
2. *Late Flattening*
    A. Infant asymmetrically grown
    B. Incidence of perinatal asphyxia and neonatal hypoglycemia high
    C. Associated with such diseases as chronic hypertension, postmaturity, severe diabetes, placenta previa
    D. Low maternal urinary estrogens, positive oxytocin challenge test, meconium in amniotic fluid-frequently present

infants with BPD growth failure in utero. They showed that if the growth failure occurred prior to 34 weeks, there was an increase in children whose height, weight and head circumference were below the 10th percentile. If the growth failure occurred before 28 weeks, there was an identifiable lower mean development quotient.

Other indirect fetal study techniques are available. These are discussed elsewhere[2,4] and include: a) Placental changes using Grey Scale echography[16]; b) measurements of maternal blood flow[14]; c) measurement of maternal blood B_1 glycoprotein[22]. The last named is a pregnancy protein that is depressed in IUGR. In view of its practicality, this method, if further developed, could become widely used.

Management

The current management of IUGR takes into account the related increased perinatal morbidity and mortality, the high rate of intrapartum fetal distress, and the thesis that the welfare of the fetus is better served outside, rather than within the uterus once pulmonary maturity is achieved. These observations form the basis for careful and meticulous prepartum and intrapartum fetal monitoring. The other aspect of management addresses itself to the improvement of fetal welfare. Basically this falls into two broad categories:

1. Attempts to improve delivery of nutrients to the fetus
    1. Rest in bed
    2. Use of Beta mimetic agents
    3. Decompression
2. Attempts to increase quantitatively the nutrients supplied to the fetus (hyperalimentation)

    1. Hypertonic glucose to mother

    2. Intraamniotic amino acids (AA)

The general principles of management as well as of fetal monitoring have been recently reviewed.[2,4] We shall discuss briefly some current developments regarding the use of Beta mimetic agents and hyperalimentation.

Fetal hyperalimentation has been tried by giving glucose or amino acids intravenously to the mother or by administering amino acids intraamniotically. There are two possible reasons why giving *glucose* I.V. to the mother may enhance fetal growth: 1) The maternal hyperglycemia will lead to elevated fetal glucose levels which in turn cause fetal hyperinsulinism. 2) Intrauterine growth retardation is sometimes accompanied by decreased placental secretion of human placental lactogen (HPL) and insulinase, while the secretion of insulin remains normal.[18] The net effect of these changes is a decrease in the availability of glucose to the fetus. Maternal glucose administration will serve to correct this deficiency. Beischer and O'Sullivan[8] and Campbell et al.[13] have administered 4 liters of 25% glucose I.V. continuously over a span of 48 hours. They reported that in some patients an improvement in fetal movement and growth and an increase in maternal urinary estrogen excretion occurred. The beneficial effects lasted about two weeks. At present it seems reasonable to recommend that under properly controlled conditions, maternal I.V. glucose therapy may be utilized in certain cases of IUGR especially in those mothers with low glucose tolerance test (GTT) curves.

The rationale underlying the administration of amino acids intraamniotically is based on the following facts[19,37]: a) The fetus swallows large amounts of amniotic fluid (AF). On the average, about 342 ml of amniotic fluid are cleared of protein per day. b) The fetus is capable of digesting and absorbing the proteins. c) The amount of protein swallowed could theoretically represent up to 18 percent of the daily protein need of the fetus.

Manzanilla and co-workers[27] attempted to feed the fetus via intraaminotic proteins by injecting[131] I albumin. Since then, there have been other attempts using a mixture of amino acids.[28,37] The results are preliminary and may be summarized as follows:

The intraaminotic injection of amino acids causes a marked increase in amino acid (AA) concentration. Within one hour, 1/3–2/3 of the amino acids have left the AF and by 48 hours, the amniotic fluid AA level has returned to normal. The amino acids leave the AF at differing rates and hence must clear by mechanisms in addition to deglutition, e.g., via the umbilical cord. They reach the fetal blood quite rapidly, with a maximum concentration in 1½-2 hours. Small amounts reach the maternal circulation. In view of their rate of disappearance, the AA should be given once every 24–48 hours.

With this mode of therapy, acceleration in the growth of the fetal BPD and improvement in fetal size has been observed. In addition, disappearance of late decelerations after an oxytocin challenge test and a return of maternal urinary estriol and plasma HCG (human chorionic gonadotropin) to normal was noted. There were no apparent adverse fetal effects.

There are as yet insufficient data to recommend the routine use of intraaminotic AA or to lay down firm guidelines. However, further research is warranted to assess the risk-benefit ratio.

The use of adrenergic Beta mimetic agents is still controversial. The variation in results may, at least partially, be explained by patient selection and the variation in dose and duration of treatment. The objective is to improve intervillous perfusion by increasing cardiac output and/or vasodilation of the uterine vessels. Positive results in the form of increased birthweight, BPD, and elevated estriol excretion levels have been reported.[17,29,38]

In summary, rational management of IUGR must await a thorough understanding of the factors controlling normal fetal growth and those factors that could adversely affect it. Our knowledge in this area is fragmentary, hence the treatment remains empirical and incomplete to a large extent. It is hoped that with time this state of affairs will be corrected.

"I have yet to see any problem, however complicated, which when you looked at it the right way did not become still more complicated." (Anderson)

BIBLIOGRAPHY

1. Abdul-Karim, R. W. The clinical significance of deviations in fetal growth. *Int. J. Gynaecol. Obstet.* **13:** 257, 1975.
2. Abdul-Karim, R. W. Retarded and accelerated fetal growth. *In* H. A. Kaminetzky and L. Iffy (Eds.) Progress In Perinatology. Philadelphia, George F. Stickley Co., 1977, p. 105.
3. Abdul-Karim, R. W. and Beydoun, S. N. Growth of the human fetus. *Clin. Obstet. Gynecol.* **17:** 37, 1974.
4. Abdul-Karim, R. W. and Beydoun, S. N. Fetal growth retardation. *In* L. Iffy and A. Langer (Eds.) Perinatology Case Studies. Garden City, N.Y., Medical Examination Publishing Co., 1978, p. 141.
5. Abdul-Karim, R. W. and Haviland, M. E. Unpublished data.
6. Abdul-Karim, R. W., Nesbitt, R. E. L., Jr. et al. The regulatory effect of estrogens on fetal growth. I. Placental and fetal body weights. *Am. J. Obstet. Gynecol.* **109:** 656, 1971.
7. Abdul-Karim, R. W., Pavy, M. et al. The regulatory effect of estrogens on fetal growth. Part IV. Brain development in growth accelerated fetuses. *Biol. Neonate* **29:** 89, 1976.
8. Beischer, N. A. and O'Sullivan, E. F. The effect of rest and intravenous infusion of

hypertonic dextrose on subnormal estriol excretion in pregnancy. *Am. J. Obstet. Gynecol.* **113:** 771, 1972.

9. Beydoun, S. N., Abdul-Karim, R. W. et al. The regulatory effect of estrogens on fetal growth. Part III. Placental deoxyribonucleic acid, ribonucleic acid, and proteins. *Am. J. Obstet. Gynecol.* **120:** 918, 1974.

10. Campbell, S. Fetal growth. *Clinics Obstet. Gynecol.* **1:** (No. 1): 41, 1974.

11. Campbell, S. Physical methods of assessing size at birth. *In* Size at Birth. Ciba Foundation Symposium 27. New York, Associated Scientific Publishers, 1974, p. 275.

12. Campbell, S. Fetal Growth. *In* R. W. Beard and P. W. Nathamielz (Eds.) Fetal Physiology and Medicine. London, W. B. Saunders Co., Ltd., 1976, p. 271.

13. Campbell, S. N., Andrew, J. D. et al. Maternal hypertonic dextrose infusion in a patient with idiopathic recurrent placental insufficiency and low urinary oestrogens. *In* B. Salvadori (Ed.) Therapy of Feto-Placental Insufficiency. Berlin, Springer-Verlag, 1975, p. 236.

14. Chatfield, W. R., Rogers, T. G. H. et al. Placental scanning with computer linked gamma camera to detect impaired placental blood flow and intra-uterine growth retardation. *Brit. Med. J.* **2:** 120, 1975.

15. Fancourt, R., Campbell, S. et al. Followup study of small-for-dates babies. *Brit. Med. J.* **1:** 1435, 1976.

16. Fisher, C. C., Garrett, W. et al. Placental aging monitored by Gray scale echography. *Am. J. Obstet. Gynecol.* **124:** 483, 1976.

17. Flynn, M. J. The effect of ritodrine on infant weight. *In* B. Salvadori (Ed.) Therapy of Feto-Placental Insufficiency. Berlin, Springer-Verlag, 1975, p. 142.

18. Friedman, S. and Goldman, J. A. The insulin tolerance test (I.T.T.) as a basis for the therapy of placental insufficiency. *In* B. Salvadori (Ed.) Therapy of Feto-Placental Insufficiency. Berlin, Springer-Verlag, 1975, p. 53.

19. Gitlin, D., Kumate, J. et al. The turnover of amniotic fluid protein in the human conceptus. *Am. J. Obstet. Gynecol.* **113:** 623, 1972.

20. Gohari, P., Berkowitz, J. C. et al. Prediction of intrauterine growth retardation by determination of total intrauterine volume. *Am. J. Obstet. Gynecol.* **127:** 255, 1977.

21. Goldstein, H. and Peckham, C. Birth weight, gestation, neonatal mortality, and child development. *In* Roberts, D. F. and Thomson, A. M. (Eds.) The Biology of Human Fetal Growth. New York, Halsted Press, 1976, p. 81.

22. Gordon, Y. B., Grudzinskas, J. G. et al. Concentrations of pregnancy-specific B_1-glycoprotein in maternal blood in normal pregnancy and intrauterine growth retardation. *Lancet* **1:** 331, 1977.

23. Hill, D. E., Holt, A. B. et al. Alterations in the growth pattern of fetal rhesus monkeys following the in-utero injection of streptozotocin. *Pediatr. Res.* **6:** 336, 1972.

24. Hopkins, P. S. and Thorburn, G. D. The effects of foetal thyroidectomy on the development of the ovine foetus. *J. Endocr.* **54:** 55, 1972.

25. Liggins, G. C. The influence of the fetal hypothalamus and pituitary on growth. *In* Size at Birth, Ciba Foundation Symposium 27. New York, Assoc. Scientific Publ., 1974, p. 165.

26. Liggins, G. C. The drive to fetal growth. *In* R. W. Beard and P. W. Nathanielsz (Eds.) Fetal Physiology and Medicine, Philadelphia, W. B. Saunders Co., 1976, p. 254.

27. Manzanilla, S. R., Suarez, C. M. et al. Intra-uterine fetal oral feeding: Basic research using intra-amniotic albumin I[131]. *Internat. J. Gynaecol. Obstet.* **8:** 238, 1970.

28. Massobrio, M., Margaria, E. et al. Treatment of severe feto-placental insufficiency by means of intra-amniotic injection of amnio-acids. *In* B. Salvadori (Ed.) Therapy of Feto-Placental Insufficiency. Berlin, Springer-Verlag, 1975, p. 296.

29. Melchior, J. and Bernard, N. Early trials in the treatment of placental insufficiency with ritodrine. *In* B. Salvadori (Ed.) Therapy of Feto-Placental Insufficiency. Berlin, Springer-Verlag, 1975, p. 137.
30. Morton, N. E. The inheritance of human birth weight. *Ann. Hum. Genet.* **20**: 125, 1955.
31. Nathanielsz, P. W. Fetal endocrinology monographs in fetal physiology. Vol. I. New York, North-Holland Publ. Co., 1976, p. 107.
32. Ounsted, C. and Ounsted, M. Effect of Y-chromosome on fetal growth rate. *Lancet* **2**: 857, 1970.
33. Ounsted, C. and Ounsted, M. Familial factors on fetal growth rate. *In* Clinics Dev. Med., No. 46. Philadelphia, Spastic Internat. Med. Publ., J. B. Lippincott, 1973, p. 57.
34. Picon, L. Effect of insulin on growth and biochemical composition of the rat fetus. *Endocrinology* **81**: 1419, 1967.
35. Polani, P. E. Chromosomal and other genetic influences on birth weight variation. *In* Size at Birth, Ciba Foundation Symposium 27. New York, Associated Scientific Publ. 1974, p. 127.
36. Potter, E. L. Bilateral absence of the ureters and kidneys. *Obstet. Gynecol.* **25**: 3, 1965.
37. Renaud, R. Kirstetter, L. et al. Intra-amniotic amino acid injections. *In* B. Salvadori (Ed.) Therapy of Feto-Placental Insufficiency. Berlin, Springer-Verlag, 1975, p. 265.
38. Scommegna, A., Dmowski, W. P. et al. Effect of an adrenergic-B-mimetic compound (Ritodrine Hydrochloride) on the feto-placental unit in chronic fetal distress. *In* B. Salvadori (Ed.) Therapy of Feto-Placental Insufficiency. Berlin, Springer-Verlag, 1975, p. 111.
39. Sherwood, W. G., Chance, G. W. et al. A new syndrome of pancreatic agenesis. *Pediatr. Res.* **8**: 360, 1974.
40. Smidt, D., Steinbach, J. and Scheven, B. Die beeinflussung der prä-und postnatalen entwicklung durch grösse und korpergewicht der mutter, largestellt an ergebnissen reziproker eitransplantatonen zwischen Zwergschweinen und grossen hausschweinen. *Monatsschr Kinderheilkd* **115**: 533, 1967.
41. Tato, L., Marc, V. L. et al. Early variations of plasma somatomedin activity in the newborn. *J. Clin. Endocr. Metab.* **40**: 534, 1975.
42. Taurog, A., Tong, W. et al. Thyroid ^{131}I metabolism in the absence of the pituitary: The untreated hypophysectomized rat. *Endocrinology* **62**: 646, 1958.
43. Thomson, A. M. and Billewicz, W. Z. The concept of "light-for-dates infants." *In* Roberts, D. F. and Thomson, A. M. (Eds.) The Biology of Human Fetal Growth. New York, Halsted Press, 1976, p. 69.
44. Thorburn, G. D. The role of the thyroid gland and kidneys in fetal growth. *In* Size at Birth, Ciba Foundation Symposium 27. New York, Associated Scientific Publ. 1974, p. 185.
45. Thorburn, G. D. and Hopkins, P. S. Thyroid function in the foetal lamb. *In* Foetal and Neonatal Physiology. Procedures of the Sir Joseph Barcroft Centenary Symposium. Cambridge, University Press, 1973, p. 488.
46. Thorburn, G. D., Nicol, D. H. et al. Effect of bilateral nephrectomy of the foetal lamb on growth and development. *Proc. Endocr. Soc. Aust.* **13**, Abstr. 1, 1970.
47. Walton, A. and Hammond, J. The maternal effects on growth and conformation in shire horse-Shetland pony crosses. *Proc. Roy. Soc. Lond.* **128**: 311, 1938.

8

Intrapartum Electronic Fetal Monitoring: Is It All Worthwhile?

ROBERT C. GOODLIN, M. D.

Soon after Laennec invented the stethoscope in 1818, physicians began auscultation of the fetal heart, and fetal monitoring became an established obstetric technique. By the end of the 19th century, it was generally agreed that the signs of fetal distress included: a) tachycardia, or a fetal heart rate (FHR) of more than 160 beats per minute (bpm); b) bradycardia, or FHR of less than 100 bpm; c) "irregularity of FHR" which was never precisely defined; d) passage of meconium when the fetus was in the vertex presentation; and e) gross alterations of fetal movements, again which were never precisely defined.[1] In European and American cities in 1910, 3 to 5 percent of normal fetuses died in labor,[2] and obstetricians' major concern remained with maternal welfare through the 1950's.

After the problems of maternal mortality had been largely resolved, physicians began to express a major interest in the fetus's welfare. The fetal monitoring experience of Cox of Australia in the 1950's was representative of that era, in that if only one sign of fetal distress was present, the perinatal rate and morbidity rates were unaltered, but if two or more signs were present, the perinatal rate and morbidity rates were increased.[3] Then, as now, obstetricians often assumed that the newborn morbidity and mortality associated with these signs of fetal distress were related to the underlying fetal illness and not to any obstetrical interference.

My own prior efforts with intrapartum fetal monitoring included the use of many different modalities, such as maternal aorta and vaginal pulse (plethysmographic) monitoring, fetal and maternal ballistocardiograph recordings, fetal scalp oxygen saturation determinations, fetal scalp pulse measurements, relative placental Doppler flow, and so forth.[4] While such applications challenged my plodding zeal, they were never demonstrated to be of benefit to the fetus.

Only the electronic recording of the instantaneous fetal heart rate (FHR) and uterine contractions, pioneered by Hon in America and Hammacher and Sureau in Europe, has been widely accepted. However, the definition of abnormal FHR has not had universal acceptance, despite more than 15 years' use. As Sureau noted in 1975, "The pathophysiological criteria of Hon's are not convincing. This is true particularly because the subjective determination of each individual pattern is so variable, and also, there are so many unclassifiable patterns present."[5]

My own studies have indicated that FHR techniques, while precise indicators of instantaneous heart rate, are subject to much misinterpretation. The fetus readily evokes the baroreflex and the associated vagal type of bradycardia is often difficult to interpret and without clinical significance, except when associated with decreased fetal cardiac output. Many of the vagal fetal heart rate decelerations (variable and early) have an obscure etiology.[6] Even the occurrence of late deceleration, when checked by fetal scalp pH determination, is often of no untoward significance. Short-term beat-to-beat variability (BBV) can reflect: a low fetal arousal level (sleep), maternal medications (particularly those with an atropine effect), tachycardia, and of course, asphyxia.[7] The number of indices of BBV appears limited only by the imaginations of investigators.

The problems of routine fetal electronic monitoring have been well documented. Their cost is substantial, although one case of malpractice lost for not using the fetal monitor would negate any consideration of this factor. The theoretical risks of Doppler radiation are well recognized, and the occurrence of fetal scalp infections from the scalp electrode has now become widely documented.[8] Perhaps the most significant "complication" of routine fetal monitoring in the low-risk gravida is the increase in cesarean section rates.

In 1968, Benson and colleagues interpreted auscultated FHR data from nearly 25,000 deliveries of the Collaborative Project, with regards to the prediction of fetal distress. These authors, in part, concluded that "no reliable auscultation indicator of fetal distress exists in terms of fetal heart rate, save in an extreme degree."[9] Their paper and this statement have been repeatedly used as an indication for more precise fetal electronic monitoring. However, reports from both Denver, Colorado in 1976[10] and Sheffield, England in 1978[11] have indicated that the abandonment of fetoscopic (stethoscopic) auscultation of fetal heart rate as a means of detecting fetal distress was perhaps a bit premature. Actually, Benson et al. showed that abnormal FHR's were associated with low Apgar scores. Perhaps it was their honest statement that the FHR detection of fetal distress "is much too complex for such an easy appraisal," which caused many to turn to apparently more precise techniques.

For the "non-high-risk" parturient, Johnstone and colleagues of Aberdeen, Scotland, suggest from their study that "the percentage of babies whose lives will be saved by continuous electronic monitoring is small, perhaps one baby in every thousand deliveries." These investigators still consider valid the use of routine electronic monitoring of low-risk parturients.[12] While prospective studies of both low and high-risk parturients have failed to demonstrate clearly the benefits of routine electronic fetal monitoring, retrospective studies appear to demonstrate its value. Indeed, if the perinatal mortality rate is compared before the introduction of electronic fetal monitoring or increased use of cesarean section (or any other changing technique in the past few years)—because perinatal mortality rates have been decreasing everywhere during the past 15 years—a "benefit" could be shown. After an organized national effort was made to improve perinatal care in France in the early 1970's it was discovered that the projected improvement of perinatal rates actually occurred between the time-interval of inception of the concept and its implementation. Nevertheless, the effort had a positive effect on perinatal care in France.[13]

Benefits from other fetal parameters have been equally difficult to demonstrate when monitored in the intrapartum period. For instance, Curron in 1975 noted that "the intuition of every obstetrician and parent cries out that surely good oxygenation at birth is the object of most obstetric practices, yet there is no evidence that this need be so." Curron went on to question whether the all-or-nothing phenomena is operative in most cases of intrapartum asphyxia. He and several others believe that it does so, that the fetus either dies or fully recovers from any intrapartum asphyxial insult.[14,15]

It is difficult to design and carry out any controlled obstetrical study, particularly when it must include large numbers of patients followed over several years' time. When Walker of South Africa reported in 1959 that responding to apparent fetal distress (especially with mid-forceps delivery) only increased the perinatal mortality rates.[16] Eastman offered him faint praise for his study. However, Eastman noted how difficult it is to carry out controlled studies of therapy for fetal distress if due deference is given to fetal welfare. He suggested that electronic fetal monitoring would be more precise.[17]

An argument for routine electronic fetal monitoring is in the prevention of cerebral dysfunction. However, in Sweden, cerebral palsy has virtually been eliminated, except for that occurring in the growth-retarded fetus.[18] This improvement occurred despite the relative absence of electronic fetal monitors. In addition, neonatal intensive care is reducing the incidence of cerebral palsy in the tiny newborns.[19] Parmelee and colleagues quote 12 papers to the effect that even though it is possible to predict mean outcome differences for groups of infants at risk for cerebral dysfunction, it is difficult to predict individual outcome. They also note that environmental factors can have a stronger influence on the expression of cerebral dysfunction than do earlier biological events.[20]

Unless prematurity is considered an obstetrical complication, recent studies suggest that obstetrical factors have a minor role in the etiology of most cases of cerebral palsy. This is not to deny that traumatic deliveries or episodes of fetal hypoxia are occasionally the cause of subsequent cerebral dysfunction.

Correlated with concepts of the need for intrapartum fetal monitoring is a recognition of the monitor's limitations, or the tendency to circumvent the intrapartum period by abdominal delivery. In California, private hospitals are now approaching a cerarean section rate of 30 percent. In the California data (available through 1976), there has been a lack of identifiable positive effects of the increased cesarean section rates on perinatal mortality rates (Table 1). While the perinatal mortality rate has decreased as the cesarean section rate has increased, the selective increase in cesarean sections in certain age, ethnic groups and classes of perinatal care has not been accompanied by a concomitant selective decline in perinatal mortality rates in the same groups. An exception has been the post-date pregnancy, where cesarean section rates have increased significantly, as perinatal rates have decreased.

Among women delivered by cesarean section in California hospitals, only two of the eight variables (Table 2) which determine rates in various hospitals were related to characteristics of the women delivering at the hospitals. These were the percentage of primigravida over 35 years of age and the percentage of white gravida. All of the other six factors (Table 2) were related to characteristics of the hospital, and especially from the standpoint of this chapter, to the presence of a fetal monitor.[21] Indeed, a superficial inspection of the California data would indicate that a pregnant woman in California wishing both a vaginal delivery and a low perinatal mortality should select delivery by a non-specialist in a small, rural hospital. The routine use of electronic fetal monitoring and the associated

Table 1. Percent Change of Cesarean Section (C.S.) Rates and Perinatal Mortality Rates by Selected Maternal Characteristics in California, 1965–1974.

CHARACTERISTICS	% C.S.	PERINATAL MORTALITY
A. *Ethnic Group*		
Black	+ 160.0	− 48.1
White (Non-Spanish)	+ 134.1	− 38.9
White Spanish	+ 100.0	− 46.6
B. *Maternal Age*		
< 20	+ 184.8	− 28.3
20–24	+ 137.2	− 25.9
25–29	+ 116.7	− 33.7
30–34	+ 104.5	− 34.4
35–39	+ 87.1	− 27.4
40 +	+ 96.2	− 13.1

Source: State of California, Department of Health, Birth Cohort Records.

high cesarean section rates have turned many gravida towards home delivery—a high-risk situation for both mother and infant. The families and communities often pay a heavy price whenever anything unforeseen occurs during such delivery.

Except for the 1950's California's perinatal and infant mortality rates have steadily improved from 1930 through 1976. This has been especially so during the last 15 years (Fig. 1). Unexpectedly, the introduction of statewide neonatal intensive care units or the widespread use of fetal monitoring has not affected the rate of improvement. By contrast, Westin with the

Table 2. Hospital Variables Determining Cesarean Section Rates, California, 1976*.

	SIGN OF COEFFICIENT
Private nonprofit status	+
Percent parturients monitored	+
Percent deliveries by specialists	+
Size of delivery service	+
Kaiser affiliation	−
Percent parturients white	+
Percent elderly gravida	+
Urban location	+

* In order of entry in final regression equation at a significant level.
Source: State Department of Health Survey, 1977.

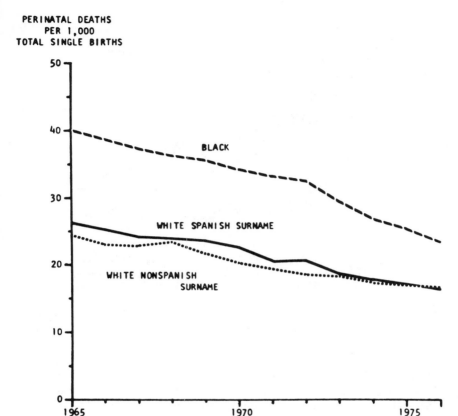

Fig. 1.   Direct method of adjustment to 1960 California single total births by age of mother. Source: State of California of Health, Maternal and Child Health, Birth Cohort Records.

Danderyd Hospital in Sweden, could show that perinatal mortality was apparently influenced by the introduction of specific obstetrical techniques (Fig. 2). Unlike the European experience, where the improvement in perinatal mortality rates has largely been due to fewer deliveries of tiny prematures,[22] the improvement in California has been strongly influenced by the improvement in perinatal rates of the large newborn (Table 3). The percentage of gravida over age 35 has decreased from 13 percent to 6 percent during the past 10 years. The reduction in this high-risk group, as gravidas suggest, could be due to the substantial contributions of contraception and therapeutic abortion to the recent decline in perinatal mortality rates.

The surprising improvement of newborns weighing 3501 to 4250 grams is

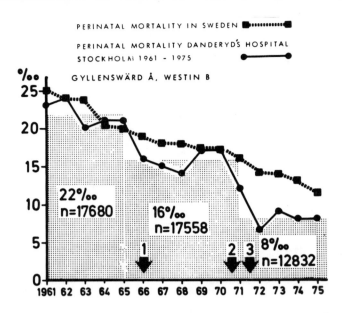

Fig. 2. Perinatal mortality in Sweden and Danderyd Hospital 1961-1975. 1. Partogram introduced. 2. Intrapartum auscultogram introduced. 3. "Gravidogram" introduced. (Reproduced with permission from Westin, B.: *Acta Obstet. Gynecol. Scand.* **56:** 273, 1977.)

unexpected. This weight category represents Gruenwald's optimal development group,[23] perhaps explaining their low perinatal rate despite longer labors and higher incidence of cephalopelvic disproportion. The improved perinatal rates of this weight group suggest improved obstetrical care, since this category should be free of illness and anomalies and, barring obstetrical accidents, should live.

The improvement in perinatal mortality rates occurring after the introduction of MediCal in 1965 is also consistent with the hypothesis that increased availability of medical services for the poor gravida improves perinatal mortality rates. However, in 1975, hospitals caring for the poor black gravida still had a divided pregnancy population. Fifty-one percent received MediCal benefits and 49 percent did not. Those receiving MediCal benefits had significantly better perinatal mortality rates (25/1000), although they presumably received the same degree of care as those without MediCal (34/1000 perinatal mortality rate).[24] It is hypothesized that those receiving MediCal benefits were better educated and more highly motivated. The importance to perinatal outcome of patient motivation and education are also illustrated by the excellent results reported from the Alternate Birth Centers.[25]

In our Alternate Birth Center, no electronic fetal monitoring is done and

Table 3. Perinatal Death Rates Among Total Births Occurring in California by Birthweight, 1974.

BIRTHWEIGHT (GRAMS)	PERCENT OF BIRTHS	PERINATAL DEATHS PER 1000 BIRTHS	PERCENT CHANGE 1965–1974
< 500		995.2	+ 1.8
500 – 750		960.3	+ 2.1
751 –1000	1.2	790.5	+ 11.9
1001–1250		515.9	+ 24.5
1251–1500		344.7	+ 29.3
1501–1750		207.7	+ 34.0
1751–2000	4.9	119.2	+ 34.0
2001–2250		67.2	+ 32.0
2251–2500		34.6	+ 28.4
2501–2750		15.0	+ 30.7
2751–3000		8.4	+ 27.0
3001–3250	93.9	6.1	+ 23.8
3251–3500		4.6	+ 27.0
3501–3750		3.5	+ 38.6
3751–4000		3.6	+ 37.6
4001–4250		4.0	+ 33.5
4251–4500		5.5	+ 30.4
4501 +		18.1	+ 17.8

Source: State of California, Department of Health, Birth Cohort Records.

fetal heart rate auscultation is optional. Pain relief is minimal and the mothers and the newborns are discharged from the Alternate Birth Room some four to six hours after delivery. Approximately 20 percent of the multigravida and 50 percent of the primigravida "risk out" of the Alternate Birth Center prior to the time of delivery. However, even considering the total group, the incidence of newborn depression, meconium staining of the amniotic fluid, congenital anomalies, toxemia, and premature delivery has been significantly less than similar low-risk parturients delivered in our regular delivery suite with routine electronic fetal monitoring (Table 4). This is a small series and the regular low-risk gravida do not serve as an adequate control because of different socioeconomic classes and inadequate follow-up. It does, however, suggest that the fetus is probably not at increased risk when delivered in our Alternate Birth Center. This may not be true for the mother.

While there is no explanation for the apparent decrease in anomalies among those delivering in the Alternate Birth Center, the reduced incidence of newborn depression and meconium staining may be related to maternal psychological preparation and resulting tranquility during labor. It seems reasonable that intravenous fluids, electronic fetal monitoring, and the

Table 4. Homestyle Delivery. (Goodwin Score < 2)

	300 HOMESTYLE	300 REGULAR LOW RISK
Perinatal mortality	0	0
Congenital anomalies	0	3
Meconium stained fluid	6 (1.5%)	28 (9.1%)
Newborn admitted	10 (3%)	—
Prolonged nursery stay	—	7
Newborn readmitted	13 (4.3%)	2 (?)
Serious maternal complications	4	2
Postpartum mastitis	4	1 (?)
Cesarean section	8/430 (1.8%)	14 (4.6%)

general atmosphere in the standard labor room contribute to the anxiety of a parturient and can lead to fetal distress through reduced uterine blood flow, abnormal labor, and so forth. A true controlled study of the benefits of an Alternate Birth Center would probably require the use of drugs in the control group to assure tranquilization so as to negate the possible detrimental effects of maternal anxiety.

While Westin found that 11 percent of perinatal deaths occurred in the intrapartum period,[26] we found (since the introduction of fetal intensive care) only 2 percent. It is traditionally accepted that birth was a very hazardous event for us all. What has not been demonstrated is that this danger of birth exists for the healthy, well-developed fetus delivered in a modern facility. Our own studies suggest that in screening out the "non-low-risk" gravida, the remaining fetuses are at minimal risk of intrapartum death except that associated with such accidents as umbilical cord prolapse or abruptio placenta. Antenatal screening is not necessarily complicated and often involves nothing more than making certain that the gravida is in good health, that the symphysis-fundus height is increasing at a normal rate, and that fetal movements appear normal. If abnormalities occur in any of these three areas of simple screening, then more detailed and expensive tests for fetal well-being are indicated. Figure 3 indicates that antenatal care is very important in regard to perinatal mortality. However, Figure 4 shows that while white Spanish gravida enjoyed the benefits of antenatal care less than did other groups, their perinatal rates were (as in Fig. 1) equal to or better than any other group.

The increased survival of the large newborn perhaps demonstrates the importance of assuring optimal in utero development. This is not to imply that we should recommend "forced feeding" for all gravida in order to achieve the 4 kg newborn, but rather to assure with every technique available to us, optimal in utero conditions. It seems reasonable to assume

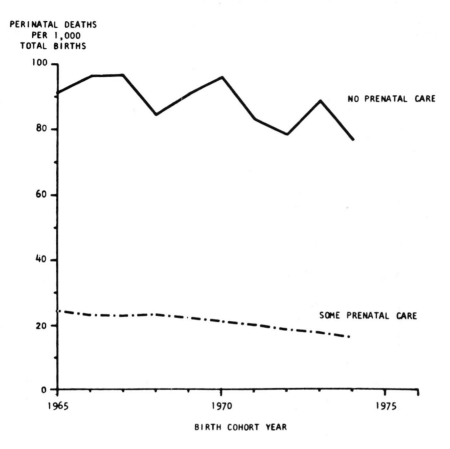

Fig. 3.   Perinatal deaths per 1,000 total births by prenatal care received. Source: State of California Department of Health, Maternal and Child Health, Birth Cohort Records.

that adding mass to the fetus otherwise destined to weigh only 2500 g, through a high caloric maternal diet, might add to its perinatal mortality rate by increasing its duration of labor and the likelihood of shoulder dystocia, and so forth. On the other hand, by assuring an adequate environment through careful antenatal monitoring the entire in utero individual is brought to optimal development.

It is postulated that antenatal monitoring can determine the need for added maternal nutrients, rest, and fluid intake as well as the assurance of tranquility, all necessary for the optimal in utero environment. If these fail, then perhaps these relatively underdeveloped fetuses should be the 20 percent delivered by cesarean section rather than those whose only high-risk problem is their mother's prior low transverse cesarean section.

PERCENT NO
PRENATAL CARE

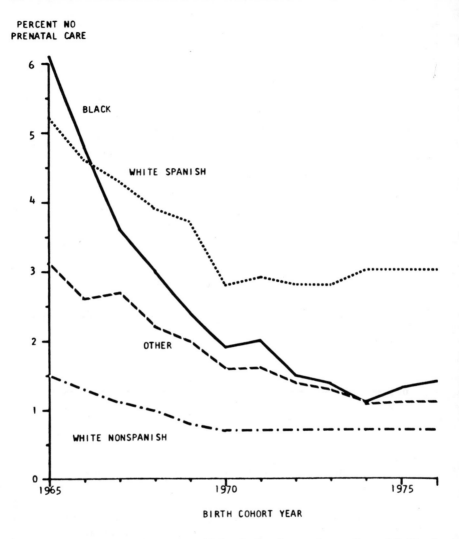

Fig. 4.   Percent no prenatal care among births of selected races. Source: State of California Department of Health, Maternal and Child Health, Birth Cohort Records.

   As Curran has suggested, either the baby is fit to withstand delivery and survive, or it is not, and dies.[14] If this is so, then the die is cast before the onset of labor and antenatal monitoring assumes a greater importance than does intrapartum monitoring. The electronic fetal monitor was originally introduced with the suggestion that it would reduce the number of cesarean sections. This concept very quickly disappeared and instead, the monitor is often used to discover the low-risk fetus who becomes high-risk during labor. As noted, this concept seems to assume that certain events regularly occur during the intrapartum period which jeopardize the normal fetus's health. The present information indicates that adequate antenatal monitoring will screen out those unfit for intrapartum risk. It is possible that routine monitoring of low-risk gravida may produce more problems than it solves.

Admittedly, there are differing viewpoints regarding the fetal hazards of the intrapartum period. Nelson and Broman recently reviewed the Collaborative Project data on children with cerebral palsy, and suggested that obstetric factors previously considered relatively minor and frequent, such as secondary arrest or prolonged second stage, was associated with a higher incidence of cerebral palsy.[27] McManus et al. have similarly suggested that many cases of cerebral palsy are preventable.[28]

Painter, Depp and O'Donoghue followed the neurological development of 50 high-risk infants for up to 12 months of age. Those with normal FHR patterns had statistically better development. However, intervention in cases of abnormal FHR patterns did not necessarily prevent subsequent abnormal neurological development.[29] In our own clinic, approximately 40 percent of the fetuses demonstrating severe fetal distress had serious anomalies or illnesses prior to the onset of labor. There is a need to repeat Walker's 1958 study to determine if response to the modern signs of fetal distress improves the newborn's subsequent development.

Even though pregnancy and delivery are natural phenomena, the achievement of optimal perinatal mortality and morbidity rates probably involves more than nutritional or psychological answers. However, it does not seem likely that our goals will be achieved with more intensive intrapartum monitoring and/or higher cesarean section rates.

ACKNOWLEDGMENT

I am indebted to Diana Petitti, M.D., of the Maternal and Child Health Branch, California Department of Health, for both data and consultation.

REFERENCES

1. Von Winckel, F. Handbook der Gebertschulfe. Weisbaden, Bergmann, 1903.
2. DeLee, J. B. Principles and Practice of Obstetrics. Philadelphia, W. B. Saunders, 1913.
3. Cox, L. W. Aust. N. Z. *J. Obstet. Gynecol.* 1: 99, 1961.
4. Goodlin, R. C. and Lowe, E. W. *Am. J. Obstet. Gynecol.* 119: 341, 1974.
5. Sureau, C. L. *In* Z. K. Stembera, Polacek, K. and Savata, V. (Eds.) Perinatal Medicine. Stuttgart, George Thieme, 1975.
6. Goodlin, R. C. and Haesslein, H. C. *Am. J. Obstet. Gynecol.* 128: 440, 1977.

7. Hellman, L., Donald, I. et al. *Lancet* **1**: 1133, 1970.
8. Okada, D., Chow, A. and Bruce, V. *Am. J. Obstet. Gynecol.* **129**: 185, 1977.
9. Benson, R. C., Shubeck, F. et al. *Obstet. Gynecol.* **32**: 259, 1968.
10. Haverkamp, A. D., Thompson, H. E. et al. *Am. J. Obstet. Gynecol.* **125**: 310, 1976.
11. Kelso, I. M., Parsons, R. J. and Lawrence, G. F. *Am. J. Obstet. Gynecol.* **131**: 526, 1978.
12. Johnstone, F. O., Campbell, D. and Hughes, G. J. *Lancet* **1**: 1298, 1978.
13. Sureau, C.: *Brit. Med. J.* **2**: 400, 1973 (Abstract).
14. Curron, J. T. Fetal Heart Monitoring. London, Butterworth, 1975.
15. Goodlin, R. C. and Haesslein, H. C. *Am. J. Obstet. Gynecol.* **128**: 440, 1977.
16. Walker, N. *Brit. Med. J.* **2**: 1221, 1959.
17. Eastman, N. J. *Obstet. Gynecol. Surv.* **15**: 351, 1960.
18. Sabel, K. G., Olegard, R. and Victoria, L. *Pediatrics* **57**: 652, 1976.
19. Andrews, B. F. and Franco, S. *Pediat. Clin. of Am.* **24**: 639, 1977.
20. Parmelee, A. H., Signon, M. et al. Infants and Young Children. Baltimore, University Park Press.
21. Williams, R. Community Organization Institute (Unpublished data).
22. Gordon, R. R. *Brit. Med. J.* **2**: 1302, 1977.
23. Gruenwald, P. *Am. J. Obstet. Gynecol.* **94**: 1112, 1966.
24. Norris, F. and Jackson, E. Impact of MediCal on Perinatal Mortality in California Bureau of Maternal and Child Health, State of California, 1973.
25. Kerner, J. and Ferris, C. B. *Obstet. Gynecol.* **57**: 371, 1978.
26. Westin, B. Acta *Obstet. Gynecol. Scand.* **56**: 273, 1977.
27. Nelson, K. B. and Broman, S. H. *Ann. Neurol.* **2**: 371, 1977.
28. McManus, F. et al. *Obstet. Gynecol.* **50**: 71, 1977.
29. Painter, M. J., Depp, R. and O'Donoghue, P. D. *Am. J. Obstet. Gynecol.* (In press).

9

Aggressive Obstetric Neonatal Management: Longterm Outcome

LULA O. LUBCHENCO, M.D.,
GAIL A. McGUINNESS, M.D.,
ALAN L. TOMLINSON, M.D.
AND DOUGLAS P. PUGH, M.D.

Data compiled throughout the United States and Europe over recent years indicate that neonatal mortality is being reduced, and that associated with this reduction is a lower longterm morbidity.

When we reviewed our follow-up data on infants born at the University of Colorado Medical Center, we could demonstrate an improved outcome in preterm infants with birth weights between 1500 and 2000 grams who were cared for in an intensive care nursery. However, there was no change in the outcome of infants < 1500 grams, or was mortality changed in infants with birth weights < 1500 grams (Table 1).

Beginning in January 1975, W. A. Bowes, an obstetrician, and M. A. Simmons, a neonatologist, began to investigate reasons for the persistence of this high mortality rate. As part of their investigation, they were present for the labor and delivery of every infant estimated to be < 1500 grams. The marked reduction in mortality in 1975 is obvious.

To achieve these results, Doctor Bowes approached the delivery of these small infants as though all were viable: thus, what was good for an 1800-gram infant was also good for a 600-gram fetus. He realized that most of the neonatal losses occurred because the fetuses were not deemed viable

Table 1. **Reduction of Neonatal Mortality In Very Low Birth Weight Infants. Birth Weights 500–1500 Grams.**

YEAR	N, ADMS	N, DEATHS	ACTUAL RATE (%)	PREDICTED RATE (%)
1970–1971	27	17	63.0	64.0
1971–1972	26	19	73.1	60.9
1972–1973	33	17	51.5	54.7
1973–1974	46	19	41.3	48.3
1974 (July–Dec)	29	20	69.0	71.8
1975 (Jan–Dec)	84	21	25.0	56.8

or worthy of an all-out effort to save them. Follow-up data from the 1950's were compared with that of the 1970's; the improved long-term outcome is clearly shown in Fig. 1.

Moreover, Bowes established that the weight of the fetus in this weight range was inevitably underestimated. A fetus estimated at 700-800 grams usually turned out to be 900-1000 grams.

These two factors, i.e., good outcome with intensive care and realization that the fetus was usually larger than estimated, resulted in a change of attitude on the part of the obstetric staff to one of optimism. Furthermore, by managing labor and delivery in the best interest of the fetus, asphyxia was prevented.

Simmons organized a neonatal team to be present at the deliveries which consisted of himself, pediatric housestaff and intensive care nursery nurses. If multiple births were expected, a team for each baby was present. The team gave immediate and continuous attention to:

1) warmth and ventilation (special intubation skills were often necessary in this weight group);
2) perfusion and blood pressure;
3) toward the end of 1975, continuous positive airway pressure (CPAP) was frequently used with intubation.

Simmons points out from his two years' experience that: (1) Apgar scores are not related to asphyxia and should not be used as a guide to resuscitation (Fig. 2 and 3). Recent data on cord blood gases verify this impression. (2) Resuscitation efforts do not result in greatly prolonged life. The mean time of death in these infants can be seen in Table 2.

Bowes and Simmons found a break in mortality rates at 900 and 1300 grams, rather than at 1000 and 1500 grams (Table 3).

Our role in this study was to determine the outcome of the infants being saved. We chose two adjacent years for comparison: 1974, before intrapartum intensive care (when mortality was high) and 1975, when the improvement in mortality occurred. The population consisted of all liveborn in-

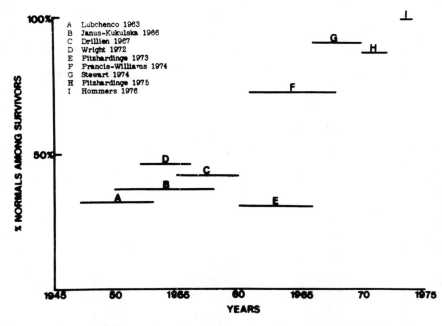

Fig. 1.   Comparison of normal survivors, various investigators, 1950 - 1975. (From Bowes, Proc. 5th Study Group, Royal College of Obstetricians and Gynaecologists. Anderson et al., Eds., London, 1977.)

Table 2.   Neonatal Deaths < 1500 Grams Mean Time of Death (1/1/74–12/31/75).

	1974		1975	
< 24 hours	21 ⎫		11 ⎫	
24–48 hours	2 ⎬ 96%		3 ⎬ 86%	
3–7 days	4 ⎭		4 ⎭	
7–14 days	1*		1**	
> 14 days			2***	

*   NEC
**   IV hem
*** BPD, IC hem

fants with birth weights < 1500 grams born at the University of Colorado Medical Center in 1974, compared with those born in 1975. The surviving children were evaluated at approximately one year of age (Tables 4–7). There was some concern on our part that the population may have been different in the two years because of the admission of slightly larger infants in 1975 (Tables 5,6).

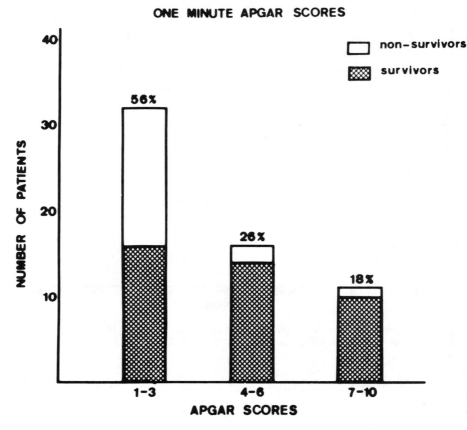

Fig. 2. Apgar scores at one minute, University of Colorado Medical Center newborns with birth weights < 1500 grams. (From Bowes, Proc. 5th Study Group, Royal College of Obstetricians and Gynaecologists. Anderson et al., Eds., London, 1977.)

Tests involving the effect of distribution of birth weights showed that the lower mortality in 1975 was a significant change. (Table 7)

In reviewing the outcome data, our hypothesis was that preterm infants who receive intensive intrapartum care will have less asphyxia and, hence, a less complicated neonatal course and better long-term outcome than infants cared for prior to the time when intensive intrapartum care was begun.

The following determinations were to be made:

1. Was there a difference in cause of death in 1974 versus 1975?
2. Was there a difference in the neonatal course in the 2 years?
3. Was there a change in longterm outcome?

Table 3. Perinatal and Neonatal Mortality January 1975-December 1976. (501-1500 Grams)

					MORTALITY RATE	
B WT (GRAMS)	TOTAL DEL.	FETAL DEATHS	NEONATAL DEATHS	NEONATAL SURVIVAL	PERI-NATAL	NEO-NATAL
501- 600	7	3	4	0	100%	100%
601- 700	9	1	6	2	78	75
701- 800	20	4	10	6	70	63
801- 900	13	4	6	3	77	67
901-1000	20	1	6	13	35	32
1001-1100	19	3	5	11	42	31
1101-1200	20	0	8	12	40	40
1201-1300	29	1	7	21	28	25
1301-1400	27	2	1	24	11	4
1401-1500	24	2	1	21	13	5

Table 4. Population to be Followed: Neonatal Survivors with Weights < 1500 Grams. (1/1/74-12/31/75)

	1974	1975
# Survivors	22(44%)	60(74%)
Mean birth weight	1191	1206
Mean gest age	29.9	29.7

Table 5. Distribution of Birth Weights by Risk Groups All Live Births < 1500 Grams. (1/1/74-12/31/75)

	1974	1975
NUMBER OF INFANTS	50	81
≤ 900 gms	23 (46%)	20 (25%)
≤ 1300 gms	16 (32%)	39 (48%)
1301-1499 gms	11 (22%)	22 (27%)

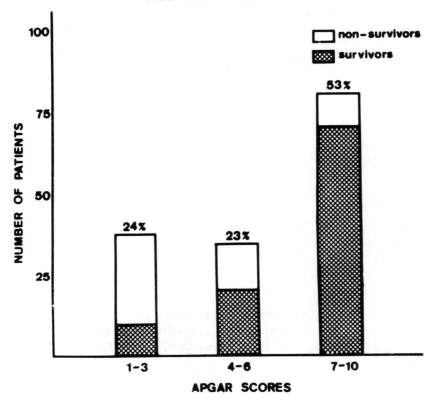

Fig. 3.   Apgar scores at 5 minutes, University of Colorado Medical Center newborns with birth weights < 1500 grams. (From Bowes, Proc. 5th Study Group, Royal College of Obstetricians and Gynaecologists. Anderson et al., Eds., London, 1977.)

Table 6.   Birth Weights <1500 Grams All UCMC New-Borns. (1/1/74-12/31/75)

	1974	1975
Number of Births	50	81
Mean birth weight	1003	1112
Mean gest age	28.8	29.0
NMR	56%	26%

Data from the neonatal course of the infants who died showed that larger infants died in 1974 (more infants > 1000 grams) (Table 8).

Nearly all neonatal deaths occurred in the first week—96 percent in 1974 and 86 percent in 1975 (see Tables 2 and 9). Those dying later encountered complications of the neonatal course such as necrotizing enterocolitis, intracranial hemorrhage or bronchopulmonary dysplasia. The cause of death was hyaline membrane disease in 78 percent. All of the others died within 3 hours of birth. Intracranial hemorrhage was suspected clinically and/or documented in 18 of the infants—10 in 1975 (48 percent), an increase over

Table 7. Predicted Mortality Rate UCMC Birth Weights < 1500 Grams. (1/1/74-12/31/75)

	1974	1975
Actual rate	28/50 = 56%	21/81 = 26%
Predicted by Birth weight-gest age	33.5/50 = 67%	46/81 = 57%
Predicted by 1974 Rate	56%	46%

Table 8. Neonatal Deaths < 1500 Grams by Birth Weight and Gestational Age. (1/1/74-12/31/75)

	1974	1975
n =	28/50	21/81
Mean birth weight	856	843
Mean gest age	27.	26.
# $\geq$ 900 grams	11	6
# $\geq$ 1000 grams	9 (32%)	4 (19%)

Table 9. Delivery Complications Neonatal Deaths < 1500 Grams. (1/1/74-12/31/75)

	1974	1975
Breech presentation	9	7
Cesarean section	0	3
Other Abn presentation	2	4
Multiple Birth	12	7
Cesarean section	0	3
Total cesarean sections	1	8

1974 (29 percent). The neonatal course gave indications of being milder initially, but complications (especially central nervous system complications) occurred later.

The surviving infants were similar in birth weight and gestational age (Tables 10–16).

Table 10. Neonatal Survivors Birth Weights < 1500 Grams. (1/1/74–12/31/75)

	1974	1975
Survivors	22/50	60/81
Mean birth weight	1191	1206
Mean gest age	29.9	29.7

Table 11. Delivery Complications Neonatal Survivors Birth Weights < 1500 Grams. (1/1/74–12/31/75)

		1974	1975
Survivors		22	60
Breech presentation		5	8
Cesarean section		2	3
Other Abn presentation		2	6
Multiple births		3	8
Cesarean section		0	3
Total number Cesarean sections		6 (27%)	14 (23%)
Fetal distress	3		1
Abn presentation	3		6
Multiple births	0		3
Other*	0		4

* Amnionitis, preeclampsia, Rh.

Table 12. Resuscitation At Birth Neonatal Survivors Birth Weights < 1500 Grams. (1/1/74–12/31/75)

	1974	1975
n =	22	60
None or mask O_2	11 (50%)	25 (42%)
Ambu	7	10
Intubation	4	9
CPAP	0	15 (25%)

Table 13. Days on Respirator Neonatal Survivors Birth Weights < 1500 Grams. (1/1/74–12/31/75)

	1974	1975
Survivors	22	60
Number of respirator care	8 ⟍	33 ⟍
≥ 3 days	4—(55%)	10—(72%)
3–7 days	1	4
7–14 days	0	3
14–21 days	0	4
> 21 days	8 ($\bar{x} = 56d$)	7 ($\bar{x} = 33d$)

Table 14. Incidence of PDA* Neonatal Birth Weights < 1500 Grams. (1/1/74–12/31/75)

	1974	1975
Survivors	22	60
Number with PDA	15 (68%)	35 (58%)
PDA ligation	5 (23%)	12 (20%)
Medical Rx	10 (46%)	23 (38%)

* Patent ductus arteriosus.

Table 15. Incidence of BPD* Neonatal Survivors Birth Weights < 1500 Grams. (1/1/74–12/31/75)

	1974	1975
Survivors	22	60
Number with BPD	8 (36%)	9 (15%)

* Broncho-pulmonary dysplasia.

Table 16. Incidence of NEC* Neonatal Survivors Birth Weights < 1500 Grams. (1/1/74–12/31/75)

	1974	1975
Survivors	22	60
Number with NEC	10 (45%)	11 (18%)
Surgical Rx	5	3
Medical Rx	5	8

* Necrotizing enterocolitis.

Seizures during the neonatal course were frequent in both years: 5 out of 22 in 1974 (23 percent) and 9 of 60 in 1975 (15 percent).

The longterm outcome was evaluated at approximately one year of age. By this time, a significant infant mortality had occurred: 6 infants died before one year in 1974 and 2 died in 1975. Three were due to the Sudden Infant Death Syndrome. Four died after 28 days of age, but had never left the nursery; all of these infants had bronchopulmonary dysplasia and seizures, plus other complications such as sepsis. One died of neglect and abuse.

A summary of the incidence of handicapped children is presented in Table 17.

Approximately the same percentage of the surviving population in the two periods was normal or only mildly handicapped at one year of age (69 versus 62 percent). The number of normal patients is impressive, especially in 1975, as are the number of handicapped children. The children with "Other" handicaps included a child with Down's syndrome and two who were neurologically sound, but were abused or neglected.

The neurologic diagnoses are detailed in Table 18.

Of interest is the absence of spastic diplegia and hemiparesis in 1974 or the emergence of neurologic problems in 1975 (spastic diplegia, hemiparesis and hydrocephalus). There is concern about the relationship of temporal artery catheter usage and hemiparesis. However, two of the infants did not have temporal artery lines.

Developmental delays occurred in a significant number of 1975 children (Table 19).

Retrolental fibroplasia is not a long term complication in these children (Table 20).

It may be that it is the small for gestational age infants who will profit most by intensive intrapartum care. First of all, small for gestational age in-

**Table 17. Summary of Outcome Survivors to One Year Birth Weights < 1500 Grams.
(1/1/74–12/31/75)**

	1974	1975
Number of survivors to 1 year	16	58
Number followed	16	55
Number handicap	9 (69%)	20 (62%)
Mild handicap	2	16
Moderate-severe handicap	3	18
Other*	2	1

* 2 were abused and 1 Downs Syndrome.

**Table 18.   Neurologic Problems Neonatal Survivors Birth Weights <1500 Grams.
(1/1/74-12/31/75)**

	1974	1975
n =	22	60
Number followed	22	57
Nml/borderline	15 (68%)	35 (61%)
Spastic diplegia/quadriplegia	0*	11 (19%)
Hemiplegia/hemiparesis	0	3**(+1)
Hypotonia	2	2
Microcephaly	0	1
Seizures	5	2 (+8)***
Hydrocephalus	0	2
Other (Down's Syndrome)	0	1

*   1 treated for spastic diplegia - Nml neurol at 27 months.
**   1 with primary Dx of hydrocephalus.
*** 8 with seizures during neonatal course.

**Table 19.   Development Survivors to One Year Birth Weights < 1500 Grams.
(1/1/74-12/31/75)**

	1974	1975
Number survivors to 1 year	16	58
Number followed	16	55
Nml test or reported Nml	10	28
Not done	0 (69%)	2 (71%)
Mild delay	1	9
Abnormal	3 (19%)	16 (29%)

**Table 20.   Retrolental Fibroplasia* Survivors to One Year Birth Weights <1500 Grams.
(1/1/74-12/31/75)**

	1974	1975
Number of survivors to 1 year	16	58
Number followed	16	55
No RLF	10	38*
RLF, stages I - II	1	3
No eye examination	5	14

* 4 without RLF have other eye disease.

fants constitute a significant portion of the low birth weight population (approximately one-third to one-half of survivors). Second, it is known that they do not tolerate labor and delivery well. Furthermore, Fitzhardingel[1] has identified the small for gestational age infant of < 1500 grams as being at very high risk for longterm neurologic handicap—in the same category as infants who have intracranial bleeds. This is not true in our inborn population (Table 21). Fitzhardinge's population was entirely outborn in hospitals without neonatal intensive care and transported to her service.

The most severely handicapped small for gestational age infants are those who have congenital viral infections. The infant < 1500 grams at birth is also at risk for a type of handicap not usually considered in longterm outcome—that of battering, or its milder form of neglect and inadequate mothering (Table 22).

Those of us who subscribe, in theory, to Marshall Klaus'[2] concepts stressing the importance of early contact (the crucial first hours after birth)

Table 21.   **Small for Gestational Age Infants Survivors to One Year Birth Weights <1500 Grams. (1/1/74–12/31/75)**

	SGA	AGA
Number of survivors to 1 year	22 (30%)	52
Nml/mild handicap	16 (73%)	33 (64%)
Moderate-severe handicap	5	16
Other (not followed, Downs)		4

Table 22.   **Other Problems Neonatal Survivors Birth Weights < 1500 Grams. (1/1/74–12/31/75)**

	1974	1975
Number =	22	60
Number followed	22	57
Neglect/abuse	1	2
Behavior problems	2	1
Medical problems		
SIDS	2	1
BPD—continuing	4*	0
NEC	0	2
Cardiac cath/surg	0	1

* 3 infant deaths.

to the maternal bonding process, are uneasy about the disruption of this process caused by high-risk delivery. We identified lack of attachment and/or overt child abuse in 6 such children in the 82 neonatal survivors in our study. Not only is early separation a deterrant factor, but even when contact is present, the awesome sight of respirators, monitors, intravenous therapy, etc., is enough to discourage contact with the most precious infant As a general rule, immediate bonding does not occur even under the most supportive conditions of empathic nursing, medical and social care. Not only is there separation and awesome intensive care, but usually the birth of a small "premie" is unexpected and the dreams of having a healthy term infant are shattered. In other words, the parents must deal with grief for the loss of an anticipated healthy infant before the more positive bonding process can occur with the premie. There are two exceptions:

1. Bonding does take place later—after the crucial first hours.
2. Not all parents experience grief. After several pregnancy losses, the birth of a viable infant is, in fact, a triumph!

The most frequent response to our "attachment questions" (When did you really feel that he was yours?" and "When did he recognize you?") is "After I got him home."

Another very difficult situation for parents is multiple birth, especially when one dies. We have excellent mothers who, after two years, are not able to resolve the grief process, especially when the living child has a handicap. Triplets are even more complicated. One mother readily informed us, "I feel closest to Anne—Tommy is his father's boy." But, whose parent is Mary's?

Mrs. G, though a concerned and experienced mother, did not feel close to Eugene even after his discharge from the nursery. Eugene was scheduled to return to the hospital for hernia repair. Only after that hospitalization did she feel he was hers. By this time, he was 4 months old and beginning to smile. The social smile has been documented as a powerful infant behavior which induces attachment. On the other hand, attachment occurs under conditions which seem almost unbearable.

Mrs. W. was referred for delivery to our medical center for placenta previa, premature rupture of membranes, amnionitis and footling presentation. A cesarean was done (father present), during which a major vessel was severed. The mother required 8 units of blood during the day, but survived. Three days later, she was taken by wheelchair to see her 1340-gram infant who was in the intensive care nursery. Her attachment was immediate. She visited frequently each day and, after her discharge, remained in Denver to be near her infant (Fig. 4). At one year, this is one of the closest family units we have observed. This was a precious pregnancy,

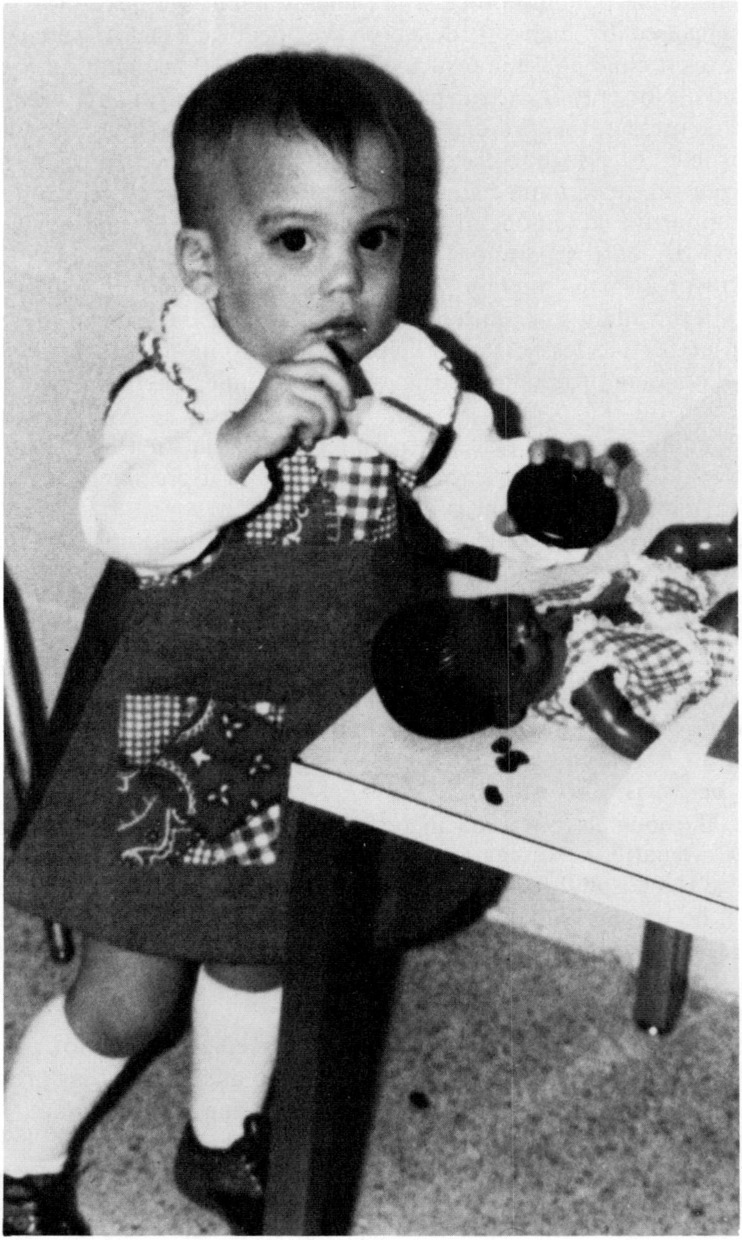

Fig. 4. 1340-gram, 31-week gestational age infant at 15 months' corrected age.

following several pregnancy losses, of a wanted child. The delivery of a 1200-gram infant was a success!

We face a dilemma in reporting the incidence of handicaps. Data, so far, indicate that the two years studied (though very different in mortality) are not significantly different in longterm outcome. However, if one looks at the total number of births (Fig. 5), it is apparent that there were many more normal children, both in numbers and percentage of total births, in 1975 than there were in 1974. Because the handicap rate in survivors is the same, there is also a larger number of handicapped children present.

We have concluded from these data that the excess of neonatal survivors in 1975 over 1974 are at no higher risk of experiencing handicapping condi-

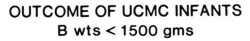

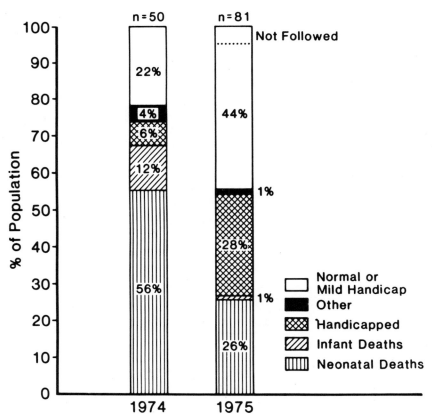

Fig. 5. Outcome of infants with birth weights < 1500 grams at 1 and 2 years of age.

tions than occurred previously. Obviously, we are not satisfied with this outcome because it appears that we were given healthier babies in 1975, but that during the neonatal period some of these infants developed intracranial bleeds, hypoxic episodes, or some other morbidity which affected their outcome.

10

Hemorrhagic Diseases of the Fetus

ALVIN LANGER, M.D.

HEMORRHAGIC DISEASES OF THE FETUS

Evaluation of risks to the well being of a fetus includes consideration of the potential of hereditary or acquired disease which may have serious adverse effects upon the long-term outcome for that fetus. Recognition of possible susceptibility to a hemorrhagic diathesis as one of the serious threats to the fetus or newborn may aid in the prevention of morbidity and mortality from that problem. A predisposition to this problem arises from a variety of causes.

The affected fetus may suffer serious consequences of birth trauma, possibly resulting in intracranial hemorrhage, or it may bleed unexpectedly and profusely at the site of insertion of a monitoring electrode or scalp blood sampling incision.[1] In certain instances the affected newborn may bleed after surgical procedures, most commonly after circumcision, or there may be spontaneous hemorrhage from the gastrointestinal tract or other organs; this poses diagnostic difficulties for the neonatologist, particularly if he or she is unaware of the obstetric background underlying the hemorrhage.

NORMAL COAGULATION MECHANISM IN THE FETUS

The coagulation cascade, depicted in Fig. 1, is well known and begins with both an intrinsic and extrinsic mechanism. (Clotting factors are listed in Table 1.) In the intrinsic coagulation mechanism, a platelet plug adheres to the site of a vascular injury, triggering an activation of clotting factors. Substances released from the platelet plug include adenosine diphosphate (ADP) which further promotes the cohesion and aggregation of platelets and also platelet factor 3 (PF-3), a phospholipid, which is an essential element in both the intrinsic clotting system and the ultimate conversion of prothrombin to thrombin. Tissue thromboplastin released as a response to tissue injury initiates the extrinsic coagulation mechanism. Both the intrinsic and extrinsic mechanisms result in the eventual activation of Factor X which in turn causes the conversion of prothrombin to thrombin. The latter is responsible for the conversion of fibrinogen to a fibrin polymer. As a

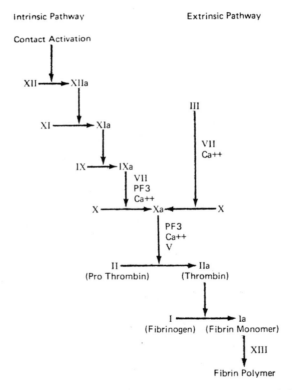

Fig. 1.   Intrinsic and extrinsic coagulation pathways, both of which result in activation of factor X and follow the same mechanism for ultimate production of the fibrinogen polymer.

Table 1.　Coagulation Factors

I	Fibrinogen
II	Prothrombin
III	Tissue thromboplastin
IV	Calcium
V	Labile factor, pro-accelerin
VII	Stable factor, pro-convertin
VIII	Antihemophiliac factor A
IX	Christmas factor, antihemophiliac factor B
X	Stuart - Prower factor
XI	Plasma thromboplastin antecedent (PTA)
XII	Hageman factor
XIII	Fibrin stabilizing factor

protective mechanism in response to the coagulation process, fibrinolysis is initiated with the activation of plasminogen to plasmin, which splits the fibrin and fibrinogen into degradation products (FDP). Plasmin also acts as a proteolytic enzyme on other plasma proteins such as Factors V and VIII, leading to inactive products and therefore also acts as a coagulation inhibitor.

Hemostatic factors develop at varying rates in the fetus.[2] Fibrinogen is first detectable at five weeks' gestation. Platelets and the Vitamin K dependent factors (II, VII, IX and X) are first demonstrable at approximately ten weeks. Platelet adhesiveness appears at 12 to 15 weeks but remains somewhat diminished until term. Megakaryocytes become fully active in producing adult numbers of platelets by 30 weeks' gestation. Although all factors are present at relatively early stages of gestation, the rate of synthesis varies, which reflects differing rates of organ maturation. Factors I, V, VIII and XIII usually reach adult levels in utero, as does the platelet count. However, the concentration of the contact factors (XI and XII) and the Vitamin K dependent factors (II, VII, IX and X) do not reach adult levels even by term, and the preterm newborn demonstrates decreased platelet aggregation as well as decreased coagulation factors. The amount of variation below adult levels depends upon the gestational age at the time of birth, with the more premature babies having greater impairment of their coagulation abilities.

HEREDITARY COAGULATION DISORDERS

Coagulation Factor Deficiency.　Deficiency of any of the numbered co-agulation factors may be inherited as a result of a genetic mutation. Fortunately, deficiencies of most factors are without significant clinical consequence to either the fetus or neonate, even though the normal coagulation factors are not transferred from mother to fetus. The exceptions to the innocuousness of the deficiencies are those of factors VIII, IX and XIII.

Factor XIII (fibrin stabilizing factor) deficiency is inherited as an autosomal recessive disease and results in bleeding of moderate severity. This factor is necessary for the normal stabilization of the fibrin molecule and is thus a prerequisite for adequate scar formation. This deficiency occurs rarely.

Deficiencies of factors VIII and IX occur much more frequently and cause, in different individuals, mild to severe bleeding. Usually bleeding does not occur as a result of birth trauma, but in the previously unsuspected case, circumcision may be accompanied by severe bleeding. Both deficiencies are inherited as x-linked recessive disorders and therefore both are usually passed from the "normal" carrier mother to her male offspring.

Hemophilia.   The identification of carriers of hemophilia remains a problem, particularly for those gravidas who would not choose to continue a pregnancy in which the fetus was likely to have the disease. Certain individuals can be identified as obligatory carriers—i.e., those whose fathers are hemophiliacs, those who have given birth to more than one hemophiliac offspring (except monozygotic twins), or those with one hemophiliac son and the appropriate affected relative. Women who are possible carriers include those who have an appropriate maternal relative with hemophilia but have had no affected son, or those who have no family history but have produced a hemophiliac son. In either instance, the gene may have been present in previous generations but there were no male births, or the gene may have been present in previous generations but the males, by chance, had not inherited the mutant gene. It appears in at least two-thirds of these instances of isolated cases of hemophilia that the mother is a carrier of a mutant gene, and that only about one-third of the time does the disease result from a de novo mutation.[3]

It would be fortunate if all carriers could be positively identified so that the "possible" carrier who is, in fact, a non-carrier would no longer have a cause for concern. Since the female carrier has one X chromosome with a normal gene for factor VIII and another X chromosome carrying a mutant gene, one might expect the carrier to have 50 percent of normal factor VIII activity. This is true if one studies population groups of carriers. However, any individual carrier may have factor VIII activity ranging from completely normal down to hemophiliac levels.[4] This is due to inactivation of one X chromosome at random, with the net effect depending upon to what extent the mutant gene is expressed or inactivated.

It has long been recognized that serum factor VIII clotting activity which measures functional factor VIII is not necessarily equivalent to immunologically detectable factor VIII antigen, which measures total factor VIII, both normally functioning and otherwise.[5] Hemophiliacs have been shown to have normal levels of factor VIII antigen, but a reduction in clotting activity. A similar reduction in clotting activity in the presence of normal antigen levels can indicate the carrier state with a greater than 90 percent accuracy.

In counseling either a known or suspected hemophilia carrier, it has traditionally been possible to determine via amniocentesis only whether the fetus is male or female, with the knowledge that 50 percent of the males will be affected and 50 percent will be unaffected, whereas female offspring should be no more than carriers. It was impossible to separate the males into affected and unaffected. Currently a higher degree of accuracy is occasionally possible, using the close linkage on the X chromosome between the genetic loci of factor VIII activity and G6PD (glucose 6 phosphate dehydrogenase). There are two distinct electrophorectic types of G6PD and if the heterozygous carrier is also heterozygous for these two types, and the appropriate affected relatives are studied to determine which type is found in association with the mutant gene for factor VIII, one may be able to predict that a fetus is likely to be or not to be affected by hemophilia. This is done by determination of G6PD type on amniotic fluid cells.[6] The recombination frequency between the two genes is less than 6.7 percent at a 95 percent confidence level, making for only a small but definite possibility of error. This margin of error will be acceptable for some gravidas, while for others any possibility of error would be too much for continuation of pregnancy. Amniocentesis performed on hemophiliac carriers has not been demonstrated to have higher risk of hemorrhagic complications than otherwise expected.[7]

Other Inherited Conditions. There are a number that may be associated with some risk of fetal bleeding. *Von Willebrand's disease,* which occurs with moderate frequency, is inherited as an autosomal dominant disease. Therefore, 50 percent of the offspring of an affected parent will have the disease, regardless of sex of parent or fetus. The disease is characterized by deficiency of factor VIII antigen together with abnormal platelet function. Even the affected fetus, however, rarely suffers from a hemorrhagic problem, so that careful management of labor and delivery should be sufficient. No method of prenatal diagnosis currently exists.

Thrombocytopenia with absent radaii (TAR) is a rare but severe syndrome of autosomal recessive inheritance.[8] There may be severe, occasionally fatal, hemorrhage shortly after birth. Bone marrow examination reveals a decrease in number of megakaryocytes. There are a variety of possible associated skeletal anomalies, usually involving the forearm, which are amenable to prenatal recognition by x-ray examination or ultrasound. Approximately one-third of those affected also have cardiovascular abnormalities. Since there is no successful treatment, the importance of the diagnosis lies in the need for genetic counseling, since 25 percent of siblings will be similarly affected.

The Wiskott-Aldrich syndrome is a sex linked recessive disorder which causes mild to moderate hemorrhage usually beginning after birth.[9] It is associated with eczema and a predisposition to recurrent infection due to a partial combined immunodeficiency. Bleeding is due to thrombocytopenia. Cases of isolated thrombocytopenia may occur by autosomal dominant, autosomal recessive, or sex-linked recessive inheritance. These cases are usually mild and are rare. Occasionally they result in neonatal purpura. They are anticipated only in the event of previous family history.

There are a number of other genetic disorders which occasionally are associated with a hemorrhagic diathesis in the fetus and newborn. The most severe of these are autosomal recessive metabolic disorders in which severe hepatocellular damage occurs in utero, resulting in inability to produce the Vitamin K dependent factors (factors II, VII, IX, X). Examples are hereditary fructose intolerance and galactosemia.[10] Diagnosis, if possible in utero, is made by specific tests for the suspected disorder. Suspicion of an affected fetus is usually on the basis of family history and/or tests for carrier detection, if they are available.

DRUG-INDUCED COAGULATION DISORDERS

A number of drugs administered to the mother are capable of producing a coagulation disorder in the fetus after crossing the placenta. An example is the oral anticoagulant, warfarin. A pregnant woman occasionally requires anticoagulation for management of deep vein thrombosis and/or pulmonary embolism, or because she has a heart valve prosthesis. Two categories of anticoagulants are available for administration to such patients. Although heparin is the safer because its molecular weight of 15,000 does not allow placental passage, long-term use is inconvenient because it must be given parenterally. Warfarin derivatives, of which Coumadin is the most commonly used, have a molecular weight of 500 to 5,000, and cross the placenta with ease, but their oral route of administration makes them much more practical for long-term use. Oral anticoagulants are contraindicated during the first trimester because of their potential teratogenic effect.[11] The gravida who requires anticoagulation at that time should be managed only with heparin. In the second trimester, oral anticoagulation may be given, and it may be continued until 37 weeks' gestation. After that, oral agents should be discontinued, and anticoagulation with heparin resumed. Such management does not appear to increase fetal risk.[12] However, should the patient begin spontaneous labor while still being anticoagulated with oral agents, then there is fetal risk. Avoidance of birth trauma is exceedingly important. Vitamin K or specific procoagulants may be administered if needed. It should be remembered that these compounds have a half-life of approximately 50 hours, so the effect is prolonged after stopping ingestion.

Although the warfarin derivatives are secreted in breast milk, the amount is probably not sufficient to injure most nursing newborns. However, if the baby of a mother being so treated must be subjected to surgery, evaluation of coagulation is mandatory prior to that surgery.[13]

Diphenylhydantoin (Dilantin) may exert a similar anti-Vitamin K effect on the fetus, and offspring of mothers given this medication during the latter part of pregnancy should be administered Vitamin K.[14]

DRUG-INDUCED THROMBOCYTOPENIA

A number of medications administered to the mother are capable of altering platelet function in the fetus. The most commonly used of these is probably aspirin, which has been demonstrated to impair platelet function in the fetus after maternal ingestion of as little as 650mg two weeks prior to delivery. The mechanism of action is via an alteration of the platelet membrane, inhibiting release of ADP, and thereby interfering with the secondary phase of platelet aggregation. This altered platelet function has resulted in minor bleeding complications such as cephalohematoma, purpura or melena. Therefore, the use of aspirin during the last trimester should be discouraged. Similar actions have been attributed to promethazine (Phenergan) and alphaprodine hydrochloride (Nisentil). The clinical significance of the in vitro alterations in platelet function which can be demonstrated in reaction to the latter drugs is not known at present.[15] They have not been shown to lead to hemorrhagic problems in the newborn, but their use in the laboring patient should be instituted with that potential in mind.

A number of drugs are also potentially responsible for platelet destruction by an immunologic mechanism. It is postulated that in the susceptible individual, such a drug interacts with the platelets at the time of an initial exposure, producing a drug-platelet combination which is antigenic and evokes an antibody response. Subsequent administration of that drug results in platelet destruction via an antigen-antibody reaction. This may occur in a fetus even if the mother is not affected. Drugs that have been implicated in causing this action include quinine, quinidine, and tolbutamide.

In addition, other drugs may directly suppress the bone marrow of the fetus, causing decreased production of platelets. The thiazide diuretics have been suspected of this type of action, and it is also known to occur in certain instances when the mother is receiving chemotherapy for a malignant disease.[16] While each of these medications is thought to be a potential cause of hemorrhage in the fetus or neonate, one cannot categorically state that all are contraindicated during pregnancy. In each instance, the indication for the choice of medication must be balanced against the potential risks, with recognition of the possibility of fetal problems after usage. Where obvious indications are present and there are no reasonable alternative methods of therapy, the fetal risk may be justifiable.

IMMUNOLOGIC THROMBOCYTOPENIA

Maternal ITP (idiopathic thrombocytopenic purpura), which is active during pregnancy or in which the effects of circulating antibodies have been obscured by splenectomy, is associated with thrombocytopenia in 30 to 50 percent of offspring. This occurrence in the fetus is due to transplacental transmission of the IgG type antibody produced by the mother. The platelet count may remain low for weeks after birth. The danger of hemorrhage is maximal during labor and delivery and is usually intracranial. Therefore, it is imperative to avoid birth trauma and many have advocated cesarean section for delivery in any such gravida.[17] After birth, acute hemorrhage in the fetus may be treated by either exchange transfusion, which removes antibodies from the serum of the newborn and/or by transfusing platelets. This neonatal thrombocytopenia is a self-limited, passively acquired disease which does not require splenectomy and does not respond to drug suppression. Recently, it has been felt that perhaps all affected gravidas do not need to be delivered by cesarean section since the majority of fetuses are unaffected. A platelet count on the fetus during labor obtained from scalp blood may allow one to deliver unaffected babies by the vaginal route unless other indications for cesarean section exist.[18]

Similar passive transfer of autoantibodies has been demonstrated to occur occasionally in gravidas with systemic lupus erythematosus. Such cases are similarly managed.

Isoimmune thrombocytopenia is a condition affecting platelets which is analogous to the red cell antigen incompatibility resulting in hemolytic disease of the newborn. It is due to incompatibility of platelet antigens, with the mother having an antibody to a fetal platelet antigen. It occurs in 1 to 2 of every 10,000 births, and differs from the red cell antigen incompatibility in that half of the affected infants are first-born. Therefore, it is not possible to anticipate the first affected progeny. Platelet antigens are inherited as autosomal dominant traits of which three types are known. About 98 percent of the population are positive for the antigen Pl^{Al}, whereas only 46 and 30 percent are positive for the antigen $PlGrLy^{Bl}$ and $PlGrLy^{Cl}$, respectively.[19] However, in spite of the fact that the occurrence of incompatibility between mother and fetus involving Pl^{Al} is rare, almost all cases of isoimmune thrombocytopenia are due to that antigen. This suggests that it is a much more potent antigen than are the others. Severely affected newborns develop a petechial rash which is present at birth or soon thereafter. These infants have a mortality of 10 to 15 percent, most often due to intracranial hemorrhage. Thus, risk to the offspring is very high. The disorder is often unsuspected. Treatment of the newborn consists of transfusion of compatible maternal antigen negative platelets and/or immediate exchange transfusion with fresh whole blood, which would both remove circulating passively acquired antibodies and provide large numbers of viable platelets. Diagnosis could be expected by maternal platelet antibody levels, but such determinations are rarely available to the obstetrician.

DISSEMINATED INTRAVASCULAR COAGULATION (DIC)

Intravascular consumption of platelets and factors I, II, V and VIII may lead to a serious risk of hemorrhage. This consumption occurs in disseminated intravascular coagulation. Initiating factors in the fetus include those obstetric complications which are associated with disseminated intravascular coagulation in the mother. Fetal DIC has been reported to occur with abruptio placentae, preeclampsia and eclampsia, amniotic fluid embolism, and the dead twin fetus syndrome and must be considered when such obstetric complications are present.[20] It also may result from birth asphyxia.

A variety of infections affecting the fetus and the newborn occasionally initiate disseminated intravascular coagulation. These include bacterial infections, cytomegalovirus, rubella, herpes simplex, toxoplasmosis and syphilis. Fortunately, serious hemorrhage in these infections is rare, and the potential of hemorrhage is not sufficient to influence the obstetric management.

DIC in the newborn may be initiated by a variety of other conditions, including the respiratory distress syndrome, severe acidosis, hypoxemia, renal vein thrombosis, and severe hemolytic disease.[20,21] In the presence of a giant hemangioma (Kasabach-Merritt syndrome) there may be a local consumption of coagulation factors in the lesion itself. One should not attempt to inhibit such coagulation, since it is this coagulation which ultimately reduces the size of the lesion. Diagnosis of the hemangioma is not made before birth.

In most conditions associated with disseminated intravascular coagulation, prevention of the underlying abnormality, if possible, is the most important factor in obstetrical management.

CONCLUSIONS

A variety of maternal and fetal conditions may predispose the fetus to increased risk of death or disability from hemorrhage. Although such cases occur infrequently, the obstetrician should be aware of the possibility, and should be able to identify some of the high risk babies. When possible, appropriate management of labor and delivery may significantly influence the outcome. Emphasis should be placed upon minimizing the possibility of hemorrhage induced by traumatic delivery, and upon counseling before conception for certain maternal diseases or hereditary defects. Communication between the obstetrician and neonatologist is mandatory for accurate diagnosis and prompt treatment in the neonate.

REFERENCES

1. Hull, M. G. R. and Wilson, J. A. Massive scalp haemorrhage after fetal blood sampling due to hemorrhage disease. *Brit. Med. J.* **4:** 321, 1972.
2. Bleyer, W. A., Hakami, N. and Shepard, T. H. The development of hemostasis in the human fetus and newborn infant. *J. Pediatr.* **79:** 838, 1971.
3. Bennet, B. and Ratnoff, O. D. Detection of the carrier state for classic hemophilia. *New Eng. J. Med.* **288:** 342, 1973.
4. Graham, J. B., Miller, C. H. et al. The phenotypic range of hemophilia A carriers. *Am. J. Hum. Genet.* **28:** 482, 1976.
5. Ratnoff, O. D. and Jones, P. K. The detection of carriers of classic hemophilia. *Am. J. Clin. Path.* **65:** 129, 1976.
6. Edgell, C. J. S. Kirkman, H. N. et al. Prenatal diagnosis by linkage: hemophilia A and polymorphic glucose - 6 - phosphate dehydrogenase. *Am. J. Hum. Genet.* **30:** 80, 1978.
7. Spiro, R. and Lubs, M. L. Survey of amniocentesis for fetal sex determination in hemophilia carriers. *Clin. Genet.* **10:** 337, 1976.
8. Hall, J. G., Levin, J. et al. Thrombocytopenia with absent radius (TAR). *Medicine* **48:** 411, 1969.
9. Wolff, J. A. Wiskott-Aldrich syndrome: clinical, immunologic, and pathologic observations. *J. Pediatr.* **70:** 221, 1967.
10. Raju, L. Chessells, J. M. and Kemball, M. Manifestation of hereditary fructose intolerance. *Brit. Med. J.* **2:** 446, 1971.
11. Shaul, W. L., Emery, H. and Hall, J. G. Chondrodysplasia punctata and maternal warfarin use during pregnancy. *Am. J. Dis. Child.* **129:** 360, 1975.
12. Pridmore, B. R., Murray, K. H. and McAllen, P. M. The management of anticoagulation therapy during and after pregnancy. *Brit. J. Obstet. Gynaec.* **82:** 740, 1975.
13. Eckstein, H. B. and Jack, B. Breast-feeding and anticoagulant therapy. *Lancet* **1:** 672, 1970.

14. Mountain, K. R., Hirsch, J. and Gallus, A. S. Neonatal coagulation defect due to anticonvulsant drug treatment in pregnancy. *Lancet* 1: 265, 1970.
15. Corby, D. G. and Schulman, I. The effects of antenatal drug administration on aggregation of platelets of newborn infants. *J. Pediatr.* 79: 307, 1971.
16. Rodriguez, S. U., Leikin, S. L. and Hiller, M. C. Neonatal thrombocytopenia associated with ante-partum administration of thiazide drugs. *New Eng. J. Med.* 270: 881, 1964.
17. Gowda, V. V., Apuzzio, J., Langer, A., Li, T. S., Devanesan, M. and Harrigan, J. Pregnancy complicated by refractory thrombocytopenic purpura and diabetes mellitus. *J. Rep. Med.* 19: 147, 1977.
18. Pitkin, R. Autoimmune Diseases in Pregnancy. Presented at the Fourth Memorial Ignatz Semmelweis Seminar. McAffee, N. J., Sept. 1978.
19. Pearson, H. A., Shulman, N. R. et al. Isoimmune neonatal thrombocytopenia purpura: clinical and therapeutic considerations. *Blood* 23: 154, 1964.
20. Lascari, A. D. and Wallace, P. D. Disseminated intravascular coagulation in newborns: survey and appraisal as exemplified in two case histories. *Clin. Pediatr.* 10: 11, 1971.
21. Chessells, J. M. and Wigglesworth, J. S. Haemostatic failure in babies with rhesus isoimmunization. *Arch. Dis. Child.* 46: 38, 1971.

11

Telegony Updated

SIR CYRIL A. CLARKE, M.D.

In the last century there was much experimental work carried out on telegony, the theory that characters derived from the male of a previous mating appear in the offspring of a subsequent mating with a different male. The scientific work to test this ancient hypothesis was carried out in Scotland (the Penycuik Experiments) and reported by Professor J. C. Ewart in 1899.[7] He mated a mare to a zebra male, and the mother and the Fl hybrid are shown in Fig. 1. The mare was mated subsequently to a stallion, and Fig. 2 shows the second offspring, which appears to have some zebra-like stripes. This seemed to support telegony, but Ewart was quick to point out that not infrequently, foals from normal mare X stallion matings have faint stripes when they are newborn.

So the idea of telegony lost ground, but it still lingers on among pedigree stock breeders. For example, "Southdown ewes which have been mated with rams of another breed cannot be considered eligible to produce pure-bred sheep, and will be excluded from the Flock Book" (Southdown Breed Society, By-law 3b, 1950).

It is not a bad plan to review ancient beliefs periodically, because they have an awkward habit of having some foundation, and while telegony in

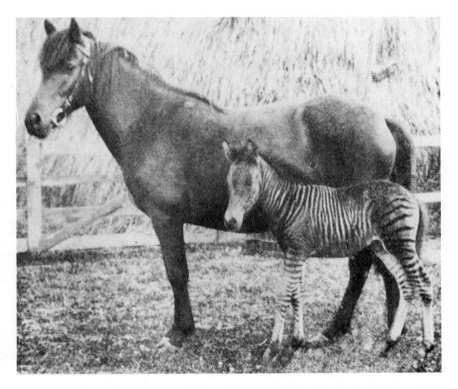

Fig. 1.   The Penycuik experiments (1899). a) The mare with her first foal, which was sired by a zebra. (Royal Society of Medicine)

its original concept remains dead and buried, yet there is no doubt that "the baby before" can sometimes influence its succeeding sib. This is clearly so in Rhesus haemolytic disease of the newborn and may have some relevance in anencephaly and spina bifida. In this chapter some recent findings are reported.

PREVENTION OF RHESUS HAEMOLYTIC DISEASE

There is now general agreement that anti-D gammaglobulin is an effective method of preventing the immunization of Rhesus negative women, but the extent of the protection is difficult to assess.

Because women are having fewer children, and also because of improvements in treatment, the death rate from haemolytic disease of the newborn (HDN) started to fall long before the introduction of anti-D. However, as shown on the logarithmic scale in Fig. 3, the death-rate from

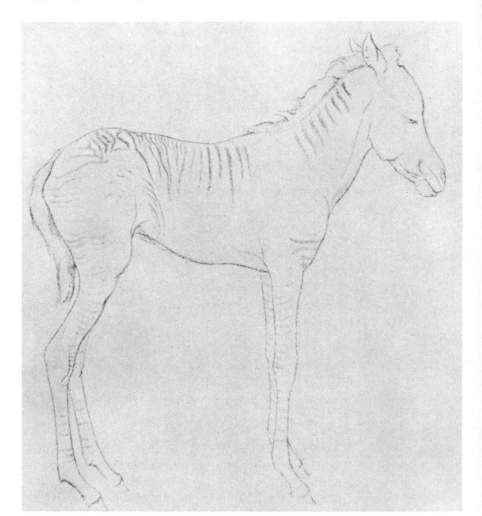

Fig. 2. The Penycuik experiments (1899). b) Second offspring of the same mare as in Fig. 1. This foal was sired by a stallion. (Royal Society of Medicine)

the disorder per 1,000 live births strongly suggests that something happened soon after 1968, which was the year when anti-D was introduced in England and Wales. The graph, however, only relates to neonatal deaths, and there remain for consideration the stillbirths. These are probably in the region of twice the neonatal deaths, but there are difficulties, because stillbirths born to Rhesus negative women tend to be classified as Rhesus deaths, whereas in fact this may not always be the case, and autopsies, par-

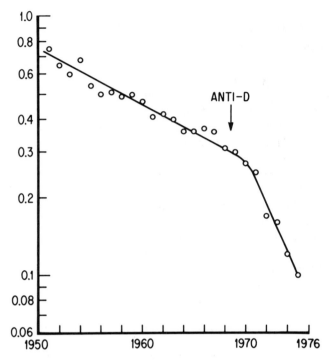

Fig. 3. The rate of deaths from hemolytic disease of the newborn per 1,000 live births in England and Wales before and after the introduction of active anti-D immunization.

ticularly when the fetus is macerated, are not always helpful. There is no ready answer to this problem, but it seemed to me there was a worthwhile subject for investigation by the Medical Service Study Group (MSSG) of which I am Director of the Royal College of Physicians of London. This was to try to find out the circumstances in which mothers became immunized to Rh when they either had a stillbirth or a death from RhHDN in 1977, according to the death certificate. These were kindly supplied by the Office of Population and Census Surveys, and I received 52 for liveborns and 100 for stillbirths.

INTERIM RESULTS OF THE MSSG STUDY

Through the cooperation of many obstetricians and gynecologists in England and Wales, I was able to scrutinize the actual case notes of the mothers and their babies. In a few cases there was a hospital rule that "Notes must not leave the premises," and where this was so, I paid a special visit to look at them.

It will be seen from Tables 1 and 2 that at the time of writing (November 1978), I have nearly finished the neonates and am about two-thirds through the stillbirths. The data as shown are raw, and the exact form of analysis has yet to be decided because occasionally patients fall into more than one category. However, in approximately one-quarter of the cases the mother had clearly been immunized before anti-D was available, and in another quarter there was no record of anti-D having been given when in my view it should have been (about 1968 onwards for neonates and 1971 et seq. after abortions). In a further quarter of the total, the notes had shown that there was no question of Rhesus or any other haemolytic process being involved, the hydrops (which was usually what was stated on the death certificate) being due to other causes—of which there are many.[3] The fourth quarter contains a miscellaneous group, including eight failures of prophylaxis.

It must be pointed out that these results came from different types of hospitals with different standards and that in some areas the prophylaxis had evidently not become routine for some years after 1968 (or 1971).

It is of interest that we have data from the U.S. which enable us to make

Table 1. RhHDN 1977.

NEONATAL DEATHS 47/52	NO.
Immunized before anti-D became available for full-term deliveries (1968)	7
Immunized by an abortion before anti-D became available after abortions (1971)	2
Antibodies found during the immunizing pregnancy: a) before the 28th week	1
b) after the 28th week	5
Immunized by c and E — mother D positive (therefore no prophylactic anti-D given)	2
Failures of anti-D prophylaxis	2
No record of anti-D having been given after immunizing fetus	17
Non-Rhesus Causes of Death	
1. Hemolytic disease, possibly due to non-Rhesus antibodies	1
2. Hydrops fetalis with no hemolysis and no antibodies found	8
3. Cytomegalovirus infection, no hemolysis	1
4. Atelectasis. "No question of Rhesus iso-immunization." Mother O Rh-positive. Baby born jaundiced and kernicterus found at post-mortem.	1
	47

Table 2. RhHDN 1977.

STILLBIRTHS 72/100	NO.
Immunized before anti-D became available for full-term deliveries (1968)	20
Antibodies found during immunizing pregnancy: a) before 28th week	1
b) after 28th week	6
Immunized by blood transfusion	2
Immunized by c and E—mother D-positive (therefore no prophylactic anti-D given)	4
Failures of anti-D prophylaxis	8
No record of anti-D having been given after immunizing fetus	17
Non-Rhesus Causes of Death	
1. Hydrops fetalis with no hemolysis and no antibodies found	6
2. Stillbirth not due to Rh (mother Rhesus negative but correctly treated and no antibodies)	5
3. Pre-eclamptic toxemia	1
4. Septicemia	1
5. Hereditary congenital spherocytosis	1
	72

some comparisons. In Connecticut, where 98.8 percent of the women have their babies in the hospital, the dedicated research analyst Mrs. Gustafson has organized the prophylaxis so well that in 1977 RhoGAM was given to 99.6 percent of the cases in which it was indicated. Deaths from RhHDN in 1977 were three, two of the women having been immunized before RhoGAM was available and the third having developed antibodies during the pregnancy in which the baby died (a stillbirth).[9] The population of Connecticut is about 3.5 million and the number of births in 1977 was 35,000. These figures are about 1/16th of those in England and Wales, and by extrapolation there would have been around 50 deaths instead of 150 if mothers there had had the same organized care that they had in Connecticut. This statement must be modified to some extent because, as will be seen from the tables, a proportion of the patients in England and Wales whose death certificates were sent to me did not in fact have Rhesus haemolytic disease at all. Again, because we are ascertaining from deaths there will be an unduly high proportion of mothers not given anti-D, and of failures of prophylaxis. Nevertheless, we clearly need to put our house in order, and this was also the opinion of Tovey et al.[15] who had similar information from Yorkshire, and in Finland, where there was failure to treat 15 percent of women at risk.[6]

ANTENATAL ANTI-D

It is well known that there exists a small failure rate for anti-D prophylaxis, the main reason for this being that a few mothers become immunized during the later weeks of pregnancy and when this happens, post-natally administered anti-D will be too late.

Extensive studies have been carried out in Canada, Australia and Sweden to see if antenatal anti-D, given usually at the 28th and 34th weeks, as well as post-natally, could reduce the number of failures. Table 3 gives the results from Sweden.[2] The whole matter was discussed by a working group at McMaster University in the fall of 1977. There was general agreement that this newer type of prophylaxis was more effective than the old. However, as far as England and Wales are concerned, we feel that before embarking on any project, we should close the gaps in our present procedure which (as has been seen) are very considerable.

ANTI-D AFTER ABORTIONS

At present, it is probably more important than the administration of antenatal anti-D to ensure that all Rhesus negative women who have had an abortion, either spontaneous or induced, should receive anti-D, since it is well known that even early abortuses can immunize. Table 4 gives some information from Hungary in this respect.[14]

HEMOLYTIC DISEASE OF THE NEWBORN FOAL (HDNF)

In the horse, there are both similarities and differences compared to the disease in man. Thus the first foal is not usually affected, and the assumption is that the mare is immunized by a feto-maternal hemorrhage (FMH). Because no staining differences have been detected between fetal and adult hemoglobin in this species, the Kleihauer-Betke technique is useless. However, we have been able to show that fetal cells are present by means of a minor cell population technique.[5] As in man, immune antibodies are formed by the mare, but they reach the foal via the colostrum and not by the placenta. The colostrum is highly toxic to the foal for about 36 hours but after that time, the antibody is no longer absorbed because of metaplasia in the gut epithelium. HDNF is not of great practical importance, because if it is known that a mare is immunized, her teats can be covered or the foal muzzled and colostrum given from a non-immunized

Table 3. Prevention of Rh-immunization by Injection of 250 mg Anti-D During Pregnancy and Post-partum, Göteborg and Växjö 1968-1976.

TRIAL	TOTAL NO. OF MOTHERS	NUMBER OF Rh-IMMUNIZED MOTHERS			
		AT DELIVERY	AT DELIVERY AND 6-8 MONTHS LATER	ONLY AT 6-8 MONTHS POST-PARTUM	TOTAL AT 6-8 MONTHS POST-PARTUM
Post-partum					
Primigravidae	625	6	2	2[a]	4
Multigravidae	652	13	8	3	11
Total	1277	19	10	5	15
Ante-partum + post-partum					
Primigravdae	369	—	—	1[b]	1[b]
Multigravidae	191	—	—	0	0
Total	560	—	—	1	1

[a] Weak Rh-antibodies by the papain method 8 months after delivery (see text).
[b] Weak Rh-antibodies by the papain method 8 months after delivery. Twenty months post-partum antibodies were not detectable.

Table 4.   Rh Immunization in Second Pregnancies in Relation to Therapeutic Abortion of First Conceptus. (Simonovits, Budapest,
Personal Communication, 1977.)

	CONTROLS (No anti-D given after therapeutic abortion)	
NO. OF WOMEN	NUMBER IMMUNIZED DURING SECOND PREGNANCY	IMMUNIZATION RATE
308	11	3.6%

	TREATED (50 μg anti-D given after therapeutic abortion)	
NO. OF WOMEN	NUMBER IMMUNIZED DURING SECOND PREGNANCY	IMMUNIZATION RATE
3,080	13	.42%

mare. Nevertheless, HDNF is of considerable theoretical interest. The
following is an account of some joint work between the University of
Liverpool and the Equine Research Station at Newmarket.[5]

By analogy with our experiments in man, we first injected 10 to 20 ml
chromium—51 labelled red cells into nonimmunized ponies in which no
antibodies were demonstrable by routine cross-matching, and the experiment was controlled by also injecting the ponies' own chromium—51
labelled red cells. The results were very different from those in man, the
allogeneic cells always (on 12 separate occasions) being largely eliminated
(probably mainly to the spleen) within a matter of hours, whereas the
autologous cells persisted much longer.

These initial findings have to be related to the fact that there is no need
to cross-match before giving a horse a first blood transfusion, and any
available animal can be used.[7] The reason for this is that naturally-
occurring antibodies are 'very weak, very rare and seem to have no effect
on transfusion.'[1] Though this explanation is clearly true for a transfusion, it may not hold for small quantities of blood such as presumably
usually occur in FMH, and we think that the rapid elimination of the
small quantities of cells we gave is probably due to the presence of
naturally-occurring antibodies, detectable by special methods but not by
routine cross-matching. Thus, in Liverpool, we tested the neat serum of
17 ponies against a panel of cells obtained from 6 other ponies. The tests
were made in saline at 10°C, and a 2% suspension of sodium chloride
obviated rouleaux formation. The serum of only 3 ponies agglutinated
none of the cells, and most sera agglutinated all the cells.

It is also of interest that we failed to immunize 6 of the ponies which had naturally-occurring antibody when 10–20 ml of blood was given intravenously, though immunization did occur on one occasion when a larger volume (40 ml) was injected intramuscularly, and it may be that naturally-occurring antibodies are absent from the tissue fluids.

To test the 'big volume versus small volume' hypothesis, we gave 400 ml of unlabeled blood with 10 ml labeled cells to see whether naturally-occurring antibodies would be 'swamped' and the chromium-51 labeled cells therefore survive much longer. Some support for this view was obtained. If valid, it would be interesting to find out in man, by *in vitro* experiments, whether using a larger volume of incompatible blood diminishes the rate of destruction of the red cells, as it appears to do in the horse.

Our tentative suggestion is that naturally-occurring antibodies are protective against small FMHs and that this is why the disease is rare in ponies. It remains to be discovered whether the prevalence of the naturally-occurring antibodies is different in different breeds of horse.

In relation to the protection afforded by ABO incompatibility in man against Rhesus sensitization, it is important to remember that the anti-A or anti-B need only have a very weak titer in order to protect, since in hypogammaglobulinemia, where the production of antibody is greatly reduced, ABO incompatible cells are removed experimentally in a few hours.[12]

WHY DON'T NEWBORN RHESUS MONKEYS GET HAEMOLYTIC DISEASE?

In a very interesting paper, Stone et al.[13] pointed out that though it is possible to immunize female Rhesus monkeys by allogeneic cells, and though this can occur in pregnancy and the newborn monkey gives a positive Coombs test, the young are never anemic. Whether this is because the concentration of the antibody is not high enough, or whether the macrophages are not properly developed in young monkeys remains to be determined.

PREVENTING ANENCEPHALY AND SPINA BIFIDA (ASB)

Here the "baby before" hypothesis is much more speculative than in RH, but no one knows why women have ASB babies; though it may be true that there is more than one cause, it seems to me more profitable to follow one line. We have noted, as have others, that the reproductive history of women who had these babies *tended* to be abnormal—they had more abortions or neonatal deaths than would be expected. We concentrated on abortions and stillbirths, and we found [4] (as shown in Figure 4) that they were about twice as likely to have had a miscarriage or a stillbirth immediately before the ASB baby as immediately afterwards. We pursued this line because Knox [10] had expounded the view some years ago that ASB might be caused by an interaction between residual trophoblast from a previous pregnancy (a "rest") with that of the current one. Although there are other explanations for our findings, they do support the "rest" theory.

THE PROSPECTIVE SURVEY

We decided to study the incidence of neural tube defects and other congenital abnormalities in babies born to 510 mothers ascertained during pregnancy. [8] The women were divided into two groups according to the outcome of their immediately preceding pregnancy. Those whose preceding pregnancy had resulted in a spontaneous abortion (256 women) formed the index cases; those in whom the outcome had been a normal baby (254 women) served as controls.

It will be seen from Tables 5 and 6 that there is a highly significant excess of congenital abnormalities in the index cases; this again could be explained on the ground of the Knox hypothesis. Another possibility is that the women are just "poor reproducers" or that aging eggs are involved, [11] but

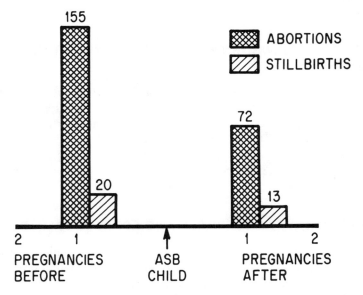

Fig. 4.   Abortions and stillbirths before and after "middle" affected children. Adapted from Dr. S. C. Rogers. (Personal communication.)

Table 5. Abnormalities Noted Among 256 Index Cases,* and Details of Previous Spontaneous Abortions and Interpregnancy Gaps.

CASE NO.	GESTATIONAL AGE AT PREVIOUS SPONTANEOUS ABORTION (WEEKS)	INTER-PREGNANCY GAP (MONTHS)	DILATATION AND CURETTAGE	ABNORMALITY (CONFIRMED AT FOLLOW-UP)	SEX
1	10	45	NK	Hypospadias	M
2	8	10	NK	Cleft lip	M
3	8	1	Yes	Sacrococcygeal dimple	F
4†	26	30	No	Hypospadias	M
5†	26	30	No	Hypospadias	M
6	8	5	Yes	Anencephaly. NND	NK
7	12	24	Yes	Sacrococcygeal dimple, brisk knee and ankle jerks, epicanthic folds, clinodactyly	M
8	8	2	Yes	Sacrococcygeal dimple	F
9	11	24	Yes	Ventricular septal defect	M
10	10	10	Yes	Sacrococcygeal dimple with hairy patch above	M
11	11	2	Yes	Spina bifida (meningomyelocele). NND	F

Table 5. (cont.)

CASE NO.	GESTATIONAL AGE AT PREVIOUS SPONTANEOUS ABORTION (WEEKS)	INTER-PREGNANCY GAP (MONTHS)	DILATATION AND CURETTAGE	ABNORMALITY (CONFIRMED AT FOLLOW-UP)	SEX
12	10	12	Yes	Rectal stricture	F
13	14	24	Yes	Hirschsprung's disease	M
14	8	5	NK	Sacrococcygeal dimple	F
15	23	6	NK	Edward's syndrome and congenital heart disease. NND	
16	7	12	Yes	Sacrococcygeal dimple	F
17	12	3	Yes	Congenital dislocation of hip	M

NK = Not known. NND = Neonatal death.

* In addition to those listed the following abnormalities were noted but not included in the analysis: clicking hips (19 cases); systolic murmur (5), later thought to be innocent; metatarsus varus (2; one with clicking hips); and positional talipes (2).

† Cases 4 and 5 were twins.

162

Table 6. Abnormalities Noted Among 254 Control Cases,* and Interpregnancy Gap.

CASE NO.	INTERPREGNANCY GAP (YEARS)	ABNORMALITY (CONFIRMED AT FOLLOW–UP)	SEX
18	10	Sacrococcygeal dimple	M
19	1	Hypospadias	M
20	1	Syndactyly	M
21	1	Congenital hemiplegia with bony abnormalities	F

* In addition to those listed the following abnormalities were noted but not included in the analysis: clicking hips (9 cases; innocent systolic murmur in one); innocent systolic murmur (1); and bilateral talipes (1).

these are difficult views to test. However, with the help of Professor K. D. Bagshowe, we have thought of a way of doing this. Women who have had hydatidiform moles must certainly be thought of as "poor reproducers," and they not infrequently have subsequent babies. We plan to examine about 150 of these to see if they have abnormalities comparable to those in Table 5 of our survey. If they have, we feel it will favor the concept of "poor reproducers" but if they have not, it might support the "rest" theory. Although moles are known sometimes to leave behind rests, great care is taken to make sure that these have been eliminated before advising a mole patient that it is safe to have another baby. On the theory of "poor reproducers" one would expect spontaneous abortions to occur just as frequently *after* the ASB child as before—which is not the case.

A final consideration concerns the inter-pregnancy gap (IPG). Because this was short in many of our index cases in the prospective survey, it would be interesting to find out whether the incidence of malformations is reduced when a subsequent pregnancy is delayed after a spontaneous abortion. It is well known that the birth rate has been falling, particularly in social classes 4 and 5, and this is probably the result of family planning campaigns with wider spacing of children. If women were advised to wait until the reproductive cycle has been entirely normal again after an abortion, then on our hypothesis the incidence of ASB—and probably of other abnormalities—would automatically fall.

REFERENCES

1. Archer, R. K. and Franks, D. *Veterinary Rec.* **73:** 657, 1961.
2. Bartsch, F. Communicated at Antenatal anti-D Conference, McMaster University, 1977.

3. Barnes, S. E., Bryan, E. et al. Oedema in the newborn. *Molec. Aspects Med.* **1:** 187, 1977.
4. Clarke, C., Hudson, D. et al. Spina bifida and anencephaly: miscarriage as possible cause. *Brit. Med. J.* **4:** 743, 1975.
5. Clark, C. A., Gimlette, T. M. D. et al. *In* Symposium on haemolytic disease of the newborn foal. *J. Roy. Soc. Med.* **71:** 574, 1978.
6. Eklund, J. Prevention of Rh immunization in Finland, a National Study. Supplement 274, *Acta Paediatr. Scandinav.,* 1969–1977.
7. Ewart, J. C. The Penycuik Experiments. Adam and Clarles Black, 1899.
8. Gardiner, A., Clarke, C. A. et al. Spontaneous abortions and fetal abnormality in subsequent pregnancy. *Brit. Med. J.* **1:** 1016, 1978.
9. Gustafson, J. A. Connecticut Rh survey. Connecticut State Department of Health, 1977.
10. Knox, E. G. Fetus-fetus interaction—A model aetiology for anencephalus. *Develop. Med. Child Neurol.* **12:** 167, 1970.
11. Mikamo, K. and Iffy, L. Aging of the Ovum. Obstetrics and Gynecology Annual. New York, Appleton-Century-Crofts, 3, 1974, p. 47.
12. Mollison, P. L. Blood Transfusion in Clinical Medicine. Oxford, Blackwell Scientific Publ. 5th Ed., 1972.
13. Stone, W. H., Blazkovec, A. A. et al. Abstract of paper presented at the 15th Int. Conf. on animal blood groups and biochemical polymorphism. Leningrad, USSR, Aug., 1978.
14. Simonovits, I. Personal communication, 1977.
15. Tovey, L. A. D., Murray, J. et al. Prevention of Rh haemolytic disease. *Brit. Med. J.* **2:** 106, 1978.

12

Corticosteroids in Induction of Labor

J.K.G. MATI, M.B.CHB., M.D., M.R.C.O.G.

AND

V.P. AGGARWAL, M.B.B.S., M.R.C.O.G.

Induction of labor may be defined as the stimulation of uterine activity by an external stimulus aimed at achieving vaginal delivery usually after 28 weeks of gestation and before spontaneous onset of labor.[1] In the past ten years or so, induction of labor has become more readily accepted and used as obstetricians have become more active in the management of pregnancy.

Labor may be induced in the interests of the mother or those of the fetus, but quite often the interests of both are served. Although a lot of progress has been made over the years in devising methods of inducing labor, a safe and effective method that would stimulate normal labor has yet to be found.

HISTORICAL REVIEW

As early as the 16th century, reports can be found of successful induction of labor. Initially mechanical methods were used for cervical dilatation, and subsequently catheters, bougies, and laminaria tents were introduced into the pregnant uterus through the cervical canal. About the 18th century, artificial rupture of membranes and ergot alkaloids were introduced.

Such remedies as castor oil, hot bath and enema have been used as methods of induction of labor for generations. Other substances that have been used over the years include quinine, sparteine sulphate and pituitary extracts. Many of these methods have gradually faded out—either they were found ineffective or their effect on the pregnant uterus could not be controlled, resulting in serious calamities—especially uterine hypertonus and uterine rupture.

MODERN METHODS OF INDUCTION OF LABOR

The methods that are widely used today are:
1. Artificial rupture of membranes (A.R.M.)
2. Intravenous oxytocin infusion with or without A.R.M.
3. Prostaglandins

Success or failure of induction of labor depends very much on the proper selection of patients. Bishop[2] introduced a scoring system based on the evaluation of cervical consistency, position, effacement and dilatation, and an estimation of the station of the fetal head. In general the patients with low scores have longer induction labor intervals, while those having high scores have easy induction and delivery.

Artificial Rupture of Membranes.

A.R.M. is a relatively effective stimulus in inducing labor. Success depends very much on the Bishop scoring system. It has the great disadvantage that patients may fail to go into labor, and prolonged rupture of membranes carries a high risk of intrauterine infection. A.R.M. combined with intravenous oxytocin therapy is certainly a more effective method.

The procedure may also act by local release of prostaglandins which then lead to the release of oxytocin and influence the myometrium contractability.[19]

Intravenous Oxytocin Infusion.

Crude posterior pituitary extract was first used in obstetrics by Bell in 1909[3] and since then oxytocin has been the most widely used hormone for induction of labor. Oxytocin has been administered by various routes— intramuscular, subcutaneous, intranasal and buccal. With these routes of administration, oxytocin absorption and action cannot be properly controlled, and serious side effects such as uterine rupture and fetal hypoxia may occur and can result in maternal and fetal deaths.

In 1948, Theobald introduced the use of an intravenous drip with low concentration of oxytocin for induction of labor.[4] The range of low "physiologic" amounts from 2 to 10 mu/min of oxytocin for IV infusion was defined as the dose necessary to sensitize the myometrium at term. For accurate infusion of oxytocin an infusion pump and later electronic infusion sets were introduced.

Oxytocin is more effective with concomitant A.R.M. All cases receiving oxytocin need to be watched carefully—ideally there should be facilities for continuous fetal heart monitoring and intrauterine pressure recording. Oxytocin infusion is not safe for highly parous patients and those previously delivered by cesarean section. It carries the dangers of uterine hypertonus, uterine rupture, postpartum uterine atony, hemorrhage and amniotic fluid embolism. Administered in large doses and in abundant fluid volume, it may cause severe water intoxication.

Prostaglandins (PG).

Karim et al.[5] were the first to use prostaglandin $F_2 \propto$ for induction of labor in patients with intrauterine fetal death. This was followed by using PGE2 and $PGF_2 \propto$ for both term and preterm labors.[6,7]

During the last few years, prostaglandins have been widely used but have not been shown to be superior to oxytocin for induction of labor. On the other hand, prostaglandins have a definite advantage over oxytocin in cases of intrauterine fetal death and midtrimester abortion. Adverse effects reported include uterine hypertonus, incoordinate uterine action, nausea, vomiting, tachycardia, and erythema along the infusion vein.

WHAT INITIATES LABOR?

The mechanisms triggering the initiation of labor are still not clear. Hippocrates believed that the fetus initiated labor when it felt that the conditions outside the uterus were better than inside.

Gestational length seems to be genetically controlled and species specific. The length of gestation is 280 days in man, 147 days in the sheep, 168 days in the rhesus monkey and 340 days in the mare.

Over the last 20 years or so, an attempt to explain the initiation of labor by means of physiological functions of the three main hormones— estrogen, progesterone, and oxytocin has had little success.

The placental production of estrogen and progesterone increases steadily throughout pregnancy, with a tenfold increase over the nonpregnant levels for progesterone and a 1000 to 10,000-fold increase for estriol alone.[8,9] Women begin labor in the absence of any abrupt change in the progesterone and estrogen levels. Thus, it is most unlikely that these hormones act as triggering mechanisms for parturition. Initially Csapo[10] postulated that progesterone maintained pregnancy ("progestene block" theory), and labor ensued when the progesterone levels fell. As no marked fall in progesterone levels has been noticed, more recently Csapo[11] suggested that the increased levels of progesterone throughout pregnancy oppose the excitatory effects of prostaglandins which are produced as a result of myometrial stretching caused by the enlarging fetus. Csapo believes that there is a slight decrease of progesterone production at term and that this hormonal imbalance is sufficient to permit the stimulatory effects of prostaglandins and allow the onset of labor. However, this theory lacks firm evidence primarily because of the logistical difficulty of collecting blood specimens during the hours preceding an undetermined onset of spontaneous labor.

The role of estrogens is also not well understood. Estriol and 17β estradiol may be the most important estrogens playing a role in the initiation of labor. A rise in plasma estradiol 17β has been observed to precede premature onset of labor.[12, 13] A study of the adrenal weights in a group of premature infants dying soon after birth suggested that an accelerated growth of the adrenals may be the cause of the rise in estrogens.[14] A shortening of induction time following injection of 17β estradiol has been reported by some; they postulate that estrogens sensitize the myometrium to oxytocin.[15] However, other studies using stilbestrol, estriol and a placebo could not confirm this finding.[16-18]

The evidence regarding the involvement of oxytocin in the initiation of labor is not clear either. Sensitive radioimmunoassays have detected oxytocin in the peripheral blood in only 10 per cent of patients at the onset of labor, and the concentration increased as labor progressed.[20, 21] It was further shown that maternal oxytocin is released in "spurts" and reaches maximum levels during the second stage of labor. It is most likely that oxytocin in the maternal circulation does not play a role in initiating labor, but that it may be important in maintaining established labor and the expulsive forces of the second stage.

The fetal membranes and decidua are uniquely suited to prostaglandin production, since all of these tissues contain glycerophospholipids that are highly enriched with arachidonic acid—the precursor of $PGF_2\alpha$ and PGE_2. The decidua is rich in lysosomes which are maintained in a stable state by the presence of stabilizers, particularly progesterone. As a result of damage to the lysosome membrane from stimuli such as ischemia during contraction or artificial rupture of membranes, lytic enzymes are released: of these, phospholipase A, acts on the phospholipids to form arachidonic acid which in turn is converted to prostaglandins.[22, 23] It is postulated that this release of prostaglandins from the uterus may promote the release of oxytocin[24] from the pituitary. Besides, prostaglandins $F_2\alpha$ and E_2

may act on the myometrial cells, sensitizing them to oxytocin[25] with the result that the effect of oxytocin on the myometrium becomes more pronounced.

THE ROLE OF CORTICOSTEROIDS

In animal experiments, the importance of an intact fetal hypothalanic-pituitary-adrenal axis for spontaneous onset of labor has been clearly demonstrated.[26] It has also been shown that secretion of cortisol by the fetal adrenal is a key factor in the initiation of labor. In man, anencephaly without associated polyhydramnios, and congenital adrenal hypoplasia may lead to a prolongation of gestation.[30] In sheep it has been shown that there is a rise in fetal cortisol at the onset of labor.[31] In human subjects, the applicability of this concept is strengthened by the investigations of Murphy[32] who noted a rise in the umbilical cord levels of cortisol between the 12th week of pregnancy and term. These levels were found to be higher in cases with spontaneous onset of labor than in those with the labor induced—irrespective of the mode of delivery. It has been postulated that the fetal rise in cortisol levels causes elevations of prostaglandins $F_2\propto$ and 17ß estradiol which in turn make the uterus more sensitive to oxytocin.[29]

In animals[27] it has also been shown that infusion of adrenocorticotropin (ACTH) or cortisol into fetal lambs could cause premature parturition. It was found that these lambs sustained respiration at a stage of development when this is normally not possible. Later it was shown[34] that single intramuscular injections of dexamethasone into the sheep fetus could induce premature labor. The resulting premature lambs also showed a degree of lung development unexpected at that stage of gestation. In veterinary practice, exogenous glucocorticoids administered to the mother have been used to induce delivery in the cow, sheep and goat.[33]

USE OF CORTICOSTEROIDS IN HUMANS

The use of corticosteroids to induce labor in the human was first reported in 1973.[34] In that study we showed that an intra-amniotic injection of 20 mg betamethasone in women beyond 41 weeks of gestation induced labor at an injection-delivery interval of 78.9 ± 10.2 (SD) hours as compared to 323 ± 62 (SD) hours in a control group treated with isotonic saline. Similar studies using intra-amniotic corticosteroids were reported by Craft et al.[35] in England and Nwosu et al.[36] In Kenya, Craft et al. showed that the injection:delivery interval was 79 hours as compared to 153 hours in the control group, while Nwosu et al. found the interval to be 86 hours as compared to 228 hours in the control group.

In another study,[37] postmature infants had low neonatal plasma cortisol levels compared to neonates delivered after spontaneous labor at term. This led to the postulation that postmaturity resulted from the inability of the fetus to initiate labor due to its adrenocorticoid insufficiency.

The experiments with intra-amniotic glucocorticoid induction of labor involved only a small number of women, all of whom had prolonged pregnancy. It was probably on this account that some authors have concluded that this method might not have a place in obstetrics.[38, 39] We now report further experience with this method. We also believe that this is the first time the method has been evaluated in pregnancies of less than 40 weeks' duration.

Material and Methods.

Thirty patients attending the antenatal clinics at the Kenyatta National Hospital, Nairobi, were studied. All were of African origin. Patients included in the study were:

1. Those for elective cesarean section.
2. Those with previous cesarean section selected for trial of labor.

The patients were admitted between 37 and 38 weeks of gestation. It is standard practice in our Unit to test L:S ratio before elective cesarean section and induction of labor except in cases of rhesus-negative mothers. Informed consent had been obtained before the procedure was carried out. In all 30 patients vaginal examination was performed to exclude impending labor.

Amniotic fluid (5 ml) was withdrawn by standard aseptic amniocentesis and replaced either with 20 mg of betamethasone in 5 ml isotonic saline or 5 ml sterile isotonic saline alone. The distribution between the control and the betamethasone-treated groups was at random.

The specimen of amniotic fluid was sent for L:S ratio using the method of Gluck et al.[40] If labor started within a week of the amniocentesis (168 hours), the patients for elective cesarean section had an emergency delivery. Those cases selected for trial of labor were managed conservatively. Patients who did not go into labor within a week of the injection, were divided into 2 groups: 1) if the L:S ratio was more than 2.0, patients for elective cesarean section had a planned operation. Spontaneous onset was waited for in the "trial of labor" group. 2) If the L:S ratio was less than 2.0 a repeat amniocentesis was performed and elective delivery delayed until the test turned positive.

Results.

Thirty patients were involved in this study. Table 1 shows their characteristics in both the bethamethasone (BM) and saline groups. Apart from differences in age and the weights of their babies which were not statistically significant, the patients were comparable in all respects.

Table 2 shows that 8 of the 15 patients (53%) in the BM group were successfully induced as compared to none among the 15 who had saline injection. The injection-onset of labor (IL) interval in those successfully induced ranged from 6 to 104 hours with a mean of 45 ± 38.7 (SD) hours. This wide standard deviation resulted from two patients having gone into labor within 6 and 8 hours and another two after 100 and 104 hours. The other four cases delivered after an interval of 14 to 53 hours.

The mode of delivery was cesarean section for all but one of those patients who had spontaneous vaginal delivery following a successful BM induction. The condition of the newborns was good as judged by Apgar scoring, with those successfully induced performing noticeably better than babies in the failed group, whether after BM or saline. All babies were examined by a pediatrician and there was no untoward effect detected.

Table 1. Patient Characteristics.

		BETAMETHASONE	NORMAL SALINE
No. of Patients		15	15
Age	Range	18–39 years	23–38 years
	Mean	25.6 ± 5.9 years	28.6 ± 5.9 years
Parity	Range	0–10	0–8
	Mode	2	2
Gestation		37–40	37–40
	Mean	38.1. ± 0.9	38.1 + 0.66
Birth Weight	Range	2370–3800	2690–3850
	Mean	2961	3266

Table 2. Outcome of Induction of Labor

	BETAMETHASONE		SALINE
No. of cases	Successful	Failed	Failed
	8	7	15
IL interval	Range 6–104 hours	One case	—
	Mean 45 ± 138.7	185 hours	—
Birth weight	Range 2650–3125	2370–3800	2690–3950
	Mean 2845 gms	3094 gms	3266 gms
Apgar score	8–10	6–10	6–10
Mode of delivery	Emergency C/S (7)		
	S.V.D. (1)	Elective C/S	Elective C/S
Sex: Male	3	5	7
Female	5	2	8
%Female	62.5	28.5	53.3

The birth weight of the babies did not seem to influence the success of the induction in that the mean weight in those successfully induced with BM was nearly 250 g less than in the group where BM had failed. One baby weighing 2370 g was born at 40 weeks' gestation with signs of intrauterine growth retardation. Surprisingly there were more female infants in the successful BM group than in the group where the drug failed, even though the distribution of the sexes in both the BM and saline groups was roughly equal (Table 2).

An analysis of the results of the induction shows that successful BM induction very much depends on the stage of pulmonary maturation. Table 3 shows that the 8 cases successfully induced had an L:S ratio ranging from 1.90 - 2.32 with a mean of 2.10 ± 0.13 S.E.M. In fact, only one of them had an L:S ratio of 2.0 or below, and it is remarkable that these are the cases with the longest IL interval of 100 and 104 hours, respectively. Scrutiny of the 7 cases where BM failed shows that the mean L:S ratio was 1.85 ± 0.3 SEM and only two had an L:S ratio of more than 2.0. One of these (L:S = 2.12) actually went into labor, but because labor started 185 hours after the injection (our limit was 168 hours) she was listed in the failed BM group. She was delivered of a female infant by emergency cesarean section. The other one (L:S = 2.56) was regarded as BM failure in the presence of pulmonary maturity. Incidentally, all of the 15 cases injected with saline had an L:S ratio of 2.0 and above. However, none of them went into labor.

Table 4 summarizes the results in those cases where the L:S ratio was 2.0 or above. In the BM group there were 9 such patients of whom 7 (78%) were successfully induced. On the other hand, all of the 15 patients in the saline group had an L:S ratio of 2.0 and above, yet none of them went into labor.

Table 3. L:S Ratio in Relation to Inducibility.

	NO. OF CASES	L:S RATIO	
		RANGE	MEAN ± SEM
Successful BM induction	8	1.9–2.32	2.10 ± 0.13
Failed BM induction	7	1.59–2.56	1.85 ± 0.3
Failed BM induction with L:S ratio 2.0	5	1.59–1.81	166 ± 0.097
Failed BM induction with L:S ratio 2.0	2	2.12–2.56	2.34 ± 0.31
Failed saline inductions	15	2.0–3.03	2.27 ± 0.30

Table 4. L:S Ratio 2.0 In Relation to Inducibility.

	BETAMETHASONE	SALINE
No. of cases with L:S ratio 2.0	9	15
Successful induction	7	0
% Success	77%	0%

FACTORS INFLUENCING SUCCESSFUL INDUCTION

Glucocorticoids are known to be involved in the maturation and biochemical differentiation of the tissues in the fetus, and there is no doubt that they play a role in the synthesis of pulmonary surfactant. Exogenous glucocorticoids have been used clinically in an attempt to prevent respiratory distress syndrome. In 1972[41] Liggins showed that following premature labor, there is a reduced incidence of respiratory distress syndrome in the infants if the mothers had received glucocorticoids at least 24 hours before delivery.

"Two Step Action" Hypothesis.

It would appear that glucocorticoids may have a double action. At first there is acceleration of lung maturation. Once the lungs are mature, a "signal" sets the events in motion which culminate in uterine contractions. The mechanism of this second step is still not clearly defined. It could be mediated through increased placental production of prostaglandins $F_2\alpha$ and estrogens which in turn makes the uterus more sensitive to oxytocin.

Recommended Dose of Betamethasone.

In the course of animal experiments and clinical trials,[34] it was found that a fetal dose of 20 mg was effective in producing early lung maturation. It is possible that a repeat injection after a week will improve the success rate of the method.

ADVANTAGES OF CORTICOSTEROID INDUCTION VERSUS CONVENTIONAL METHODS

1. This technique is comparatively simple and can be carried out easily as an outpatient procedure. The patient may be allowed home and labor usually follows a normal course. This has obvious practical, financial as well as psychological advantages since the woman is not made aware of the fact that labor has been induced.

2. The method is based on physiological principles and reduces the risk of a failed induction. In contrast, oxytocic drugs or other methods of induction may be working against the physiological mechanisms designed to maintain the pregnancy.

3. The method stimulates the maturation of normal lung function, thus reducing the risk of fetal respiratory distress.

4. The method has a particular advantage in multiparous patients and in those with a previous cesarean section in whom the use of oxytocic agents may be dangerous.

DISADVANTAGES OF CORTICOSTEROID INDUCTION

1. Amniocentesis and its dangers:
It is generally accepted that amniocentesis is a relatively safe procedure. There are several series reported where over 1000 procedures were performed without fetal or maternal complication. However, it is an invasive procedure and thus not devoid of risks and possible complications such as:
1. Unsuccessful and bloody tap.
2. Rhesus sensitization following feto-maternal hemorrhage.
3. Infection (maternal and/or fetal).
4. Amniotic fluid embolism.
2. Adverse effects of corticosteroids upon the fetus
In this series all infants were examined by a pediatrician and no untoward effects were detected. It is too early to say that there could be no harmful effect on the infant, but a five-year follow-up revealed no growth or developmental abnormality among those whose birth had been preceded by betamethasone-induced labor.[34]

REFERENCES

1. Craft. Management of Labour—Proceedings of the 3rd Study Group of the Royal College of Ostetricians & Gynaecologists, 1975.
2. Bishop E. H. Pelvic scoring for elective induction. *Obstet Gynecol.* **24:** 266, 1964.
3. Bell W. B. The pituitary body and the therapeutic value of the infundibular extract in shock, uterine atony and intestinal paresis. *Brit. Med. J.* **2:** 1609, 1909.
4. Theobald G. W., Graham A. et al. The use of posterior pituitary extract in physiological amounts in obstetrics. *Brit. Med. J.* **2:** 123, 1948.
5. Karim S. M. M., Trussell R. R. et al. Response of pregnant human uterus to prostaglandin $F_2 \propto$ induction of labour. *Brit. Med. J.* **4:** 621, 1968.
6. _____, _____ et al. Induction of labour with prostaglandin F_2 *J. Obstet. Gynaecol. Brit. Commonw.* **76:** 769, 1969.
7. _____, Hillier K. et al. *Induction of labour with prostaglandin E_2 J. Obstet. Gynaecol. Brit. Commonw.* **77:** 200, 1970.

8. Bengtsson L. P. The role of progesterone in human labour. Endocrine factors in labour. Memoirs of the Society for Endocrinology, No. 20. Cambridge University Press P37, 1973.
9. Klopper A. The Role of oestrogens in the onset of labour. Endocrine factors in labour. Memoirs of the Society for Endocrinology No. 20. Cambridge University, Press P47, 1973.
10. Csapo A. I. The progesterone block. *Amer. J. Anat.* **98:** 273, 1956.
11. _____, Knobile, E. et al. Peripheral plasma progesterone levels during human pregnancy and labour. *Amer. J. Obstet. Gynaecol.* **110:** 630, 1971.
12. Tamby, Raja R. L., Anderson, A. B. M. et al. Endocrine changes in premature labour. *Brit. Med. J.* **2:** 67, 1974.
13. _____, Turnbull A. C. et al. Predictive oestradiol surge of premature labour and its suppression by glucocorticoids Austral. *New Zeal. J. Obstet. Gynaecol.* **15:** 191, 1975.
14. Anderson A. B. M., Lawrence K. M. et al. Foetal adrenal weight and the causes of premature delivery in human pregnancy. *J. Obstet. Gynaecol. Brit. Commonw.* **78:** 481, 1971.
15. Pinto A. M. et al. Action of oestradiol 17B upon uterine contractility and the mild ejecting effect in the pregnant woman *Amer. J. Obstet. Gynaecol.* **90:** 999, 1964.
16. Klopper A. and Dennis, K. J. Effect of oestrogens on myometrial contraction. *Brit. Med. J.* **2:** 1157, 1962.
17. _____, _____ et al. The effect of intra-amniotic oestriol sulphate on uterine contractions. *Brit. Med. J.* **2:** 786, 1969.
18. _____, _____ et al. The effect of intra-amniotic oestriol sulphate on uterine contractility at term. *J. Obstet. Gynaecol. Brit. Commonw.* **80:** 34, 1973.
19. Ferguson J. K. W. A study of the motility of the intact uterus at term. *Surg. Gynecol. Obstet.* **73:** 359, 1941.
20. Chard A. T., Hudson C. N. et al. Release of oxytocin and vasopressin by the human foetus in labour. *Nature* **234:** 352, 1971.
21. _____. The posterior pituitary and the induction of labour. *In* Endocrine Factors in Labour. *Memoirs Soc. Endocrin.* **20:** 61, 1973.
22. Gustavii, B. Release of lysosomal acid phosphatase into the cytoplasm of decidual cells before the onset of labour in humans. *J. Obstet. Gynaecol.* **82:** 177, 1975.
23. _____. Sweeping of the foetal membranes by a physiologic saline solution. Effect on decidual cells. *Amer. J. Obstet. Gynaecol.* **120:** 531, 1974.
24. Gillespie, Brummer, H. C. et al. Oxytocin release by infusion of prostaglandins. *Brit. Med. J.* **1:** 543, 1972.
25. Brummer H. C., Interaction of E Prostaglandins and Syntocinon on the pregnant human myometrium, *J. Obstet. Gynaecol. Brit. Commonw.* **78:** 305, 1971.
26. Liggins, G. C., Kennedy, P. C. et al. Failure of initiation of parturition after electrocoagulation of the pituitary of the foetal lamb. *Amer. J. Obstet. Gynaecol.* **98:** 1080, 1967.
27. _____. Premature parturition after infusion of corticotrophin or costisol into foetal lambs. *J. Endocrin.* **42:** 323, 1968.
28. _____. Premature delivery of foetal lambs infused with glucocorticoid. *J. Endocrin.* **45:** 515, 1969.
29. _____, Grieves, S. A. et al. The physiological role of progesterone oestradiol 17ß and prostaglandins $F_2 \propto$ in the control of ovine parturition. *J. Reprod. Fertil. Supp.* **16:** 85, 1972.
30. Malpas, P. *J. Obstet. Gynaecol. Brit. Emp.* **40:** 1046, 1933.
31. Bassett, J. M. and Thorburn, G. D., Foetal plasma corticosteroids and the initiation of parturition in sheep. *J. Endocrin.* **44:** 285, 1969.

32. Murphy, B. E. P. Does the human foetal adrenal play a role in parturition? *Amer. J. Obstet. Gynaecol.* **115:** 521, 1973.

33. Jochle, W. Corticosteroid induction of parturition in domestic animals. *Folia Vet. Latina* **1:** 229, 1971.

34. Mati, J. K. G., Horrobin A. F. et al. Induction of labour in sheep and humans with single doses of corticosteroids. *Brit. Med. J.* **2:** 149, 1973.

35. Craft, I., Brummer, V. et al. Betamethasone induction of labour. *Proc. Roy. Soc. Med.* **11:** 827, 1976.

36. Nwosu U., Wallach E. E. et al. Possible role of foetal adrenal glands in the aetiology of postmaturity. *Amer. J. Obstet. Gynaecol.* **121:** 366, 1975.

37. _____, _____ et al. Possible adrenocorticol insufficiency in postmature neonates. *Amer. J. Obstet. Gynaecol.* **122:** 969, 1975.

38. Liggins G. C., Forster C. S. et al. Control of parturition in man. *Biol. Reprod.* **16:** 39, 1977.

39. Editorial Note. Betamethasone induction of labour. *Obstet. Gynecol. Surv.,* Sept., 1977.

40. Gluck, L. and Kulovich, M. V. Lecithin/sphingomyelin ratios in amniotic fluid in normal and abnormal pregnancy. *Amer. J. Obstet. Gynaecol.* **115:** 539, 1973.

41. Liggins, G. C. and Howie, R. N. A controlled trial of antepartum glucocorticoid treatment for prevention of the respiratory distress syndrome in premature infants. *Pediatrics* **50:** 515, 1972.

13

Premature Rupture of the Membranes and Premature Labor

R. J. PEPPERELL, M.D.

AND

LANCE TOWNSEND, M.D.

INTRODUCTION

Although improvement in obstetric and neonatal care has resulted in a dramatic fall in perinatal mortality (PNM), particularly in infants weighing between 750 and 1500 g at delivery,[12] prematurity is still associated with more than half of all perinatal deaths.[13] Many deaths are related to the cause of the premature labor (antepartum hemorrhage, intrauterine infection), others are due to hazards faced by the premature infant in labor and at delivery (fetal distress, cord prolapse, difficult delivery in breech presentation), and the remainder are due to complications of the neonatal period (particularly hyaline membrane disease, intraventricular hemorrhage and infection). Attempts to reduce the PNM further have centered around intensive fetal monitoring in labor,[8] abdominal delivery when the infant is presenting by the breech,[8,9] suppression of labor by the administration of beta-sympathomimetic drugs,[5,6] and the administration of glucocorticoid agents to improve fetal lung maturation, thereby reducing the incidence of respiratory distress syndrome.[15]

When premature rupture of the membranes occurs and labor does not follow immediately, there is considerable controversy as to the correct management. The risk of ascending infection and amnionitis,[20] associated with a policy of "watchful expectancy," must be balanced against the risk of prematurity if early induction and delivery is carried out. A conservative policy should prolong the pregnancy for an average of 14 days but is associated with infection in approximately 13 per cent of patients.[21] The role of glucocorticoid therapy is also debatable since, although several workers have reported a lower incidence of RDS if the membranes are ruptured for more than 16 to 24 hours before delivery,[1,19,23] this finding has been refuted by others.[11] The improvement in fetal lung maturity with glucocorticoids given to patients in premature labor with intact membranes[2,15] led Mead and Clapp[18] to administer these agents to patients with premature rupture of the membranes and time delivery for approximately 24 hours after the first dose of steroid. Although such a policy reduced the neonatal mortality considerably, the study and control patients were really not comparable.

In November, 1976, the Consultant Obstetric Staff at the Royal Women's Hospital, Melbourne, regionalized their obstetric care, and all patients in premature labor or with premature rupture of the membranes were transferred to the Professorial Unit. This report presents the results of treatment of the 222 patients referred during the subsequent 18-month period and details the effect of the administration of the beta-sympathomimetic drug salbutamol (Ventolin[R]) and the glucocorticoid betamethasone (Celestone[R]) to the patients in premature labor, and the administration of betamethasone to alternate patients with premature rupture of the membranes who were not in labor.

PATIENT MATERIAL

Patients in Premature Labor

One hundred and twenty-nine patients between 20 and 34 weeks of gestation were admitted in premature labor, with intact membranes, during the study period. Where a definite antepartum hemorrhage (APH) was present (> 100 ml blood loss or evidence of uterine tenderness on palpation), the patient was excluded from the study; however, in many instances only a small amount of blood loss had occurred at the time of admission to hospital, and doubt existed as to whether this was just a heavy "show" associated with cervical dilatation or a small APH. Where the blood loss continued, became heavier during labor, or was associated with evidence of retroplacental clot during placental expulsion, the patient was then classified as having had a small APH but was included in this report.

When painful contractions occurred regularly at least every 10 minutes, the patient was deemed to be in labor. Bacteriological swabs for microscopy and culture were taken from the cervix, a full blood examination was performed, and the degree of cervical dilatation was assessed on vaginal examination. Any cervical stitch present was removed.

Treatment with salbutamol and betamethasone was available for all patients, but was usually only given when the cervical dilatation was ≤ 4 cm. As approximately one-third were private patients, they remained under the care of their own consultant who decided if these drugs were to be administered.

Salbutamol was administered as follows: 5 mg of salbutamol was added to 500 ml of 5% dextrose in water and infused intravenously through a peripheral vein. The initial infusion rate was 10 drops per minute (6.7 ug salbutamol/min) and this rate was increased by 10-drop increments at 5–10-minute intervals until the contractions ceased or an infusion rate of 50 drops per minute (33 ug/min) was reached. If the contractions still had not ceased, the infusion rate was further increased by 10-drop increments at 20-minute intervals until an infusion rate of 80 drops per minute (54 ug/min) was reached. Once contractions ceased, the infusion rate was maintained steadily for one hour, then reduced by half and maintained at that rate for 6 hours, then reduced by half again and continued for a further 6 hours (Fig. 1). Thirteen hours after cessation of contractions the intravenous infusion was stopped and oral salbutamol (4 mg, 4 times daily) administered for one week.

Treatment with salbutamol was stopped if infusion at the maximum rate did not reduce the contractions in strength, duration or frequency; the cervix had dilated further after 6 hours of treatment; or a steady maternal pulse rate exceeding 140/minute was reached.

Where contractions were re-established during or after treatment, the infusion rate was increased or restarted at the previous one-hour maintenance level and subsequently reduced as above. Treatment was not repeated more than three times.

Intramuscular betamethasone was usually administered to the patients receiving salbutamol, but was also given to some other patients where suppression of labor was not attempted. A total of 24 mg was usually given over a 48-hour period (4 mg, 8 hourly) unless delivery occurred prior to completion of the course of therapy. Further courses of betamethasone were not given even when premature labor recurred a week or more after initial suppression was obtained.

Evidence of sepsis in the infants was sought diligently. Most had cultures taken from gastric aspirate, throat, and the external auditory meatus and many had urine, cerebrospinal fluid and blood cultures as well. All infants

Example of Salbutamol Treatment

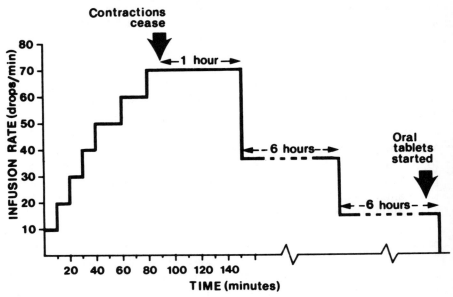

Fig. 1.   Schematic diagram of salbutamol infusion.

with respiratory distress syndrome (RDS) also had an x-ray examination of the chest.

Maternal sepsis was deemed to be present if the temperature exceeded 37.8° C prior to, or during, labor and when the cervical swabs confirmed the presence of infection. Fetal infection was considered to be present if septicemia was diagnosed on blood culture, or if all of the cultures obtained from the gastric aspirate, throat and external auditory meatus were positive. When the infant was stillborn or died within 24 hours of birth, evidence of infection was also sought at autopsy by histological examination of the lungs and culture of swabs taken from the lungs and heart. The radiographic appearance of the lungs was not taken into account when deciding if fetal infection was present, since it is impossible to be certain if the appearance is due to aspiration of infected liquor or non-infected blood or meconium, or even just a variant of hyaline membrane disease (HMD).

The condition of the infant during the neonatal period was fully documented, particular attention being paid to the clinical features, diagnosis and treatment of RDS. While many infants were given additional oxygen for a brief period in the nursery, many did not develop the classic features of RDS. When respiratory distress did develop, however, it was classified into either transient tachypnea of the newborn or mild, moderate or severe RDS. The infant was deemed to have transient tachypnea of the newborn when the RDS resolved within 24 hours, the chest radiograph did not suggest HMD, and oxygen needed to be administered in a concentration of 40 percent or less for a period of 12 hours or less. In the remainder of the patients, the clinical course and radiologic findings suggested HMD and/or pneumonia present. If oxygen administration was necessary for more than 12 hours, but less than 48 hours, the infant was said to have mild RDS. Moderate RDS was present when the oxygen concentration administered was more than 40 percent or when therapy had to be continued for more than 48 hours. Severe RDS was present when assisted ventilation in the form of continuous positive airway pressure (CPAP) or intermittent positive pressure ventilation (IPPV) was necessary to keep the arterial oxygen concentration in excess of 50 mmHg, in the presence of clinical and radiologic evidence of hyaline membrane disease (HMD).

Patients with Premature Rupture of the Membranes

Ninety-three patients between 20 and 34 weeks of gestation presented with premature rupture of the membranes, but not in labor, during the study period. Following confirmation of membrane rupture on speculum examination—at which time bacteriologic swabs were taken for microscopy and culture, and the cervical stitch removed in patients with cervical incompetence—the standard ward care patients were alternately allocated to the "steroid" or "no steroid" groups. Patients in the "steroid" group were given betamethasone 4 mg intramuscularly at 8 hourly intervals until a total of 24 mg had been given, unless delivery occurred prior to completion of the course of therapy. Further courses of betamethasone were not given even when premature labor did not ensue for many weeks after the time of membrane rupture. Salbutamol was only administered to inhibit labor when this began spontaneously during the 48 hours of steroid administration, and was not continued after the course was completed. Approximately 40 percent of the patients were private patients; they remained under the care of their own consultant who decided if steroids were, or were not, to be administered. Except at gestations of 33–34 weeks, when the private consultants preferred not to administer steroids, they generally accepted that alternate patients should be treated, however.

Cervical swabs for microscopy and culture were collected again if the patient became febrile, the vaginal loss became purulent, or labor commenced. Antibiotics were administered routinely in labor, and to all infants after delivery, but were rarely given prior to the onset of labor. The condition of the infant during the neonatal period and the incidence of sepsis were documented the same as for the patients in premature labor.

RESULTS

Premature Labor

The etiology of the premature labor during the 18-month period under review is shown in Table 1. No apparent cause was found in 43.4 percent of the patients; however, 30.2 percent had had a small antepartum hemorrhage and 14.0 percent had cervical incompetence.

With the exception of the 18 patients with cervical incompetence—all of whom had previous history of a pregnancy termination and–or midtrimester abortion or premature labor—only 23 of the remaining 111 patients (20.7%) gave any indication that they might labor prematurely from an analysis of their past obstetric performance.

Seventy-six of the 129 patients were treated with salbutamol and betamethasone in an attempt to inhibit labor and improve lung maturation, respectively. Thirty-one of the patients who were not treated with these agents had significant cervical dilatation (> 4 cm) at the time of admission to hospital and were not considered suitable for treatment. However, the other 22 patients, including 14 with small episodes of antepartum hemorrhage, would have qualified for treatment had the consultant in charge requested this.

1. Effectiveness of Salbutamol and Betamethasone in Inhibiting Labor. Labor was suppressed for at least 48 hours in 64 percent of patients (Table 2), and suppression was more likely if the cervical dilatation at the com-

Table 1. Etiology of Premature Labor at The Royal Women's Hospital, Melbourne.

ETIOLOGY	NUMBER OF PATIENTS	PREVIOUS OBSTETRIC PERFORMANCE		
		TOP ALONE	MID-TRIM. AB OR PREMATURE LABOR	TOP AND MID-TRIM. AB OR PREMATURE LABOR
No apparent cause	56	7	7	—
Antepartum hemorrhage	39	4	4	—
Cervical incompetence	18	4	11	3
Multiple pregnancy*	14	—	1	—
Hydramnios	2	—	—	—
Total	129	15	23	3

* One of these was a triplet pregnancy; the remainder were twin pregnancies. TOP = termination of pregnancy; Mid-trim. AB = mid-trimester abortion (14–26 weeks gestation); prem. labor = premature labor (27–34 weeks gestation).

Table 2. Effectiveness of Salbutamol and Betamethasone in Inhibiting Labor.

ETIOLOGY OF PREMATURE LABOR	CERVICAL DILATATION AT START OF TREATMENT	NUMBER OF PATIENTS		
		TOTAL	LABOR SUPPRESSED FOR ≤ 48 HOURS	LABOR SUPPRESSED FOR > 48 HOURS
No apparent cause	≤ 2 cm	27	3 (11%)	24 (89%)
	3-4 cm	10	3 (30%)	7 (70%)
	> 4 cm	4	4 (100%)	—
Antepartum hemorrhage	≤ 2 cm	9	3 (33%)	6 (67%)
	3-4 cm	6	4 (67%)	2 (33%)
Cervical incompetence	≤ 2 cm	7	4 (57%)	3 (43%)
	3-4 cm	3	3 (100%)	—
	> 4 cm	3	2 (67%)	1 (33%)
Multiple pregnancy (all twins)	≤ 2 cm	4	1 (33%)	3 (75%)
	3-4 cm	1	—	1 (100%)
Hydramnios	≤ 2 cm	1	—	1 (100%)
	3-4 cm	—	—	—
	> 4 cm	1	—	1 (100%)
All causes	≤ 2 cm	48	11 (23%)	37 (77%)
	3-4 cm	20	10 (50%)	10 (50%)
	> 4 cm	8	6 (75%)	2 (25%)
	All dilatations	76	27 (36%)	49 (64%)

mencement of treatment was less than 2 cm ($X^2 = 7.61$, $p < 0.01$). The highest rate of suppression (89%) was achieved in patients with no apparent cause for their premature labor; however, the increased suppression rate in this group of patients over those with small antepartum hemorrhages or with cervical incompetence did not reach statistical significance ($\leq$ 2 cm dilatation, $X^2 = 1.07$ and 3.66, respectively; > 2 cm dilatation, $X^2 = 0.03$ and 0.80, respectively). Eighteen of the patients with no apparent cause for their premature labor, and five of those who had had an antepartum hemorrhage, had their labor suppressed until the gestation of the pregnancy exceeded 37 weeks.

Where the cervical dilatation exceeded 2 cm at the start of treatment, suppression of labor for at least 48 hours was achieved in 12 of the patients (42.8%) and was also more likely when no apparent cause for premature labor was evident. Five of these patients delivered in the succeeding 24 hours, but the remainder were not delivered until 7, 8, 31, 35, 36, 56 and 84 days after admission, respectively.

When salbutamol and betamethasone were not administered, only six of the 53 patients were undelivered 24 hours after admission to hospital; each of these six patients had had a small antepartum hemorrhage and the cervical dilatation on admission was 2 cm or less.

2. Incidence of Respiratory Distress Syndrome. The incidence of RDS in patients delivered at gestations, varying between 26 and 33 weeks inclusive, is shown in Table 3. Only patients with no apparent cause for their premature labor or those with a small antepartum hemorrhage have been included in the assessment. Patients delivered prior to 25 weeks or after 34 weeks of gestation have been excluded, as have patients with lethal congenital abnormalities and those where the infant was stillborn.

The overall incidence of RDS was not significantly different ($X^2 = 0.41$, N.S.) in the patients who were treated with betamethasone and salbutamol than in those who received no treatment at all. Except when the gestation at delivery was 25 or 26 weeks, treatment with betamethasone and salbutamol was associated with a less severe form of RDS, especially when the labor was suppressed for more than 48 hours and the full course of betamethasone could be given.

3. Risk of Infection. Eight of the 129 infants were severely infected at delivery. One stillborn infant and another who died neonatally one hour after birth showed evidence of bacterial pneumonia at autopsy. The other six had positive blood cultures when this procedure was performed within six hours of birth (Table 4). Maternal infection was evident in four of the mothers who had infected babies (patients 1, 3, 4 and 6); however, the maternal infection was readily controlled in all except one patient (no. 3)

Table 3. Incidence of Respiratory Distress Syndrome.

GESTATION AT DELIVERY (WEEKS)	TREATMENT	NUMBER OF PATIENTS				
		TOTAL	NO RDS	MILD RDS	MODERATE RDS	SEVERE RDS
25–26	B & S	6	—	1	1	4
	None	4	—	—	1	3
27–28	B & S	5	2	1	1	1
	None	5	—	1	1	3
29–30	B & S	3	—	2	1	—
	None	5	3	—	—	2
31–32	B & S	12	11	1	—	—
	None	11	7	2	1	1
33–34	B & S	6	4	1	—	1
	None	6	3	—	1	2
25–34	B & S	32	17	6	3	6
	None	31	13	3	4	11

RDS = respiratory distress syndrome; B = betamethasone; S = salbutamol.

Table 4. Details of Patients in Whom Fetal Infection was Present.

PATIENT NUMBER	ETIOLOGY OF PREMATURE LABOR	TREATMENT	TIME INTERVAL FROM ADMISSION TO DELIVERY	INFECTION	BIRTHWEIGHT AND OUTCOME
1	No apparent cause	B and S	7 days	E. Coli septicemia	970 g, survived
2	No apparent cause	—	12 hours	E. Coli septicemia	1400 g, N.N.D.
3	Cervical incompetence	S only	12 hours	E. Coli pneumonia	1040 g, S.B.
4	Cervical incompetence	S only	24 hours	E. Coli septicemia	570 g, N.N.D.
5	Cervical incompetence	B and S Antibiotics	14 hours	Pseudomonas septicemia	1100 g, survived
6	Cervical incompetence	B and S	56 days	E. Coli septicemia	1100 g, survived
7	Cervical incompetence	B and S	36 hours	Intrauterine pneumonia	640 g, N.N.D.
8	Cervical incompetence	B and S	26 hours	Staphylococcal septicemia	1800 g, survived

B = betamethasone; S = salbutamol; S.B. = stillbirth; N.N.D. = neonatal death.

who almost died due to endotoxic shock complicating the gram-negative septicemia.

In patients with cervical incompetence, fetal infection occurred in six of 13 (46.2%) given salbutamol (four of these were also given betamethasone), but not in the five patients in whom these drugs were not used. Where no apparent cause for the premature labor was identified, only two patients showed evidence of fetal infection—one of these patients had received treatment with salbutamol and betamethasone, whereas the other had not.

Because of the high incidence of fetal infection in patients with cervical incompetence, and the effect the infection had on respiratory function in the neonatal period, it was not possible to determine if the betamethasone and salbutamol-treated patients had a lower incidence of RDS than would have been expected had this treatment been withheld.

4. Perinatal Mortality. The overall perinatal mortality was 22 percent; however, the mortality of those given salbutamol and betamethasone was significantly less than those not so treated (X^2 = 4.07, $p <$ 0.05). The reduction in perinatal mortality was achieved principally by a reduction in the number of neonatal deaths (X^2 = 6.08, $p <$ 0.02), since the incidence of stillbirths was not changed (Table 5). Nineteen of the 31 deaths were associated with delivery occurring at or before 26 weeks of gestation. Only seven of the infants who died weighed in excess of 1000 g; two had congenital abnormalities incompatible with life; two died of infective complications already considered; one died of complications resulting from ill-advised breech extraction, and two died of severe RDS.

5. Other Side Effects of Treatment. The only other side effects noted were the irritability and jitteriness which accompanied the administration of salbutamol, especially when large amounts were required to inhibit labor, and maternal tachycardia was present. Most patients were prepared to cope with these side effects when the need for continuing the treatment was explained, and many had a recurrence of symptoms when the intravenous salbutamol was discontinued altogether and oral therapy began.

Premature Rupture of the Membranes

Ninety-three patients presented with premature rupture of the membranes between 20 and 34 weeks of gestation. In most of these patients no predisposing cause for membrane rupture was identified (Table 6); however, this complication followed a small antepartum hemorrhage (less than 100 ml) in 18 patients and was associated with cervical incompetence in 18 others. Apart from the patients with cervical incompetence, all of whom had previously had a termination of pregnancy or spontaneous mid-

Table 5. Perinatal Mortality.

ETIOLOGY OF PREMATURE LABOR	TREATMENT GROUP* NUMBER OF PATIENTS					NO TREATMENT GROUP+ NUMBER OF PATIENTS			TOTAL PNM (%)
	TOTAL	SB	NND	PNM (%)	TOTAL	SB	NND	PNM (%)	
No apparent cause	41	2	1	3 (7%)	15	1	2	3 (20%)	6 (11%)
Antepartum hemorrhage	15	—	—	—	24	1	2	3 (13%)	3 (8%)
Cervical incompetence	13	1	3	4 (31%)	5	1	1	2 (40%)	6 (33%)
Multiple pregnancy	5 (10 infants)	2	2	4 (40%)	9 (19 infants)	—	11	11 (58%)	15 (52%)
Hydramnios	2	—	1	1 (50%)	—	—	—	—	1 (50%)
All causes	76 (81 infants)	5	7	12 (15%)	53 (63 infants)	3	16	19 (30%)	31 (22%)

* Given salbutamol ± betamethasone.
+ Not given salbutamol ± betamethasone.
SB = stillbirth; NND = neonatal death; PNM = perinatal mortality.

Table 6. Predisposing Factors to Membrane Rupture.

FACTOR	NUMBER OF PATIENTS	(%)
None identified	48	(51.6%)
Antepartum hemorrhage	18	(19.4%)
Cervical incompetence	18*	(19.4%)
Multiple pregnancy	8*	(8.6%)
Hydramnios	2	(2.2%)
Total	93*	(100.0%)

* One patient with cervical incompetence also had a twin pregnancy.

trimester abortion, only 12 of the remaining 75 patients had had these complications in previous pregnancies.

Thirteen of the 93 patients were given intravenous salbutamol in an attempt to inhibit labor during the period of steroid administration. In nine of these patients such treatment allowed the full course of betamethasone to be given. Having had their labor suppressed with intravenous salbutamol, 5 of the 9 subjects remained out of labor for periods varying between 6 and 18 days following discontinuance of this agent.

1. Interval between Membrane Rupture and Delivery. Two patients were electively delivered soon after the membranes ruptured. One had severe pre-eclampsia at 32 weeks of gestation and was delivered by elective cesarean section before labor commenced. The other was shown to have an anencephalic infant and labor was initiated with a syntocinon infusion. The remaining 91 patients were allowed to labor spontaneously, and the time interval between membrane rupture and delivery is shown in Table 7.

Only 2 of the 8 patients with a multiple pregnancy were not delivered within 48 hours of membrane rupture, and the 2 patients with hydramnios not associated with multiple pregnancy were delivered at 16 and 60 hours, respectively. The time interval was virtually identical in patients with no apparent predisposing cause for their membrane rupture or when this complication followed a small antepartum hemorrhage, but was shorter in patients with cervical incompetence; this reduction did not reach statistical significance, however. In the former group of patients, 22 percent were delivered within 48 hours, 40 percent within 96 hours, and 72 percent were delivered within a week of membrane rupture. Labor tended to occur earlier, the more advanced the gestation; if this trend continues, it will reach significance when the number of patients in each of the gestation categories is trebled.

Twenty-two patients (24 percent) were not delivered within one week of

Table 7. Interval Between Time of Membrane Rupture and Delivery.

GESTATION AT MEMBRANE RUPTURE (WEEKS)	NUMBER OF PATIENTS	NUMBER DELIVERED		
		< 48 HOURS	< 96 HOURS	≤ 7 DAYS
No predisposing cause				
20–24	—	—	—	—
25–27	10	—	1	8
28–30	16	4	6	10
31–33	20	9	12	16
Antepartum hemorrhage				
20–24	2	—	—	1
25–27	4	1	2	2
28–30	7	2	4	6
31–33	5	1	2	3
Cervical incompetence				
20–24	2*	1*	2*	2*
25–27	8	3	4	7
28–30	4	—	1	2
31–33	4	1	2	4
Multiple pregnancy				
20–24	1*	1*	1*	1*
25–27	1	1	1	1
28–30	3	1	2	2
31–33	3	3	3	3
Hydramnios				
28–30	1	—	1	1
31–33	1	1	1	1
All causes				
20–24	4*	1*	2*	3*
25–27	23	5	8	18
28–30	31	7	14	21
31–33	33	15	20	27
All gestations	91	28	44	69

* One patient had a twin pregnancy and cervical incompetence.

membrane rupture; 14 of these delivered at 8 to 14 days, 3 more were delivered at 17 to 21 days, and the remaining 5 delivered at 27 (2), 28, 35 and 46 days, respectively, after the membranes ruptured.

Treatment with betamethasone had no effect on the time interval between membrane rupture and delivery, except in patients with cervical incompetence where infection and premature delivery proved to be a major problem (see later).

2. Incidence of Respiratory Distress Syndrome. The incidence of RDS at the varying gestations at delivery is shown in Table 8. Patients delivering before 25 weeks, when all infants died, or after 34 weeks, when none developed RDS, have been excluded from this analysis. Also excluded were patients with cervical incompetence, where the high incidence of infection made determination of the severity of any RDS due to HMD almost impossible, and patients with multiple pregnancies, because the second twin is often known to be in a poorer condition at birth and this predisposes to the subsequent development of RDS.[23]

The time interval between membrane rupture and delivery had no effect on the incidence or severity of RDS, except where prolonged membrane rupture allowed the patient to deliver at a more advanced gestation, nor did the administration of betamethasone. As can be seen in Table 9 which compares the incidence of RDS in this series with that seen in infants who had been delivered prematurely—but where the membranes were still intact at the onset of labor except at gestations of 25 to 26 weeks and 31 to 32 weeks—the incidence of RDS following premature rupture of the membranes was less than that following premature labor where the membranes were still intact. This reduction applied whether the latter patients were, or were not, treated with betamethasone, but did not reach statistical significance in any of the gestation categories (possibly due to the small number of patients involved).

(c) Risk of Infection. Maternal infection occurred in 18 patients (19 percent); however, only one patient was severely ill with a septicemia due to a gram-negative organism. The usual organisms identified were the anerobic streptococci, anerobic gram-negative bacilli, or E. coli, although one patient had a klebsiella infection.

Fetal infection was found on 16 occasions (17 percent), and 5 of these infants died. The usual organisms identified were E. coli or the anerobic streptococci and gram-negative bacilli; however, 4 infants had klebsiella, serratia, pseudomonas and bacteroides septicemias, respectively.

Fetal infection was more common in patients with cervical incompetence (Table 10) and occurred in 67 percent of such patients when steroid therapy was given. When this therapy was withheld, however, the incidence of fetal infection (11 percent) was virtually identical to that of the other patients in the series, whether they were given steroids or not (14 and 11 percent, respectively). Fetal infection was uncommon where delivery occurred within 48 hours of membrane rupture—except in patients with cervical incompetence—and was also unusual when delivery was delayed for more than 8 days.

Table 8. Relationship of Gestation at Delivery and Betamethasone Therapy to the Incidence of Respiratory Distress Syndrome.

GESTATION AT DELIVERY (WEEKS)	TREATMENT	TOTAL	NUMBER OF PATIENTS			
			NO RDS OR TTN	MILD RDS	MODERATE RDS	SEVERE RDS
25–26	No steroids	1	—	—	—	1 (5*)
	Steroids	2	—	—	—	2 (4*, 6)
27–28	No steroids	8	2 (4, 7)	4 (0.7, 1, 3, 4)	2 (6, 17)	—
	Steroids	6	1 (2)	1 (2)	3 (4, 4, 11)	1 (0.6*)
29–30	No steroids	8	5 (0.3,1,2,4,21)	2 (0.3, 5)	1 (8)	—
	Steroids	4	2 (3, 5)	—	1 (18)	1 (4)
31–32	No steroids	9	3 (1.5,2,11)	2 (4, 7)	1 (28)	3 (0.3,0.8,11)
	Steroids	8	5 (0.4,0.6,2,3,4)	3 (1.2, 7, 22)	—	—
33–34	No steroids	10	5 (0.3,0.8,1,14,14)	4 (0.2,8,12,14)	—	1 (6)
	Steroids	1	1 (14)	—	—	—

* Neonatal death.
TTN = transient tachypnea of the newborn; RDS = respiratory distress syndrome.
Figures in brackets are the number of days between membrane rupture and delivery.

Table 9. Effect of Premature Membrane Rupture on Incidence of Respiratory Distress Syndrome.

GESTATION AT DELIVERY (WEEKS)	PATIENT CATEGORY	RESPIRATORY DISTRESS SYNDROME NUMBER OF PATIENTS (%)	
		NONE, TTN + MILD	MODERATE + SEVERE
25–26	PRM	—	3 (100%)
	Premature labor (+ S)	1 (17%)	5 (83%)
	Premature labor (− S)	—	4 (100%)
27–28	PRM	6 (75%)	2 (25%)
	Premature labor (+ S)	3 (60%)	2 (40%)
	Premature labor (− S)	1 (20%)	4 (80%)
29–30	PRM	7 (87%)	1 (13%)
	Premature labor (+ S)	2 (67%)	1 (33%)
	Premature labor (− S)	3 (60%)	2 (40%)
31–32	PRM	5 (56%)	4 (44%)
	Premature labor (+ S)	12 (100%)	—
	Premature labor (− S)	9 (82%)	2 (18%)
33–34	PRM	9 (90%)	1 (10%)
	Premature labor (+ S)	5 (83%)	1 (17%)
	Premature labor (− S)	3 (50%)	3 (50%)

TTN = transient tachypnea of the newborn; PRM = premature rupture of membranes; (+ S) = betamethasone given;
(− S) = betamethasone not given.
Note: All patients were treated in the same Unit during the same 18-month period.

Table 10. Relationship between Maternal and Fetal Infection, Duration of Ruptured Membranes and Steroid Therapy.

| | PATIENTS WITH CERVICAL INCOMPETENCE | | | | | | ALL OTHER PATIENTS | | | | | |
| DURATION OF RUPTURED MEMBRANES (HOURS) | STEROIDS GIVEN | | | STEROIDS WITHHELD | | | STEROIDS GIVEN | | | STEROIDS WITHHELD | | |
	TOTAL	MAT. INF.	FETAL INF.	TOTAL	MAT. INF.	FETAL INF.	TOTAL	MAT INF.	FETAL INF.	TOTAL	MAT. INF.	FETAL INF.
< 24	—	—	—	3	—	—	5	—	—	15	—	1
24–48	2	1	2	2	2	—	4	2	—	4	1	—
49–96	2	—	—	3	—	1	10	3	2	6	1	2
97–192	3	—	3	1	—	—	4	1	1	9	4	2
> 192	2	1	1	—	—	—	6	1	1	12	1	—
Total	9	2	6*	9	2	1*	29	7	4	46	7	5

* X^2 = 3.74, 0.05 < p < 0.10.
Mat. Inf. = maternal infection; Fetal Inf. = fetal infection.

4. Perinatal Mortality. The overall perinatal mortality was 23.7 percent. Six of the 22 deaths (27 percent) were due to lethal congenital abnormalities, 4 (18 percent) were due to intrauterine infection, and 8 (36 percent) resulted from severe hyaline membrane disease (Table 11). On all four occasions when the membranes ruptured before 25 weeks of gestation, the infant was lost. When membrane rupture occurred after 30 weeks of gestation, however, all infants, except those with lethal congenital abnormalities, survived.

DISCUSSION

Even though the increased risk of premature labor can be predicted in patients who have had previous premature labor, mid-trimester abortions or first trimester pregnancy terminations,[7] and is still likely even after cervical ligation has been performed,[14] the majority of patients who labor prematurely do not give the obstetrician warning that this complication is likely to occur. Prevention of premature labor by the prophylactic administration of appropriate drugs would thus only be possible if all antenatal patients were treated, and there is some doubt if such treatment would be effective.[17]

The beta-sympathomimetic agent salbutamol is certainly effective in inhibiting premature labor whether given intravenously[16] or orally,[10] but inhibition of labor is more likely if the cervix is not dilated more than 2 cm. Although some of these patients probably would have stopped laboring even if salbutamol not been given, the therapy has minimal side effects, so delay in initiating therapy to see if labor ceases spontaneously cannot be justified. Even when cervical dilatation exceeds 2 cm at the start of treatment, suppression of labor for at least 48 hours can be expected in more than 40 percent of patients, especially where no apparent cause for the premature labor is evident. This delay, which permits administration of the full course of betamethasone, has no effect on the stillbirth rate, but may well reduce the severity of the RDS and result in neonatal survival when death might otherwise have occurred. It also permits transfer of the mother in premature labor to a hospital where intrapartum and neonatal intensive care facilities are available. Transfer of the mother prior to delivery is much preferred to transfer of the premature neonate ever since the advent of the neonatal emergency transport service (NETS), because expert resuscitation and supportive care are of utmost importance in keeping morbidity and mortality to a minimum.

The only serious side effect associated with treatment with salbutamol and betamethasone in patients in premature labor was evidence of increased maternal and fetal infection in patients with cervical incompetence.

Table 11. Perinatal Mortality Associated with Premature Rupture of the Membranes.

| ETIOLOGY OF PRM | NUMBER OF PATIENTS | PERINATAL DEATHS | | | | | | PNM |
| | | STILLBIRTHS | | | NEONATAL DEATHS | | | |
		IU HYPOXIA	IU INF.	CONG. ABN.	RDS	IU INF.	CONG. ABN.	TOTAL (%)
None identified	48	—	—	1	1	1	2	5 (10.4%)
Antepartum hemorrhage	18	1	—	—	2	—	2	5 (26.3%)
Cervical incompetence	18*	1	1	—	3	2	—	7 (39.0%)
Multiple pregnancy	8* (16 infants)	2	—	—	2	—	—	4 (25.0%)
Hydramnios	2	—	—	—	—	—	1	1 (50.0%)
Total	93 (101 infants)	4	1	1	8	3	5	22 (21.8%)

* Both infants of the mother with cervical incompetence and twin pregnancy survived.
PRM = premature rupture of membranes; IU Hypoxia = intrauterine hypoxia; IU Inf. = intrauterine infection; Cong. Abn. = congenital abnormalities; RDS = respiratory distress syndrome; PNM = perinatal mortality.

These patients are known to have an increased risk of infection even when these drugs are not administered, and it is now believed that the premature labor probably occurs because of the intrauterine infection[14] and suppression of labor and steroid therapy is contraindicated. Apart from patients with cervical incompetence, it would seem unlikely that unrecognized amnionitis is a common cause of premature labor,[3] since the incidence of infection was extremely low whether the patients had their labor suppressed, and steroids administered, or not.

Premature rupture of the membranes also occurs commonly in patients with cervical incompetence[14] and antepartum hemorrhage,[21] but in more than 50 percent of patients no predisposing cause for the premature rupture can be found. Although this complication is associated with a lesser incidence of RDS than when premature labor occurs with intact membranes, attempts to decrease the PNM associated with this complication must be directed toward a further reduction in the incidence and severity of RDS and the prevention of intrauterine infection.

Numerous factors influence the development of RDS in the prematurely delivered infant, but the most important of these are the gestation at delivery, fetal asphyxia and delivery by cesarean section.[6,22] This prospective study has shown that although almost one-fourth of the patients are still undelivered seven days after the membranes have ruptured, one-third are delivered within 48 hours of this event. Only 13 patients in the current series were treated with intravenous salbutamol when contractions occurred during the 48 hours of steroid administration and, despite discontinuance of this agent when the course of steroids was completed, 5 of the patients were still undelivered at least six days later.

These results suggest that if the premature labor occurring in the first 48 hours after the membrane rupture can be inhibited by salbutamol, the phase of uterine irritability accompanying the decrease in uterine volume (and/or antepartum hemorrhage) can often be suppressed for much longer than the period of administration of this drug. If the prophylactic administration of beta-sympathomimetic agents to all patients with premature rupture of the membranes was able to produce similar results, the prolongation of gestation would probably be of advantage to the infant. Although the duration of ruptured membranes does not appear to influence the severity of RDS at the various gestations of delivery considered, it does allow the infant to be delivered at a longer gestation when there is less incidence of RDS.

In contrast to patients in premature labor with intact membranes,[15] treatment with betamethasone did not reduce the incidence of RDS in the infants where membrane rupture occurred prior to the onset of labor. There would thus appear to be little justification for the administration of this drug to patients with ruptured membranes, since the increased risk of infection associated with its use, especially in patients with cervical incompetence, may be hazardous to both mother and baby.

This study has confirmed that after premature membrane rupture, the risk of maternal and fetal infection is low, except in patients with cervical incompetence. There would appear to be no real basis for the stimulation of labor in patients with premature rupture of the membranes, especially before 32 weeks of gestation, since the risk of infection was unrelated to the duration of membrane rupture. A reduction in the incidence of fetal infection can only be achieved by a "hands off" policy because prophylactic antibiotic therapy has been shown to be of no value, and cultures from the lower genital tract, although often isolating potentially pathogenic organisms, are of little predictive value as to the likelihood of maternal or fetal infection, or the organism involved if such infection occurs.[4,21]

SUMMARY

In a consecutive series of 93 patients with premature rupture of the membranes at 20–34 weeks of gestation, the perinatal mortality was 23.7 percent. One-fourth of the deaths were due to lethal congenital abnormalities, 18 percent were due to intrauterine infection, and 36 percent resulted from severe respiratory distress syndrome (RDS). Corticosteroid therapy increased the risk of infection, especially in patients with cervical incompetence, and did not reduce the incidence or severity of RDS. Almost one-third of the patients were delivered within 48 hours of membrane rupture; however, short-term treatment with salbutamol was able to delay the delivery for at least six days in 5 of the 13 patients to whom it was given. Since postponement of delivery for days or weeks after the membranes have ruptured reduces the incidence and severity of RDS, this therapy may well have a place in the treatment of this condition.

ACKNOWLEDGMENTS

We wish to thank the medical staff members of the Royal Women's Hospital for referring the patients to the Professorial Unit for investigation and management. We also wish to thank the Department of Paediatrics, without whose expertise the superb results obtained in this study would not have been possible. Allen and Hanburys kindly supplied the salbutamol used.

REFERENCES

1. Berkowitz, R. L., Bonta, B. W. et al. The relationship between premature rupture of the membranes and the respiratory distress syndrome. *Amer. J. Obstet. Gynec.* **124:** 712, 1976.

2. Block, M. F., Kling, O. R. et al. Antenatal glucocorticoid therapy for the prevention of respiratory distress syndrome in the premature infant. *Obstet. Gynecol.* **50:** 186, 1977.
3. Bobitt, J. R. and Ledger, W. J. Unrecognized amnionitis and prematurity: a preliminary report. *J. Reprod. Med.* **19:** 8, 1977.
4. Christensen, K. V., Christensen, P. et al. A study of complications in preterm deliveries after prolonged premature rupture of the membranes. *Obstet. Gynecol.* **48:** 670, 1976.
5. Dawson, A. M. and Davies, H. J. The effect of intravenous and oral salbutamol on fetus and mother in premature labour. *Brit. J. Obstet. Gynaec.* **84:** 348, 1977.
6. Desa, D. J. An analysis of certain factors in the aetiology of respiratory distress syndrome of the newborn. *J. Obstet. Gynaec. Brit. Commonw.* **76:** 148, 1969.
7. Fedrick, J. and Anderson, A. B. M. Factors associated with spontaneous pre-term birth. *Brit. J. Obstet. Gynaec.* **83:** 342, 1976.
8. Flowers, C. E. The obstetric management of infants weighing 1000 to 2000 grams. *J. Reprod. Med.* **20:** 51, 1978.
9. Goldenberg, R. L. and Nelson, K. G. The premature breech. *Amer. J. Obstet. Gynec.* **127:** 240, 1977.
10. Hastwell, G. B., Halloway, C. P. et al. A study of 208 patients in premature labour treated with orally administered salbutamol. *Med. J. Aust.* **1:** 465, 1978.
11. Jones, M. D., Burd, L. I. et al. Failure of association of premature rupture of membranes with respiratory distress syndrome. *New Engl. J. Med.* **292:** 1253, 1975.
12. Kitchen, W. H. The small baby: a short-term and long-term prognosis. *Med. J. Aust.* **1:** 82, 1978.
13. Korda, A. R. The prevention of prematurity. *Med. J. Aust.* **2:** 671, 1977.
14. Kuhn, R. J. P. and Pepperell, R. J. Cervical ligation: A review of 242 pregnancies. Aust. N.Z. *J. Obstet. Gynaec.* **17:** 79, 1977.
15. Liggins, G. C. and Howie, R. H. A controlled trial of antepartum glucocorticoid treatment for prevention of respiratory distress syndrome in premature infants. *Pediatrics* **50:** 515, 1972.
16. Liggins, G. C. and Vaughan, G. S. Intravenous infusion of salbutamol in the management of premature labour. *J. Obstet. Gynaec. Brit. Commonw.* **80:** 29, 1973.
17. Marivate, M., De Villiers, K. Q. et al. Effect of prophylactic outpatient administration of fenoterol on the time of onset of spontaneous labor and fetal growth rate in twin pregnancy. *Amer. J. Obstet. Gynec.* **128:** 707, 1977.
18. Mead, P. B. and Clapp, J. F. The use of betamethasone and timed delivery in the management of premature rupture of the membranes in the preterm pregnancy. *J. Reprod. Med.* **19:** 3, 1977.
19. Sell, E. J. and Harris, T. R. Association of premature rupture of membranes with idiopathic respiratory distress syndrome. *Obstet. Gynecol.* **49:** 167, 1977.
20. Taylor, E. S., Morgan, R. L. et al. Spontaneous premature rupture of the fetal membranes. *Amer. J. Obstet. Gynec.* **82:** 1341, 1961.
21. Townsend, L., Aickin, D. R. et al. Spontaneous premature rupture of the membranes. *Aust. N.Z. J. Obstet. Gynaec.* **6:** 226, 1966.
22. Usher, R. H., Allen, A. C. et al. Risk of respiratory distress syndrome related to gestational age, route of delivery and maternal diabetes. *Amer. J. Obstet. Gynec.* **111:** 826, 1971.
23. Worthington, D., Maloney, A. H. A. et al. Fetal lung maturity. Mode of onset of premature labor—influence of premature rupture of the membranes. *Obstet. Gynecol.* **49:** 275, 1977.

14

Factors Influencing Post-Cesarean Infection.

GYÖRGY ILLEI, M.D.

There has been considerable controversy in the literature regarding the origin of post-cesarean wound infections. It seems to be the consensus in the literature that the most frequent source of infection is from the vaginal flora, thus the prevention of postoperative infection is largely beyond control. Others feel that the vaginal flora is not a likely contaminant per se[1] and that pathogenic microorganisms are not very prone to ascend and invade the amniotic cavity, the endometrium or the wound of the operative incision unless one or both of the following circumstances facilitates their attack:

1) Replacement of the regular vaginal saprophytes by virulent microorganisms from the hospital environment;
2) Active transfer of vaginal pathogens into the uterine cervix or cavity by the hand of the physician(s) in the course of examination before or during labor.[2]

With the rate and severity of post-cesarean wound infections on the increase the world over, [3-5] it is a matter of interest whether available measures of infection control could, or could not prevent the occurrence of cesarean, as well as other postoperative wound infections, in contemporary surgical practice. The apparent inability of prophylactic antibiotics to control the development of severe wound infection[6] dramatizes the importance of the problem and the necessity for subjecting this question to appropriate clinical investigation.

METHOD OF INVESTIGATION

To determine the role of the patient's own habitual bacterial flora, the effect of unlimited vaginal examinations and the influence of surgical technique in the pathogenesis of post-cesarean infections, a study was undertaken in the Maternity Department of the Markusovsky Teaching Hospital in Szombathely, Hungary.

The observations were made in two periods: between September 1973 to January 1975 and May 1975 to January 1976, respectively. The first 16 months were characterized by unlimited vaginal examinations during labor (carried out under sterile conditions). During the 8 months of the second period rectal examination was the routine method, permitting not more than two vaginal investigations during the whole process of labor in those cases, where information obtainable only through vaginal examination was essential for the further management of labor. A change in surgical technique was also introduced in the second period. The uterine incision was sutured in one layer with interrupted O catgut sutures, instead of the previous practice of suturing the uterine wall—first with continuous catgut suture followed by a second layer consisting of interrupted single catgut stitches.

There was no change among the staff members, nor were any alterations made in the existing rules concerning asepsis in the labor ward, operating room or post-partum wards.

During the whole investigation period, after decision for a cesarean section was reached, cultures were taken from the uterine cervix under strictly sterile conditions immediately before the operation started. Only cases where maternal bleeding prevented the taking of a sample suitable for bacteriological culturing were omitted from the study.

Postoperative infection was defined by fever observed during the first postoperative week. It was regarded as moderate if the rise in temperature over 38°C lasted for 48 hours or less and was considered severe if it exceeded this time limit. The cause of pyrexia was determined as accurately as possible by all clinical and laboratory means at our disposal, including cultures taken from the lochia in every case with postoperative fever. X^2-test with Yates' correction was used for the statistical analysis. During the two investigation periods, the frequency of cesarean sections has not been changed, nor was there any major variation in the indications.

There were few induced labors, and no intrauterine monitoring was applied. Figure 1 indicates that a significant decrease occurred in the overall rate of post-cesarean infections during the second period. It is also evident, however, that this was due to the dramatic drop in the frequency of postoperative infections after repeated cesarean sections. In this group, a complete eradication of severe infections was noted. The rate of contaminated preoperative cervical culture was very high in the first period,

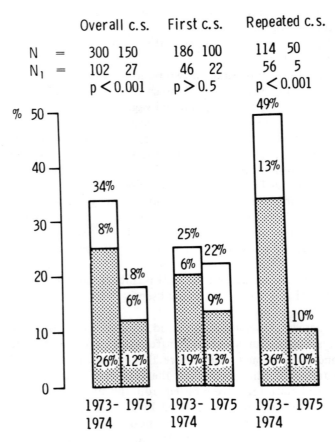

Fig. 1. The incidence and degree of severity of postcesarean infections in the two periods studied.

N = Number of operations.

N_1 = Number of operations followed by infection.

% = Relative frequency of infection related to N.

☐ severe infection   ▨ moderate infection

with a decline in the second, and the difference being highly significant statistically (Table 1). The most common bacteria were *E. coli* and *Staphylococcus albus. Monilia albicans, Klebsiella, Proteus, Streptococcus* and *Enterococcus* were among the other bacteria identified in the cultures.

Concerning the results of the preoperative cultures in patients who developed postoperative infection subsequently (Table 2), a striking difference became evident when the results of the two periods where compared. Whereas during the first period a contaminated preoperative cervical culture was identified in almost every patient, this phenomenon was significantly less frequent in the second period.

Comparing the results of the cultures taken from the lochia in patients with post-partum infections, the ratio of contaminated versus sterile

Table 1. The Results of Preoperative Cervical Bacterial Cultures in the Two Periods Studied.

PREOPERATIVE CERVICAL CULTURE	1973–1974		1975	
	N	%	N	%
Sterile†	33	11	76	50.6
Contaminated††	267	89	74	49.4
Total	300	100	150	100

†
†† P< 0.001

Table 2. Correlation Between the Results of the Preoperative Cervical Cultures and Postoperative Infections.

POST-PARTUM CULTURE (LOCHIA)	POSTPARTAL INFECTION			
	1973–1974		1975	
	N	%	N	%
Sterile	3	2.9	5	18.5
Contaminated†	99	97.1	22	81.5
Total	102	100.0	27	100.0

† P> 0.5

cultures was extremely high in the first, with a mild, statistically not significant decrease in the second period (Table 3). *E. coli* was detected in more than 90 percent of the contaminated cultures, and associated with *Staphylococci, Proteus* and *Klebsiella* (10–20%). The rate of these associations was much higher in cases of severe infections (20–40%).

The site of the infection was also analyzed (Fig. 2). No change was observed in the frequency of the urinary tract and respiratory infections between the two periods, while a comforting drop in the rate of the postoperative abdominal wound infections was apparent in the second period.

Genital (endometrial) infection was the most common postoperative complication in both periods. Detailed analysis of its occurrence (Table 4) shows that there was no significant difference in the frequency of genital infection in the two periods following the first cesarean section, in contrast to a significant decrease in its rate after repeated operations in the second period. Attention should be paid to the fact that during the second period the overall genital infection rate was only one-half of that observed in the first interval, with severe infections having been completely eradicated after repeated cesarean sections.

These results indicate that restrictions of vaginal examinations to not more than two occasions during labor, combined with the introduction of a different surgical technique, i.e. the suturing of the uterine wound in one layer instead of two, produced

1. a significant decrease in the frequency of postoperative infections

Table 3. Correlation Between Postoperative Infections and the Result of the Post-partum Cultures Taken From the Lochia in the Two Periods.

PREOPERATIVE CERVICAL CULTURE	POSTPARTAL INFECTION			
	1973–1974		1975	
	N	%	N	%
Sterile†	6	5.9	11	40.8
Contaminated††	96	94.1	16	59.2
Total	102	100	27	100

† †† P< 0.001

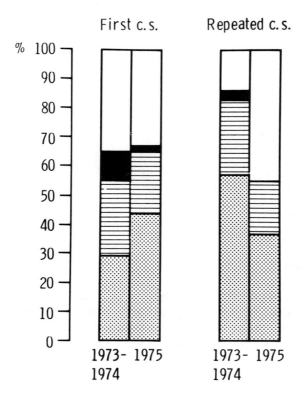

Fig. 2. The relative frequency of the most common sites of post-cesarean infection in the two-study period, related to the number of infected patients in each group (see Fig. 1).

▓ Genital tract   ▤ Urinary tract   ■ Abdominal wound

▭ Other sites

after repeated cesarean sections, due mainly to decrease in the number of infections;

2. a significant increase in the ratio of serile preoperative cervical cultures. There was, however, no significant change in the rate of contaminated postoperative cultures taken from the lochia of patients suffering from postoperative infection.

These observations may indicate that the patient's own vaginal bacterial flora could play a role in the pathogenesis of post-cesarean infections. In this study, the improvement was most conspicuous in cases of repeated cesarean section.

Table 4. The Incidence of Genital Infection After Cesarean Sections. % = Related to the Total Number of Operations of Each Group (See Fig. 1).

GENITAL INFECTIONS	1973–1974		1975	
	N	%	N	%
Total	45	15	12	8
Following first c.s.	13	7	10	10
repeated c.s.	32	28	2†	4

† P< 0.02

CONCLUSION

While it seems apparent that emphasis upon reduction in the number of vaginal examinations, along with reduction in the operating time and the amount of catgut utilized for the operation, improved postoperative infection rates, the significant difference between primary and repeated cesarean sections is not readily apparent. It is possible that because patients who were delivered eventually by primary cesarean section received two vaginal examinations almost invariably, the opportunity for contamination had not been eliminated. The avoidance of any vaginal examination prior to elective repeat cesarean sections might have been the crucial factor in the improvement obtained. While it would be of interest to identify the components in the reduction of the infection rate more unequivocally than the analysis of the presented data permit, the logical conclusion is that elimination of all potential sources of infection, including those which have not been proven conclusively as significant causative factors, offers the best results in terms of prevention of post-cesarean infection.

REFERENCES

1. Lancefield, R. C. A serological differentiation of human and other groups of hemolytic streptococci. *J. Exper. Med.* **57:** 751, 1933.
2. Reid, D. E. Lethal Intrauterine Infection. *In* D. Charles and M. Finland (Eds.): Obstetric and Perinatal Infections. Philadelphia, Lea & Febiger, 1973, p. 47.
3. Hockuli, E. Infektionen in der Geburtshilfe and Gynäkologie. *Gynäk Rundsch.* **16** (Suppl. 1): 52, 1976.

4. Ganti, J. and Sidiropoulus, D. Infektionsmorbidität nach Section caesarea an der Universitäts-Frauenklinik Bern. *Gynäk. Rundsch.* **16** (Suppl.): 96, 1976.
5. Zoltán, I., Horváth, II, S. and Illei, G. Lázas szövödmények császármetszés után. *Orv. Hetil.* **116:** 2532, 1975.
6. Ledger, W. J. Bacterial infections complicating pregnancy. *Clin. Obstet. Gynecol.* **21:** 455, 1978.

15

Myths and Facts about the Etiology of Ectopic Pregnancy

LESLIE IFFY M.D.

There is a broad spectrum of opinion regarding the etiology of ectopic gestation:

"Conditions that prevent or retard the passage of the fertilized ovum into the uterine cavity (or) . . . increase the receptivity of the tubal mucosa. . ."[1]

". . . a variety of disorders that partially obstruct the uterine tube or alter its physiology so that ovum transport is adversely affected."[2]

". . . all factors which may impede or delay the normal transport of the fertilized ovum into the uterine cavity."[3]

An extensive review of the literature identified dozens of factors that have, at one time or another, been suggested as conducive to ectopic implantation (Table 1). Few of these are supported by any direct or indirect evidence and the potential role of some of them has been disproven conclusively by experimental data. However, since the latter have been published in basic research rather than clinical journals, they have almost invariably been overlooked by writers of textbooks. Thus, against the background of an explosive growth of information regarding almost all other aspects of reproductive biology and clinical perinatology, stereotyped views pertaining to ectopic implantation can be traced back through

Table 1.   Classical Concepts of the Causes, or Predisposing Factors, of Extrauterine Implantation of the Fertilized Human Ovum.*

1. ABNORMALITIES OF THE FALLOPIAN TUBE

Congenital hypoplasia
Localized narrowing
Persistent convolution
Diverticula
Accessory lumina or ostia
Excessive length of the tubes
Compression by extrinsic tumor
Neoplasm of the fallopian tube
Constriction due to surgical trauma
Pelvic adhesions after surgery
Kinking of the salpinx
Acute infections (e.g., gonorrhea)
Chronic infections (e.g., tuberculosis)
Sterile endosalpingitis
Incomplete recanalization following antibiotic treatment of acute (gonorrheal) salpingitis
Endometriosis of the salpinx
Abnormal tubal peristalsis
Functional tubal spasm
Decreased tubal motility due to endocrine imbalance
Neuromuscular dysfunction
Tubal hypofunction due to emotional factors
Diminished ciliary action
Reversal of the direction of ciliary propulsion
Increased (genetically determined) receptivity of the tubal mucosa

2. ABNORMALITIES OF THE OVUM

External transmigration
Internal transmigration
Premature trophoblastic activity
Excessive size of the ovum

3. PATERNAL FACTORS

Morphologically abnormal spermatozoa

4. CAUSATIVE FACTORS FOR RARE TYPES OF ECTOPIC IMPLANTATION

Intrafollicular fertilization
Intrafollicular development by parthenogenesis
Superficial ovarian nidation due to endometriotic islands
Failure of the fimbriated end of the tube to pick up the ovum
Abdominal implantation after initial tubal development in the salpinx
Expulsion from the fallopian tube of the unimplanted ovum due to tubal antiperistalsis

5. CAUSES OF LOW IMPLANTATION

Destruction of healthy endometrium by endometritis or multiparity
Protracted migration due to unduly slow development of the ovum
Inadequate development of the decidua
Uterine hypoplasia
Scars of previous uterine operations
Delayed ovulation
Gravitational effect: fall of the ovum from the fundus to the lower uterine segment

generations of textbooks as far as Mauriceau[5] and Dionis.[6] Indeed, the reader who compares the recent literature on this subject with that of the early years of the century,[7-10] cannot but be impressed by the large amount of information that has seemingly been lost in the intervening decades.

While duly quoting the traditional concepts regarding the presumed causes of ectopic implantation, the authors of some current textbooks[11-14] have expressed interest in the suggestion that the relatively recently introduced". . . concept of 'late implantation' warrants consideration".[15] A review of the data upon which this theory rests[16-20] seems justifiable and timely.

THE NATURAL HISTORY OF ECTOPIC IMPLANTATION

The concept of "late implantation" as a cause of ectopic pregnancy has been referred to as follows:[1]

> "Delayed fertilization of the ovum with menstrual bleeding at the usual time, theoretically, could either prevent the ovum from entering the uterus or flush it back into the tube. Little direct support for this concept is available."

Unstated and not alluded to is the fact that the same comment could apply equally to the etiology of almost all pathological conditions of gestation since it is ethically unacceptable to set up an experimental design with the intention of producing a pathological gestation in the human species. Indeed, much of our current knowledge with regard to perinatology and prenatal pathology rests upon indirect deductions, based upon the results of retrospective studies and experiments with laboratory animals with vastly different reproductive patterns. Far-reaching conclusions have been drawn from just such data in a number of fields, including pregnancy induced hypertensive disorders, the teratogenic effect of various drugs, human placental physiology and pathology and many others. Indeed, it is proposed that the available data concerning ectopic nidation permit an almost unequivocal interpretation of several aspects of its patho-genetic background for the following reasons:

1. The causes responsible for ectopic implantation must display their effects between the time of ovulation and nidation, i.e., an interval of 6 or 7 days. Few other reproductive abnormalities exist where the time of action of the etiologic factors can be defined with a comparable degree of accuracy.
2. The events during the days that follow fertilization have been studied more extensively than those of any other stage of gestation.

Ectopic implantation frequently occurs after an episode of involuntary infertility. Thus, infertility workers have had the opportunity of observing cases of ectopic gestation that occurred at a time when the patient was under close surveillance and the cyclic events were carefully monitored.[21-30] Up to the date of this writing the author has been able to review 12 of such records. All but two contained full information relating to the cyclic events that accompanied ectopic implantation. With remarkable consistency these basal body temperature records provided evidence of the following events:

1. Prolongation of the follicular phase of the cycle beyond the usual 12 to 14 days;
2. Occurrence of an apparent "menstrual" bleeding following fertilization;
3. Shortening of the luteal phase of the cycle, i.e., the interval between ovulation and the onset of the quoted hemorrhagic phenomenon;
4. "stepwise" temperature rise during the mid-cycle for a period of time exceeding 3 days;
5. Unsustained temperature levels during the secretory phase.

The events mentioned under 1. and 3. have often been described in various publications as "delayed ovulation" whether they occurred alone or in combination. Thus, controversy and misinterpretations have developed about the term.

The basal body temperature charts depicted in Fig. 1 which were recorded by an infertile patient who subsequently developed ectopic pregnancy display all of the above-listed criteria of "luteal phase defect,"[31] an entity closely related not only to infertility but also to early abortion and its related phenomena.[32-37]

The records provided information concerning the length of the follicular phase—defined as the interval between the first day of menstrual bleeding and the elevation of the basal body temperature 0.6° F. (0.4° C) above the baseline—in 11 cases. In only three instances did ovulation take place on, or before, the 14th day of the cycle, the usual time of ovulation according to Ogino, Knaus and other proponents of the "mid-cycle theory."[38-42] In the remaining 8 cases ovulation was delayed beyond the 14th day (Fig. 2). The latter finding is of considerable import in the light of the observation of Hertig, who noted that conceptions that had occurred from such "delayed" ovulations resulted in abnormally segmenting preimplantation ova in the majority of cases (Fig. 3).[43] Thus, the phenomenon shown in Figure 2 may offer an explanation for the high rate of blighted ova, embryonic developmental defects[9] and chromosomal abnormalities[44] among ectopic products of conception.

The earlier described phenomenon of "post-conception menstrual bleeding"[45] could be demonstrated in all but one of the basal body temperature records taken during the cycles of conception that resulted in an ectopic implantation (Fig. 4). The hemorrhage seems to be a remarkably constant feature of this pathological entity; nonetheless, it has been ignored rather consistently by editors and writers of contemporary textbooks and reviews.

The occurrence of an apparent "menstruation" following conceptions

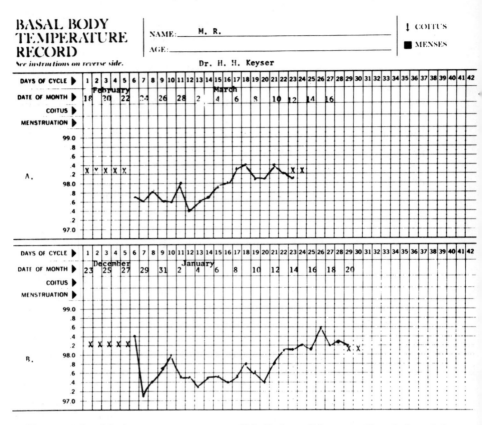

Fig. 1. A basal body temperature pattern which displays all features of luteal phase defect recognizable in a basal body temperature record. Following these 2 cycles the patient continued to present evidence of corpus luteum deficiency, and when she conceived a year later, the gestation resulted in tubal implantation. (Courtesy of Dr. Herbert H. Keyser and the Editor of *Journal of Reproductive Medicine*.)

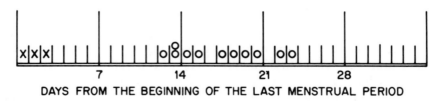

DAYS FROM THE BEGINNING OF THE LAST MENSTRUAL PERIOD

Fig. 2. The length of the follicular phase in 11 cases of ectopic pregnancy based on basal body temperature recordings taken during the cycle of conception.

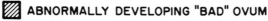

☐ NORMALLY DEVELOPING "GOOD" OVUM

▨ ABNORMALLY DEVELOPING "BAD" OVUM

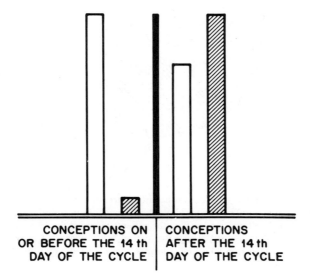

| CONCEPTIONS ON OR BEFORE THE 14th DAY OF THE CYCLE | CONCEPTIONS AFTER THE 14th DAY OF THE CYCLE |

Fig. 3.   Correlations between the time of fertilization during the intermenstrual cycle and the frequency of abnormal embryonic development, based on Hertig's retrospective study of his 34 famous preimplantation ova in 1965. Note high incidence of anomalous segmentation of early ova in those cases where conception had followed ovulations occurring after the 14th day of the cycle.

destined to result in ectopic implantation permits characterization of the luteal phase in this entity. Of the cases reviewed, in only four instances was the interval between ovulation and the ensuing vaginal bleeding longer than 11 days. In the remaining patients the length of the apparent luteal phase ranged between 1 and 10 days.

It should be pointed out that due to the occurrence of "stepwise temperature rise" in the mid-cycle, the exact time of ovulation, and thus the length of the follicular and luteal phases, is difficult to determine. However, since ectopic pregnancy so often exhibits the signs and symptoms that characterize luteal phase defect, we may assume that this condition apparently is often causally related to a deficiency of the corpus luteum. Indeed, none of the cases reviewed displayed fewer than two of the earlier listed features of this entity.

Abnormal corpus luteum function is the consequence of defective ovula-

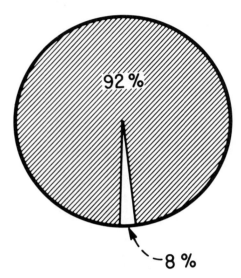

Fig. 4.   Frequency of bleeding episodes following conception in cases of ectopic pregnancy. Analysis has been based on 12 cases where basal body temperature record was taken during the cycle of fertilization. In all but one instance the patients recorded the occurrence of a vaginal hemorrhage at about the time of the expected period, a prevalence of approximately 92%. (Shaded area: post-conception bleeding episodes. Non-shaded area: no post-conception hemorrhage documented.)

tion. The latter has been shown to result from inappropriate ratios between the follicle-stimulating hormone (FSH) and the luteinizing hormone (LH) ratios during the preovulatory phase (Figs. 5 and 6).[46, 47] It has been demonstrated that such an abnormal endocrine relationship tends to result in prolongation of the follicular and shortening of the luteal phases (Fig. 7), the phenomena that have been referred to as delayed ovulation. There is no reason to assume that the identical events associated with ectopic gestation would have a different origin. Accordingly, it is suggested that the phenomena during the intermenstrual cycle related to conceptions that result in ectopic implantation are:
1. Inappropriate FSH:LH ratio during the follicular phase;
2. Frequent ill-timed and defective ovulation;
3. Inadequate function of the corpus luteum, reflected in demonstrable abnormalities of the BBT curve;
4. Failure of the corpus luteum to suppress the succeeding menstrual period leading to the occurrence of a bleeding episode that may be typical, or atypical, at the approximate time of the next expected menstrual flow.
As described in several older publications,[8, 10, 48] the patient's misinter-

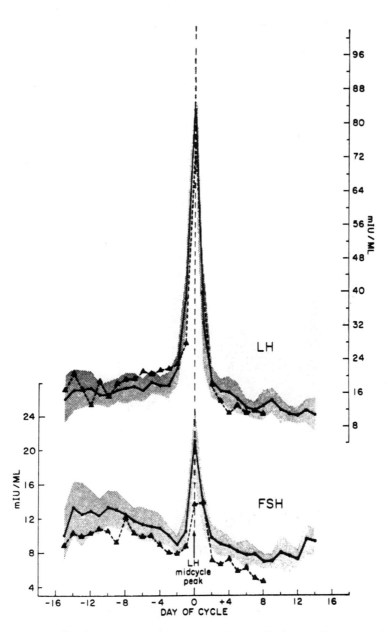

Fig. 5. Mean daily plasma LH and FSH concentrations (solid line, small points) and their 95% confidence intervals for 16 cycles with post LH peak intervals of 13 days or more (normal luteal phase cycles) compared to mean daily LH and FSH concentrations (dotted lines, solid triangles) for 7 cycles with post LH peak intervals of 8 days or less (short luteal phase cycles). All cycles are synchronized around the day of the LH midcycle peak (Courtesy of Dr. G. T. Ross and the Editor of *Recent Progress in Hormone Research.*)

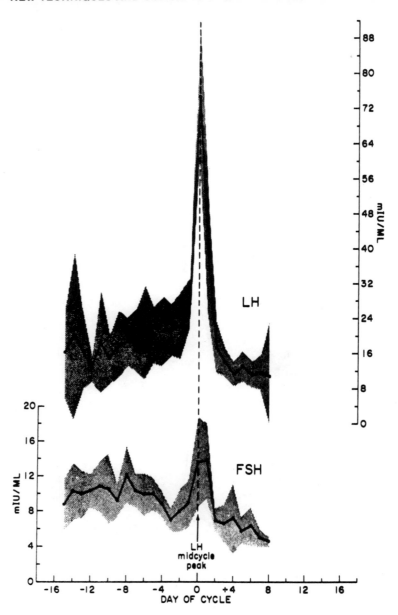

Fig. 6.   Mean (bold line) and 95% confidence limits of mean (shaded areas) daily plasma concentrations of LH and FSH during 7 cycles with post LH peak intervals of 8 days or less (short luteal phase cycles). All cycles are synchronized on day of LH peak. (Courtesy of Dr. G. T. Ross and the Editor of *Recent Progress in Hormone Research.*)

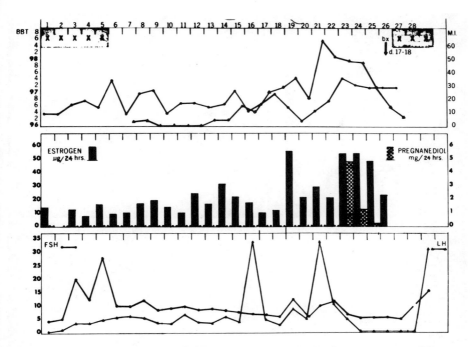

Fig. 7. Laboratory data in a case of severe luteal phase defect. Note evidence of delayed ovulation and considerable shortening of the luteal phase. Pregnanediol excretion values fell to subnormal levels three days after ovulation. The urinary estrogen excretion remained low until the day; thereafter a short secondary rise occurred before menses. The plasma FSH pattern was within normal limits in this case. The LH values remained low during the follicular phase but abrupt rises occurred on the 16th and 21st days. Apparently, the latter LH surge resulted in ovulation. Endometrial biopsy on the 26th day revealed 17 to 18-day endometrium. (from Jones and Madrigal-Castro. *Fertil. Steril.* 21:1, 1970. Courtesy of The Williams and Wilkins Co.)

pretation of this bleeding episode as a normal period is the reason for the frequently recounted fable of dramatic and unexpected early rupture of an ectopic gestation without a period of amenorrhea.

In the initial studies, the conclusion that ectopic pregnancies result from a "delayed" ovulation was based on the study of early embryonic specimens, most of which belonged to the Carnegie Institution of Washington. Their stages of development compared with the menstrual history indicated that they had originated from conceptions that had usually preceded the last menstrual period. (Figs. 8 and 9). In other words, the time of ovulation in these cases did not seem to coincide with the "midcycle", but rather with the later days of the intermenstrual interval (Fig.

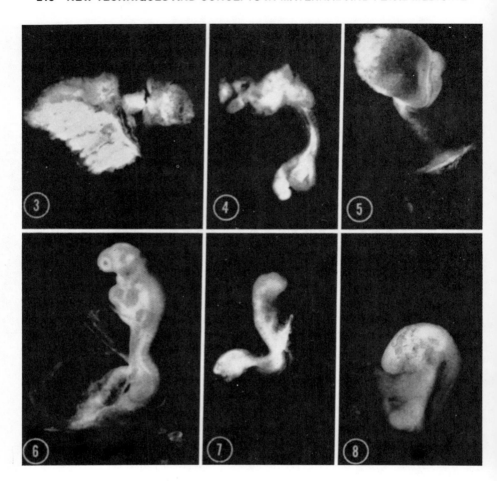

Fig. 8.   Embryos from tubal pregnancies. Fig. 3. Presomite embryo. Estimated ovulation age is 18 days. Patient had less than normal menstrual flow 9 days before operation. Symptoms and possibly fetal death occurred 3 days before laparotomy. (Grade 2 specimen; Carnegie No. 7972.) (× 22) Fig. 4. "16 somite" embryo. Estimated age is 18–19 days. Pregnancy was discovered 18 days after moderate bleeding occurred at time of expected period. (Carnegie No. 8005) (× 13) Fig. 5. Early ectopic embryo with estimated age of slightly over 3 weeks. Embryo was recovered at operation 19 days after apparently normal menstruation. (Carnegie No. 7568.) (× 20) Fig. 6. "23–24 somite" embryo. Estimated developmental age is about 3½ weeks. Embryo was recovered from tube 24 days after last, apparently normal, menstrual period. (Carnegie No. 9154.) (× 12) Fig. 7. "26 somite" embryo. Estimated age is 26 days. Embryo was found at operation 14 days after last (slighter than normal) period. (Carnegie No. 6937.) (× 12) Fig. 8. Early embryo with an estimated age of about 26 days. Patient had less than normal flow at expected time 23 days before recovery of specimen. This is a Grade 3 specimen included on account of its rarity. Embryo might have been dead for slightly more than 3 days. (Carnegie No. 5206.) (× 10)

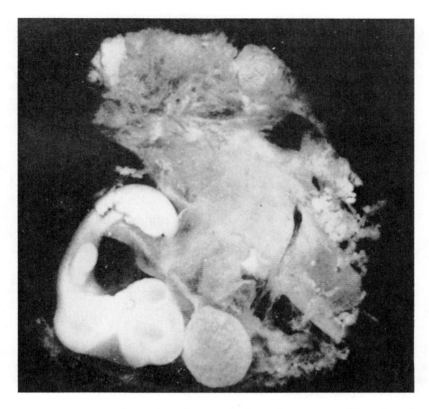

Fig. 9.   A case of early primary abdominal (pouch of Douglas) pregnancy. The estimated age of the embryo is about 5 weeks.[49,50,67] The last menstrual period began 28 days before the recovery of the specimen through laparotomy (Courtesy of the Editor of *British Journal of Obstetrics and Gynaecology.*)

10, Table 2). The evidence from BBT records supports the findings of these embryologic investigations and suggests that the occurrence of an apparent menstruation after such conceptions is more frequent than earlier investigations had suggested. It is probable that some of the physicians who submitted their specimens for inclusion in the embryologic collection of Carnegie Institution had corrected the date of the last menstrual period when they realized that there had been an obvious discrepancy between the menstrual data and the stage of development of the specimen.

In the initial studies, it was emphasized that as a result of delayed ovulation and shortened luteal phase, the subsequent "menstrual" bleeding finds an unimplanted ovum in the fallopian tube or in the uterine cavity. It was suggested that this hemorrhage, through the often demonstrated reflux

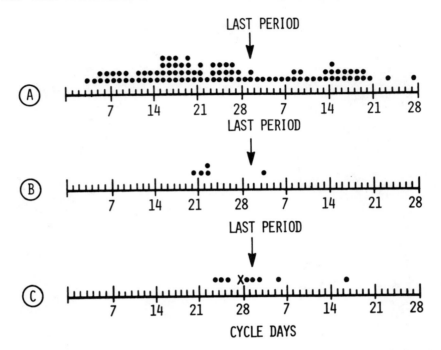

Fig. 10.   The study has been based on very early embryos, mostly from the Embryologic Collection of the Carnegie Institution in Washington. The estimated conception times represent rough approximations. (Courtesy of the Editor of *Australian and New Zealand Journal of Obstetrics and Gynaecology.*)

bleeding, misplaces the ovum into the salpinx or the abdominal cavity, or alternatively arrests its progress in the fallopian tube. It was further suggested that the same hemorrhage could also misplace the conceptus into the lower segment of the uterus or into the cervix, thus leading to placenta previa and to cervical pregnancy.[17,49] The latter suggestion has been supported by evidence which indicated frequent discrepancies between the stage of fetal development and the menstrual history and thus frequent "post-conception menstrual bleeding" in connection with this entity[50] (Fig. 11). It was on the basis of this reasoning that the name "reflux theory" was applied to the proposed etiologic concept of ectopic pregnancy.

In retrospect, the name selected for the theory was unfortunate. While the available data, as summarized in this review, provide strong support for the proposed role of ovulatory and corpus luteum defects in the pathogenesis of ectopic implantation, they offer only circumstantial evidence regarding the proposed reflux mechanism. Nevertheless, basic scientists recognized the potential importance of the proposed ovulation

Table 2.   Data on Specimens of Very Early Ectopic (Tubal) Pregnancy.

CARNEGIE NO.	LMP (DAYS BEFORE OPERATION)	STREETER'S HORIZON	ESTIMATED AGE (DAYS)	COMMENTS
8186	11	Presomite embryo	18½	Germ-disk about 1.2 mm. long; tissues are somewhat macerated showing that development had ceased, perhaps, a few days prior to the operation
8005	18*	16 somites	18–19	Menstrual cycle, 31 days
7972	9*	Presomite VIII	18	Grade 2 specimen (slightly macerated); symptoms 3 days before operation; menstrual cycle, 28 days
7568	19	XI	Slightly over 3 weeks	Chorionic cavity measures 6 × 5 × 4 mm. Menstrual cycle, 25 days; period, 3–6 days
6310	14	XI About 17 somites	19–21	Estimated length, 2.5 mm.
5206	23*	XII	26†	Length, 4mm. Menstrual cycle, 25–28 days
6097	4*	XII	26	Length, 3.43 mm. Menstrual cycle, 32 days; period 7–8 days
9154	24	XII 23–24 somites	About 3½ weeks	Length, 4 mm.
2035	30	XII	26	Length, 4 mm.
6937	14	XII 26 somites	26	Length, 3 mm.

* Duration of bleeding shorter than usual.
† Grade 3 specimen.

Table 2. Analysis of the earliest cases of ectopic pregnancy in the Embryologic Collection of the Carnegie Institution of Wahsington. Note the obvious discrepancies between the length of the amenorrhea and the stage of development of the ectopic embryos. The data suggest the occurrence of an apparent menstruation after conception, since the specimens are older than the length of time between the last recorded period and the recovery of the ectopic embryo from the abdominal cavity. (Courtesy of the Editor of *Obstetrics and Gynecology*.)

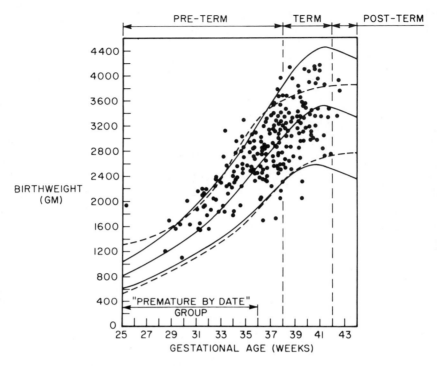

Fig. 11. Correlations between menstrual age (horizontal line) and fetal weight (vertical line) in 250 cases of placenta previa. Note considerable increase in the number of "high weight for gestational age" fetuses in the "premature by date" group. Presumably many of these patients had given erroneous menstrual history due to a "postconception" bleeding episode. (Courtesy of Medical Examination Publishing Co.)

defects in the genesis of many pathological conditions of gestation; research testing of this hypothesis has resulted in important contributions to prenatal pathology.[53-64]

An exceedingly rare observation of Falk et al.[65] has provided substantial, though still circumstantial, evidence for the reflux mechanism as the basis for ectopic implantation. In this case the age of the embryo could be determined to be 9 days with a high degree of accuracy by comparison with established standards of intrauterine growth (Figs. 12–14).[66,77] The patient's last menstrual period began six days before the recovery of the specimen from the abdominal cavity through laparotomy. Since at this stage of gestation the age of the embryo can be determined with an accuracy of about ± 1 day, it could be established with certainty that the ovum was still unimplanted at the time of the menstrual bleeding. Thus, beyond doubt, this ovum was exposed to the menstrual cataclysm prior to its implantation in the lumen of the fallopian tube.

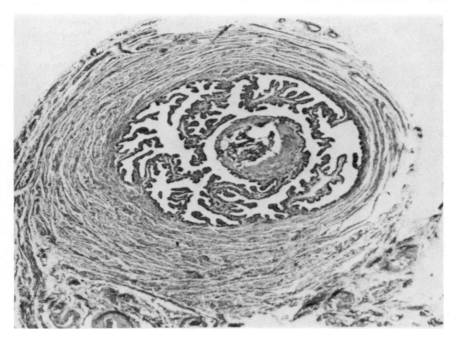

Fig. 12.   Tubal pregnancy in the lumen of the fallopian tube. The ovum is attached to one of the tree-like folds of the tubal mucosa (luminal form of tubal implantation). This case probably represents the earliest tubal pregnancy reported in the medical literature. (Courtesy of Dr. Henry C. Falk and the Editor of *Obstetrics and Gynecology*.)

Further circumstantial evidence suggesting that ectopic implantation is the result of mechanical displacement has been provided fortuitously by Steptoe and Edwards.[68] These investigators attempted to introduce into the uterine cavity an artificially fertilized, late preimplantation-stage human ovum with the intention of achieving normal gestation. Placed into a small amount of physiologic solution, the fertilized egg was introduced into the endometrial cavity through the cervix by a syringe. A tubal implantation resulted from this attempt, indicating that the ovum injected under pressure had been forced into the salpinx. Since, by design, the ovum was about ready to implant, it took root in the tube rather than on the surface of the endometrium. Obviously, the mechanism of this ectopic nidation was by reflux from the uterine cavity into the salpinx, the same process proposed as responsible for extrauterine implantation.[15]

On all these counts, and because ectopic gestation under natural conditions is practically restricted to menstruating primates[69-71] (the only species where menstruation, and thus menstrual reflux, can occur), the author still believes that the original proposition with regard to the mechanism of ec-

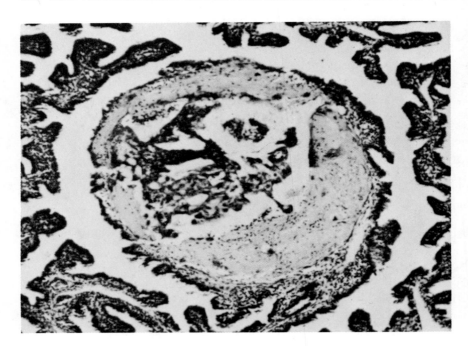

Fig. 13.   High power magnification of the ovum shown in Figure 12. Early trophoblast is attaching the ovum to tree-like folds of the tube. The trophoblast appears well developed, which places it in Stage 5 on the embryonic growth standards. Such ova are implanted, but previllous. The formation of lacunae is suggested in the micrograph which indicates that the ovum should be approximately 9 days old. (Courtesy of Dr. Henry C. Falk and the Editor of *Obstetrics and Gynecology*. The quoted interpretation is presented by courtesy of Dr. Raymond F. Gasser.)

topic implantation was correct; however, the evidence cannot be considered unequivocal. Kirby[72] has demonstrated in laboratory rodents that experimentally induced ectopic implantation fails to provide the hormonal stimulus necessary to suppress continued cyclic changes. In at least one reported case of tubal gestation,[27] the presence of the ectopic products of conception failed to prevent the occurrence of another ovulation in the course of a seemingly regular cycle. Thus, it is reasonable to argue that the bleeding episode following or accompanying ectopic implantation is the result, rather than the cause, of the extrauterine pregnancy present. There is evidence to indicate that chorionic gonadotropin production by an ectopically implanted placenta is significantly lower than that of normally implanted products of conception.[73] This could account for the almost invariable occurrence of "menstrual" bleeding after fertilization, since this is the hormone which is considered responsible for the suppression of further cyclic endocrine changes.

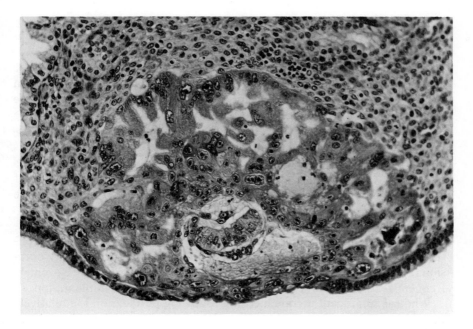

Fig. 14.   An embryo representing Stage 5 of the embryonic growth standards.[67] Note evidence of early superficial implantation, separation of the embryonic disc from the chorion and development of lacunae in the trophoblastic tissue. (Courtesy of Dr. Raymond F. Gasser.)

DISCUSSION AND CONCLUSIONS

A recent review of ectopic pregnancy involving extensive analysis of relevant experimental and clinical evidence[4] concluded that the available data decisively disproved most of the proposed etiologic hypotheses. On the other hand, possible predisposing role for certain factors such as infection in the fallopian tube, endometriosis and space-reducing conditions in general, was indicated by their relatively frequent presence in association with tubal pregnancies. However, none of these "predisposing conditions" was a *sine qua non* for tubal implantation, thus supporting the generally held belief that ectopic implantation occurs fortuitously.

In previous studies[16-20] it was pointed out that ectopic pregnancy shares many features with other reproductive abnormalities, some of them with fairly well understood pathogenetic background. Thus, ectopic implantation tends to precede, coincide with, or follow early spontaneous abortion, twinning, placenta previa, chorionic malignancy[74,75] embryonic developmental defects and chromosome abnormalities of the products of conception. Advanced maternal age, involuntary infertility, clinical evidence of endocrine dysfunction and history of nutritional deficiencies are predisposing factors for these reproductive abnormalities, suggesting a possible common etiologic background for this group of clinically rather dissimilar abnormalities of human gestation.

In search of a common denominator, attention was drawn over a decade ago to circumstantial evidence that seemed to indicate that deviations from the normal ovulatory pattern were frequently demonstrable during the cycle of conception resulting in ectopic pregnancies. Since comparable evidence pointed to the same factors in the pathogenesis of these related entities, the suggestion was made in 1962 that ovulatory and ensuing corpus luteum defects were the common denominator in the etiology of various types of ectopic gestation, early spontaneous abortion and the varieties of fetal malformation commonly associated with them ("post-mid-cycle theory").[59]

The above summary of currently available evidence on the etiology of extrauterine nidation of the fertilized human ovum concludes that, in contrast to the earlier mentioned predisposing factors recognizable only occasionally in the background of this entity, luteal phase defect is an extremely frequent feature of those cycles that result in extrauterine implantation.

Whereas significant uterine bleeding following fertilization is a relatively rare event in human reproduction, a bleeding episode which imitates a normal menstrual period is apparently the rule in those cases where the ovum implants upon an ectopic site. This event is likely to be relevant to the mechanism that causes nidation of the egg on an anatomic surface not designed by nature for the imbedding, nutrition and development of the products of conception.

Ectopic pregnancy appears more unequivocally tied to the phenomenon of luteal phase defect than do such long-recognized entities as female infertility and first trimester abortion. Since these conditions can be traced back to defective ovulatory and corpus luteum functions, the possibility exists that luteal phase defect may also be a common denominator in the pathogenesis of embryonal and chromosome defects, anomalies that correlate etiologically with early abortion and ectopic gestation. A considerable amount of experimental evidence tends to support this assumption. Ovulation defects, whether associated with natural biological variability, or artificially induced by the suppression of ovulation by drugs at a crucial time before the rupture of the graafian follicle, have been demonstrated to be conducive to fetal monstrosities and chromosome abnormalities both in amphibians and mammals.[53-58] This outcome has been attributed to pre-ovulatory overripeness of the ovum.[60] The fact that an apparently similar ovulatory dysfunction is conducive to a pathological entity which is frequently associated with identical types of embryonic damage,[9,44] suggests the potential teratogenic role of similar spontaneously occurring "ovulation defects" in the human female. The actual mechanism of ovulatory and luteal phase defects has been identified in considerable detail recently[46,47]. There is now an impressive body of indirect evidence suggesting that those endocrine events leading to *defective ovulation, over-ripeness* and *corpus luteum deficiency* deserve consideration as potentially important causes of human reproductive wastage.

The term *delayed ovulation,* frequently referred to in previous studies, has been de-emphasized purposely in the current review. The term has been interpreted in a number of ways in relevant research dealing with infertility, reproductive wastage and teratology. To some investigators it implies belated occurrence of ovulation following the 14th day of the intermenstrual cycle in the human species. Others consider ovulation delayed only if it occurs relatively close to the beginning of the next cycle. In human reproduction the latter definition postulates a luteal phase reduced to less than 12 days, in contrast to the normal "biological mid-cycle" that precedes the onset of the next period by about 14 days irrespective of cycle length. In some laboratory research "delayed ovulation" was induced in rodents by exposure to barbiturates at a critical stage of the follicular ripening: usually within 24 hours of the anticipated ovulation. Delay of ovulation by this mechanism was found highly conducive to fetal malformations and chromosome defects.[55-57] In the course of the same research it was found that spontaneous (usually age-related) prolongation of the pre-ovulatory phase increased the rate of embryonic developmental defects significantly. This finding is practically identical with Hertig's earlier quoted observation in the human female (Fig. 3).[43]

Short luteal phase (relevant to one interpretation of delayed ovulation) has been recognized as a factor in human reproductive wastage.[31-37] Thus there is little doubt that all of the cited interpretations have a measure of plausibility. In addition, the various phenomena interpreted as "delayed ovulation" tend to occur together and apparently contribute, through a mechanism not yet clearly defined, to the earlier described outcome.

The theoretical and practical ramifications of the suggested role of ovulatory and corpus luteum defects in the pathogenesis of ectopic pregnancy and other reproductive abnormalities are numerous. These implications have been discussed in other recent publications.[4,60]

REFERENCES

1. Pritchard, J. A. and McDonald, P. C. Williams Obstetrics (15th Ed.) New York, Appleton-Century-Crofts, 1976, p. 431.
2. Greenhill, J. P. and Friedman, E. A. Biological principles and Modern Practice of Obstetrics. Philadelphia, W. B. Saunders Co., 1974, p. 351.

3. Page, E. W., Villee, C. A. and Villee, D. B. Human Reproduction. Philadelphia, W. B. Saunders Co., 1972.

4. McElin, T. W. and Iffy, L. Ectopic Gestation: A Consideration of New and Controversial Issues Relating to Pathogenesis and Management. *In* R. M. Wynn: Obstetrics and Gynecology Annual (Vol. 5) New York, Appleton-Century-Crofts, 1976, pp. 241–292.

5. Mauriceau. Traité des maladies des femmes grosses. Paris, 1694.

6. Dionis, P. Traité général des accouchements. Paris, 1718.

7. Strassman, P. Placenta praevia. *Arch. Gynäk,* **67–68:** 112, 1902.

8. Champneys, F. H. A contribution towards the study of the natural history of tubal gestation. *J. Obstet. Gynaec. Brit. Emp.* **1:** 585, 1902.

9. Mall, F. P. On the fate of the human embryo in tubal pregnancy. *Contrib. Embryol. Carneg. Instit.* **1:** 1, 1915.

10. Lavell, T. E. The diagnosis of ectopic gestation. *Amer. J. Obstet. Gynec.* **18:** 379, 1929.

11. Carter, F. B. Extra-uterine Pregnancy. *In* R. A. Kimbrough: Gynecology. Philadelphia, J. B. Lippincott Co., 1965, pp. 436–438.

12. de Alvarez, R. R. Textbook of Gynecology. Philadelphia, Lea & Febiger, 1977, pp. 219–235.

13. Romney, S. L., Gray, M. J. et al. Gynecology and Obstetrics. The Health Care of Women. New York, McGraw-Hill Book Co., New York, 1975. p. 720.

14. Mc Elin, T. W. Ectopic Pregnancy. *In* D. N. Danforth: Textbook of Obstetrics and Gynecology (3rd Ed.), New York, Harper & Row, pp.

15. Novak, E. R. and Woodruff, J. D. Novak's Gynecologic and Obstetric Pathology (7th Ed.) Philadelphia, W. B. Saunders Co., 1974, p. 489.

16. Iffy, L. Contribution to the aetiology of ectopic pregnancy. *J. Obstet. Gynaec. Brit. Commonw.* **68:** 441, 1962.

17. ———. Contribution to the pathological mechanism of ovarian, abdominal and cervical pregnancies. *Gynaecologia* **153:** 188, 1962.

18. ———. The role of premenstrual, post-mid-cycle conception in the aetiology of ectopic gestation. *J. Obstet. Gynaec. Brit. Commonw.* **70:** 996, 1963.

19. ———. Embryologic studies of time of conception in ectopic pregnancy and first trimester abortion. *Obstet. Gynecol.* **26:** 490, 1965.

20. ———. Recent investigations concerning the aetiology of ectopic pregnancies. *Austral. N. Z. J. Obstet. Gynaec.* **8:** 131, 1968.

21. Benjamin, F. Basal body temperature recordings in gynaecology and obstetrics. *J. Obstet. Gynaec. Brit. Emp.* **67:** 177, 1960.

22. Stewart, H. L. Oral basal body temperatures in abortion and ectopic pregnancy. *Amer. J. Obstet. Gynec.* **59:** 563, 1950.

23. Stewart, H. L. Personal communication (1971).

24. Iffy, L., Chatterton, R. T., Jr., and Jakobovits, A. The "high weight for dates" fetus. *Amer. J. Obstet. Gynec.* **115:** 238, 1973.

25. Philippe, E., Ritter, J. et al. Grossesse tubaire, ovulation tardive, at anomalie de nidation. *Gynec. Obstet. (Paris)* **69:** 617, 1970.

26. Philippe, E. and Walter, F. X. Personal communication (1972).

27. Keyser, H. H., Iffy, L. and Cohen, J. Basal body temperature recordings in ectopic pregnancy. *J. Reprod. Med.* **14:** 37–40, 1975. (*Erratum:* **14:** 240, 1975.)

28. Keyser, H. H. Personal communication (1978).

29. Saito, M., Koyama, T. et al. Site of ovulation and ectopic pregnancy. *Acta Obstet. Gynaecol. Scand.* **54:** 227, 1975.

30. Saito, M. Personal communication (1977).

31. Jones, G. E. S. and Madrigal-Castro, V. Hormonal findings in association with abnormal corpus luteum function in the human: the luteal phase defect. *Fertil. Steril.* **21:** 1, 1970.

32. Grant, A., McBride, W. G., and Murray Moyes, J. Luteal phase defect in sterility. *Internat. J. Fertil.* **4:** 315, 1959.
33. Arrata, W. S. M. and Iffy, L. Normal and delayed ovulation in the human. *Obstet. Gynec. Surv.* **26:** 575, 1971.
34. Guerrero, R. and Rojas, O. I. Spontaneous abortion and aging of human ova and spermatozoa. *New Eng. J. Med.* **293:** 573, 1975.
35. Cohen, J., Iffy, L. and Keyser, H. H. Basal body temperature recordings in early abortion. *Internat. J. Gynaec. Obstet.* **14:** 117, 1976.
36. De Moraes-Ruehsen, M. D., Jones, S. E. G. et al. *The aluteal cycle* **103:** 1059, 1969.
37. Delfs, E. and Jones, G. E. S. Endocrine patterns in abortion. *Obstet. Gynec. Surv.* **3:** 680, 1948.
38. Ogino, K. Ovulationstermin und Konzeptionstermin. *Zbl. Gynaek.* **54:** 464, 1930.
39. Knaus, H. Periodic Fertility and Sterility in Women. Vienna, Wilhelm Maudrich Publ., 1934.
40. Hartman, C. G. Mechanism Concerned with Conception. New York, Macmillan Publ., 1963.
41. Behrman, S. J. Artificial insemination. *Internat. J. Fertil.* **6:** 291, 1961.
42. Siegel, P. W. Warum ist das Beischlaf nich befruchtend? *Dtsc. Med. Wchschr.* **41:** 1251, 1915.
43. Hertig, A. T. The overall problem in man. *In* Benirschke, K. (Ed.) Comparative Aspects of Reproductive Failure. New York, Springer-Verlag, 1967.
44. Poland, B. J., Dill, F. J. and Styblo, C. Embryonic development in ectopic pregnancy. *Teratology* **14:** 315, 1976.
45. Iffy, L., Wingate, M. B. and Jakobovits, A. Postconception "menstrual" bleeding. *Internat. J. Gynaec. Obstet.* **10:** 41, 1972.
46. Ross, G. T., Cargille, C. M. et al. Pituitary and gonadal hormones in women during spontaneous and induced ovulatory cycles. Recent Prog. *Hormone Res.* **26:** 1, 1970.
47. Ross, G. T. Preovulatory determinants of human corpus luteum function. *Europ. J. Gynec. Reprod. Biol.* **6:** 147, 1976.
48. Cope, Z. The Early Diagnosis of the Acute Abdomen. London, Oxford University Press, 1927.
49. Streeter, G. L. Weight, sitting height, head size, foot length and menstrual age of the human embryo. *Contrib. Embryol. Carneg. Instit.* **11:** 143, 1920.
50. Arey, L. B. Developmental Anatomy. Philadelphia, W. B. Saunders Co., 1954.
51. Iffy, L. Contribution to the etiology of placenta previa. *Amer. J. Obstet. Gynec.* **83:** 969, 1962.
52. Iffy, L. and Langer, A. Perinatology Case Studies. Medical Examination Publishing Co., Garden City, New York, 1978, pp. 359-368.
53. Witschi, E. and Laguens, R. Chromosomal aberrations in embryos from overripe eggs. *Develop. Biol.* **7:** 605, 1963.
54. Mikamo, K. Intrafollicular overripeness and teratogenic development. *Cytogenetics* **7:** 212, 1968.
55. Fugo, N. W. and Butcher, R. L. Overripeness and the mammalian ova. I. Overripeness and early embryonic development. *Fertil. Steril.* **17:** 804, 1966.
56. Butcher, R. L. and Fugo, N. W. Overripeness and the mammalian ova. II. Delayed ovulation and chromosome anomalies. *Fertil. Steril.* **18:** 297, 1967.
57. Butcher, R. L., Blue, J. D. and Fugo, N. W. Overripeness of the mammalian ova. III. Fetal development at midgestation and at term. *Fertil. Steril.* **20:** 223, 1969.
58. Bomsel-Helmreich, O. The aging of gametes, heteroploidy, and embryonic death. *Internat. J. Gynaec. Obstet.* **14:** 98, 1976.

59. Iffy, L. The time of conception in pathological gestations. (The scope of the reflux-theory.) *Proc. Roy. Soc. Med.* **56:** 1098, 1963.
60. Mikamo, K. and Iffy, L. Aging of the ovum. *In* R. M. Wynn: Obstetrics and Gynecology Annual (Vol. 3) New York, Appleton-Century-Crofts, 1974, pp. 47–99.
61. Witschi, E. Developmental causes of malformation. *Experientia (Separatum)* **27:** 1245, 1971.
62. Jongbloet, P. H. The intriguing phenomenon of gametopathy and its disastrous effects on the human progeny. *Maandschr. Kindergeneesk.* **37:** 261, 1969.
63. Philippe, E. Histopathologie Placentaire. Paris, Masson & Cie, 1974.
64. Guerrero, R. and Lanctot, C. A. Aging of fertilized gametes and spontaneous abortion. *Amer. J. Obstet. Gynec.* **107:** 263, 1970.
65. Falk, H. C., Hassid, R. and Dazo, E. P. Tubal pregnancy. *Obstet. Gynec.* **45:** 215, 1975.
66. Iffy, L. and Gasser, R. F. Tubal pregnancy. *Obstet. Gynec.* **47:** 380, 1976.
67. Gasser, R. F. Atlas of Human Embryos. Hagerstown, Md., Harper & Row, 1975.
68. Steptoe, P. C. and Edwards, R. G. Reimplantation of a human embryo with subsequent tubal pregnancy. *Lancet* **1:** 880, 1976.
69. Ruch, T. C. Diseases of Laboratory Primates. Philadelphia, W. B. Saunders Co., 1959.
70. Waldeyer, W. Ueber eine ectopische Schwangerschaft bei einem Mantelpavian. Zbl. Geburtsh. *Gynäkol.* **111:** 322, 1919.
71. Hansen, J. S. Ectopic pregnancy in a queen with one uterine horn and urachal remnant. *Vet. Med. Small Anim. Clin.* **69:** 1135, 1974.
72. Kirby, D. R. S. Endocrinological effects of experimentally induced extra-uterine pregnancies in virgin mice. *Reprod. Fertil.* **10:** 403, 1965.
73. Wide, L. An immunological method for the assay of human chorionic gonadotropin. *Acta Endocrin. (Suppl.)* **41:** 70, 1962.
74. Walsh, C. H. A specimen of chorion epithelioma following ectopic gestation. *J. Obstet. Gynaec. Brit. Emp.* **42:** 194, 1935.
75. Iffy, L. Contribution to the aetiology of hydatidiform mole. Common pathogenetic factors with various clinical manifestations in obstetrics. *Ann. Chir. Gynaec. Fenn.* **51:** 428, 1962.

16

Basal Body Temperature Recordings During the Cycle of Conception in Cases of Extrauterine (Tubal) Gestation

D. SCHWARTZ, M.D.[1]
AND
ANNE BOYCE, M.D.[2]

These basal body temperature charts along with up to 17 monthly temperature recordings taken during the cycles preceding the ectopic pregnancy have been provided by the authors indicated above. The following comments represent the *editors' interpretation* of these records.

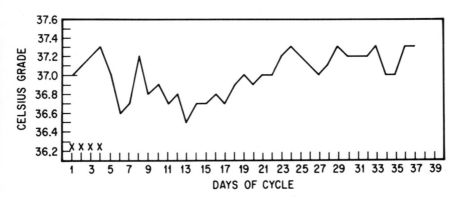

Fig. 1.

Prior to the tubal gestation this patient took her basal body temperature daily through 17 cycles. Criteria listed in the preceding chapter were used to identify the luteal phase defect—i.e., significant prolongation of the follicular phase; stepwise mid-cycle temperature rise; unsustained temperature elevation during the luteal phase; significant shortening of the luteal phase and occurrence of uterine bleeding following conception. The patient's cycle of fertilization provided evidence of luteal phase defect on at least three counts: the follicular phase was prolonged, the ovulatory temperature elevation was stepwise (reaching a peak in about 8 days) and the secretory phase temperature level was poorly sustained. The patient's record contained no data regarding bleeding or its absence. All of the preceding cycles displayed evidence of luteal phase defect except one which was probably anovulatory.

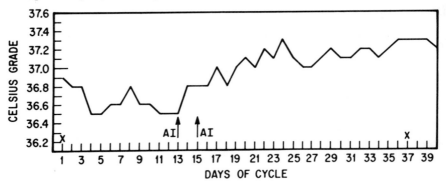

Fig. 2.

Prolonged follicular phase and gradual mid-cycle temperature rise lasting about 8 days characterized the cycle of fertilization. Uterine bleeding was noted on the 39th day. Eleven preceding cycles were recorded. All of them were ovulatory and all but one showed at least two of the criteria of luteal phase defect.

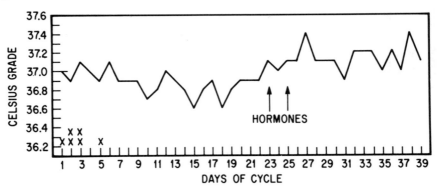

Fig. 3.

The follicular phase lasted 22 days; stepwise temperature elevation, about 5 days in duration, followed. The temperature elevation during the luteal phase was poorly sustained despite the administration of hormones (progesterone ?) on the 23rd and 25th days of the cycle. The record offered no data concerning the occurrence, or absence, of bleeding episodes after conception. Six previous cycles were recorded. All of them displayed evidence of ovulatory and luteal phase defects. In one cycle prolongation of temperature elevation well beyond 14 days and repeated vaginal bleeding episodes while the temperature was still elevated suggested "occult abortion."

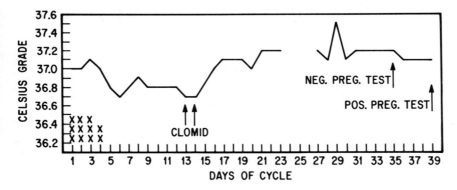

Fig. 4.

Through 11 preceding cycles BBT records displayed evidence of ovulation and luteal phase defects. During the cycle of conception ovulation was induced by Clomid. Ovulation probably occurred on the 16th day. In this case prolongation of the follicular phase (delayed ovulation) is the only recorded evidence of ovulation defect.

17

Early Tubal Ovum

A. MADRAZO, M.D.

The etiology and mechanism of tubal implantation has been a matter of controversy for centuries. The fact that destruction of the supporting anatomic structures is a predictable early result of extrauterine nidation has made the evaluation of the relevant evidence extremely difficult. The identification of primary ovarian, abdominal and cervical pregnancies as independent pathologic entities has been facilitated by careful observation and reporting of very early cases. It seems reasonable to expect, therefore, that careful description of cases of early tubal implantation may be conducive to the understanding of the pathological mechanism of tubal gestation. A recent observation made in our institution may belong to this important category of rare cases.

The patient, Mrs. G. H., was admitted for routine surgical sterilization (tubal ligation) on February 6, 1974. She had had three full-term pregnancies (last childbirth in 1969) and five spontaneous abortions. She had four years' history of irregular periods including two years on birth control medication (Demulen). Her last menstrual period began on January 15, 1974.

Physical examination and routine laboratory studies, including pregnancy tests were negative on the day of the admission. The next day, i.e. on the 23rd day of the patient's cycle, the operation was performed. The surgeon noted no deviation from normal anatomy in the course of the procedure and the presence of an implanted ovum in the middle segment of fallopian tube was an incidential finding during the routine pathological investigation of the removed section of the salpinx. Macroscopically, the specimen consisted of two portions of the fallopian tube, the left one measuring 1.3 x 0.5 cm. and the right one 1.5 x 0.7 cm. No gross abnormalities were present and no fimbria were identifiable.

The microphotographs obtained (Fig. 1 and 2) were reviewed by an expert embryologist:

"The specimen is most closely related to a stage 7 normal human embryo[1] with related membranes. This would give an estimated age of 15–17

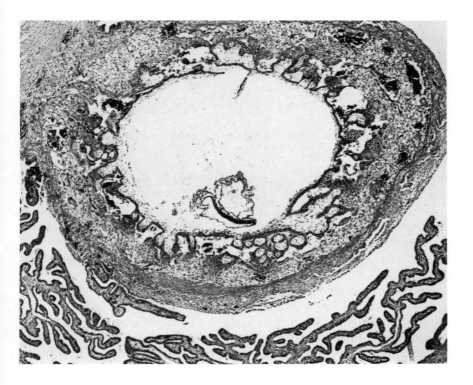

Fig. 1. Early tubal implantation. The implanting ovum has established contact with the uterine wall but the main direction of the growth is intraluminal. Note the presence of well developed chorionic villi in apparent contact with the fimbriae.

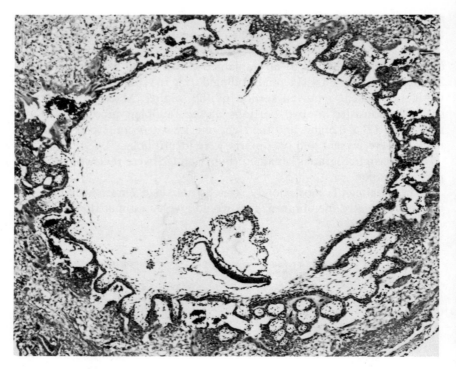

Fig. 2. Large magnification of the implanting ectopic embryo shown in Fig. 1.

days when compared to specimens implanted in the uterine wall. The chorionic villi appeared to be approximately this age.

The characteristic feature of stage 7 is the presence of the notochord process. Although this process is not evident in the section, I would classify it as stage 7 specimen based on the characteristics of its yolk sac wall (angioblastic tissue differentiating) and the advanced formation of chorionic villi.''

Another section through the embryonic disc confirmed the estimated age as approximately 17 days (Fig. 3). These data suggest that conception took place very early in the intermenstrual cycle. The significance of the time of conception with regard to the existing etiologic theories of tubal implantation has been discussed in recent editions of gynecologic textbooks.[2,3]

ACKNOWLEDGMENT

The author and the editors wish to record their gratitude to Dr. Raymond F. Gasser of New Orleans for the embryologic evaluation of the specimen presented in this paper.

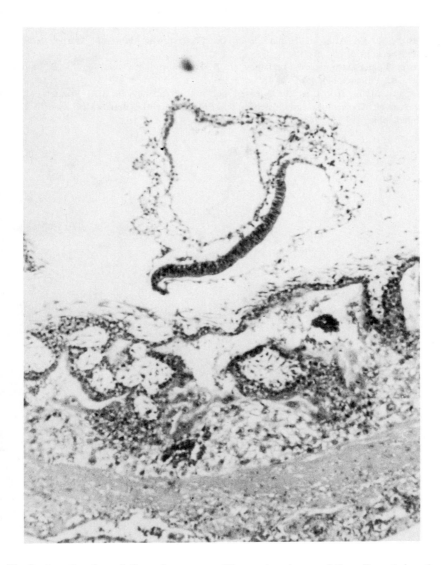

Fig. 3. A section through the embryo proper. The amnion above and the yolk sac below the mebryonic disc are well formed and clearly shown. Chorionic villi in close contact with the wall of the fallopian tube. The specimen corresponds with State 7 (Horizon VII) of early human development; probably the earliest complete tubal embryonic specimen on record.

REFERENCES

1. Gasser, R. F.: Atlas of Human Embryos. Hagerstown, Maryland, Harper & Row Publishers, 1975.
2. Carter, F. B.: Extra-uterine Pregnancy. In: R. T. Kimbrough: Gynecology, J. B. Lippincott Co., Philadelphia, 1965 (p. 435).
3. Wingate, M. B., Iffy, L. et al.: Diseases Specific to Pregnancy. In: S. L. Romney, M. J. Gray, et al.: Gynecology and Obstetrics. The Health Care of Women. McGraw-Hill Inc., Philadelphia, 1975 (p. 713).

18

Intrafollicular Ovarian Gestation

MILIVOJE MILOSEVIC, M.D.
AND
ILONA R. TOTH, M.D.

The pathological mechanism by which the fertilized ovum takes root in the ovary has been a controversial issue. It is generally believed that when the products of conception develop inside the graafian follicle, the mechanism is intrafollicular fertilization of an ovum. It has been suggested that the etiology might even involve parthenogenetic development of a retained ovum. Actually, the presumed mechanism of fertilization within the graafian follicle rests upon as yet unproved assumptions. In contrast, the alternative mechanism of ovarian implantation—superficial imbedding of an ovum fertilized presumably in the fallopian tube—has been demonstrated conclusively by the unique case of Dougherty.[1]

Cases of ovarian gestation are rare, and extensive destruction of the surrounding tissues usually obliterates all clues relevant to the mechanism of implantation. The forthcoming two cases which provide a relatively undisturbed picture of the anatomic relations of the ova developed within the graafian follicle are of obvious academic interest.

Case 1.   A 20-year-old nulligravida (H.N.) was hospitalized as an acute abdominal emergency 7 weeks after her last menstrual period. The patient's general condition in the presence of blood obtained by culdocentesis from the peritoneal cavity necessitated an immediate laparotomy on the basis of suspected ruptured tubal pregnancy. On operation the uterus and fallopian tubes were found to be entirely normal. However, the left ovary was enlarged and cystic and a bleeding point was visible on its surface corresponding to the site of the corpus luteum. The corpus luteum was removed *in toto* by wedge resection and the specimen was submitted for pathological evaluation.

Pathology Report-Case 1. Gross examination of the ovarian wedge (1.1 x 1.5 cm) exhibits the yellowish cut surface of the corpus luteum with a rim of firmer, whitish ovarian tissue. The center is formed by a collapsed blood-containing cavity. Serial sections of the submitted tissue reveal the presence of a hemorrhagic mass incorporated within partly well-preserved and avascular and partly necrotic or degenerating chorionic villi. The cyst is surrounded by decidual cells and proliferating sheets of syncytiotrophoblast. The chorionic implant is almost surrounded by pale-colored masses of cells representing the corpus luteum of pregnancy.

Neither amniotic sac nor embryo is identifiable. The diagnosis is consistent with ovarian pregnancy of the juxta-follicular type (Fig. 1).

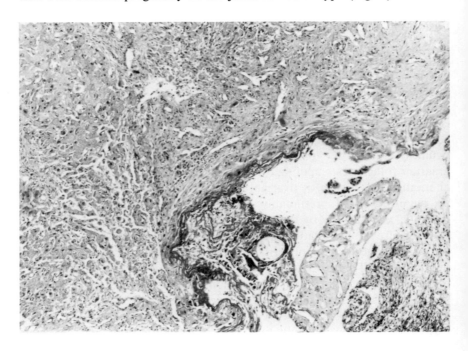

Fig. 1. Ovarian pregnancy.

Case 2. Under circumstances somewhat similar to those in Case 1, a 22-year-old nulligravida (M.A.) was admitted in a state of shock. The history indicated that she had had a normal menstrual period only 20 days prior to her admission. The culdocentesis yielded 5 ml. of bright red blood, and the general clinical picture was considered compatible with a ruptured ectopic pregnancy of a bleeding corpus luteum cyst. An emergency laparotomy revealed an intact uterus and fallopian tubes. The right ovary was enlarged and cystic in appearance and the bleeding point was recognizable on the surface of a cystic corpus luteum. The latter was removed by wedge resection.

Pathology Report-Case 2. The ruptured cystic area on the surface of the ovary is covered by decidual cells and several chorionic villi. The villi appear swollen and hyperplastic. The rest of the specimen presents the regular structure of the cystic corpus luteum. The ovarian stroma is edematous and scattered luteal cells are recognizable throughout the several sections.

Diagnosis: Ruptured ovarian (corpus luteum) pregnancy (Figs. 2 and 3).

DISCUSSION

It has been pointed out that ovarian pregnancy resembles many of the features of other types of ectopic implantation. Prominent among these is the occurrence of a menstrual bleeding episode following fertilization.[2]

Since no embryo has been discovered in these cases, the exact length of the gestation and thus the time of fertilization cannot be defined unequivocally. However, the fact that only 20 days after the occurrence of an apparently normal menstruation, well-developed chorionic villi were found inside the corpus luteum, and the chorionic invasion was extensive enough to induce profuse homorrhage (estimated as approximately 1,500 ml), makes it virtually certain that the time of conception had preceded the last menstrual episode.

The exact mechanism of nidation remains unresolved. However, the histological picture is compatible in both cases with a presumed mechanism of superficial implantation.

The cases described above fulfill all of the criteria of Spiegelberg[3] for primary ovarian pregnancy:

A. The tubes on either side were intact.

B. Chorionic invasion was restricted to the ovary.

C. The ovary maintained its connection with the uterus and with the ovarian ligament.

D. The chorionic villi were implanted upon ovarian tissue (in actual fact that of the corpus luteum) entirely.

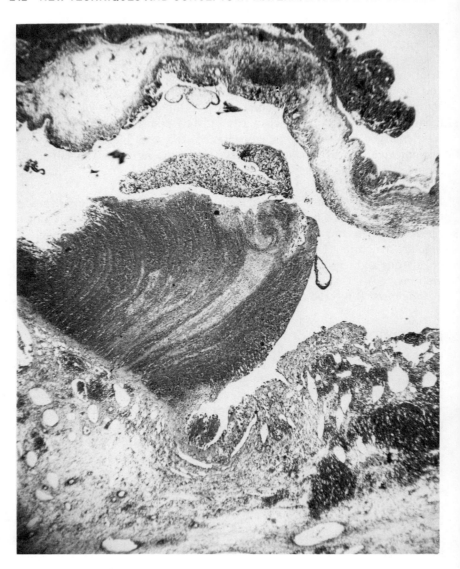

Fig. 2. Ruptured ovarian pregnancy.

While both cases fulfilled the criteria of primary follicular gestation (generally attributed to intrafollicular fertilization), we find it necessary to reiterate that the existence of this mechanism is still unproven. Indeed, there is evidence to indicate that a ruptured graafian follicle offers a *locus minoris resistentiae* to a variety of potential invaders such as: pathogen

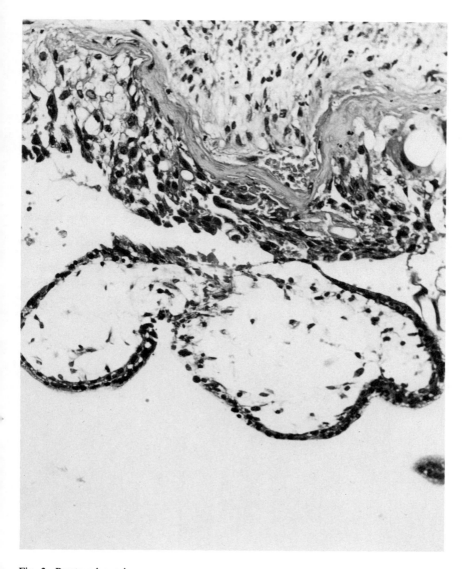

Fig. 3. Ruptured ovarian pregnancy.

microorganisms, cancer cells, as well as endometrium cells displaced from the uterine cavity by the menstrual reflux.[4] The development of ovarian implantation in the cases presented here appears conceivable by a comparable mechanism.

It is worthy of note that neither of these patients had an intrauterine device (IUD) implanted, nor did they suffer from pelvic inflammatory disease.

The standard treatment of ovarian pregnancy is salpingoophorectomy; however, it has been suggested that when the involvement of the ovary is not extensive, conservative surgery should be attempted (retention of the ovary). In the cases reported, the invasion of the chorionic villi was limited to the corpus luteum, thus permitting a limited surgery by wedge resection. Undoubtedly, this is the management of choice when circumstances permit conservation of the uninvolved ovarian tissue.

REFERENCES

1. Dougherty, C. M. *Surgical Pathology of Gynecologic Disease.* New York, Harper & Row, 1968, p. 516.
2. Iffy, L. Contribution to the pathological mechanism of ovarian, abdominal and cervical pregnancies. *Gynaecologia* (Basel) **153:** 188–204, 1962.
3. Spiegelberg, O. Zur Casuistik der Ovarialschwangerschaft, Arch. Gynäk. **13:** 73, 1878.
4. Sampson, J. A. The life history of ovarian hematomas (hemorrhagic cysts) of the endometrial type. *Am. J. Obstet. Gynecol.* **4:** 451, 1922.

19

Some Considerations in the Management of Hypertensive Disorders in Pregnancy

LEON C. CHESLEY, PH.D.

If we knew the cause of preeclampsia-eclampsia, we might be able to prevent it or evolve a rational management for it. Many treatments have been tried in the past utilizing almost every known drug, including strychnine; several surgical approaches have also been tried.

Cows sometimes develop parturient paresis: it is now known that a severe depletion of calcium is a major causative factor in this condition. In 1897 a Danish veterinarian discovered that injecting the udder with potassium iodide ameliorated the disease. Several German obstetricians promptly tried the measure in eclamptic women. One day the veterinarian was caught without his potassium iodide and instead blew air into the teats. It stopped lactation and cured the cow. Suspecting a similarity between parturient paresis and human eclampsia, Sellheim,[1] in 1910, tried variations of air insufflation in some of his patients. The breasts were resistant to inflation, so he excised them. His high prestige led several others to try bilateral mastectomy but the results, medically and cosmetically, were unsatisfactory.

At the turn of the century postpartum curettage was used in the management of puerperal psychosis, based on the hypothesis that the causative agent was contained in the decidua or retained trophoblast. In 1908 it occurred to Latzko[2] that the eclamptic toxin might have the same source, so he used postpartum curettage in the treatment of eclampsia. Papers appeared from several clinics over the next five years, but the method fell into disuse until Hunter, Howard, and McCormick[3] revived it in 1961.

In 1903 Edebohls[4] reported the use of renal decapsulation based on the hypothesis that eclamptic oliguria and disturbed renal function might depend upon edema of the renal parenchyma with compression of the kidney by its unyielding capsule. Sitzenfrey[5] reviewed the literature in 1910 and found a mortality rate of 39.6 percent in 58 recorded cases, which was about twice the prevailing rate in eclampsia at that time.

Zangemeister[6] thought cerebral edema to be the cause, and in 1911 he reported that he had opened the skulls of three living eclamptic women. Wieloch,[7] in 1927, used cisternal puncture for the same reason, and drainage of spinal fluid by lumbar puncture was in wide use when I came into the field 44 years ago. Other surgical procedures have included oophorectomy, ventral suspension of the uterus, ureteral catheterization, and implantation of the ureters into the intestine.

Bizarre as these methods may seem to us, it is important to remember that each was rational in the light of some hypothesis as to the cause and nature of eclampsia. That is more than we can say about our present management, which is empiric, too often symptomatic, and in some respects, based upon what appears to be imitative magic. As an example, recovery from eclampsia is associated with hemodilution and diuresis. Is not the obstetrician practicing imitative magic when he administers fluids to dilute the blood and gives diuretic drugs? The spontaneous hemodilution and diuresis occur because the disease is abating and not the converse.

DIURETIC DRUGS

Then as now, each new treatment was introduced with enthusiastic assertions. In 1958, Finnerty, Buckholz, and Tuckman[8] reported sensational results with chlorothiazide (Diuril[R]) and acetazolamide (Diamox[R]), although their results seem to be unconfirmed. They treated 16 women with severe preeclampsia and all responded with marked decreases in blood pressure and proteinuria; 6 became normal and were discharged from the hospital before delivery. Finnerty changed his emphasis in all of his later papers, indicating that the diuretic drugs prevent the progression of incipient preeclampsia to its hypertensive phase, but are ineffective once the blood pressure has risen.

However, several double-blind studies indicate that diuretic drugs do not prevent preeclampsia. For example, Kraus, Marchese, and Yen[9] administered hydrochlorothiazide 50 mg per day to 195 nulliparas, beginning before the 24th week of gestation and continuing until delivery. A placebo was given to 210 nulliparas in the double-blind study. The incidence of later preeclampsia in each group was 6.67 percent; one patient more or less in either group would have spoiled the beautiful symmetry.

As for the treatment of preeclampsia, MacGillivray and co-workers[10] found that thiazide diuretic agents elicited losses of sodium, water, edema and weight, but they could discern no beneficial effect upon the course of the disease. The drug did what it was designed to do and controlled a sign without modifying the basic disorder. Salerno, Stone, and Ditchick[11] observed that 11 of 24 preeclamptic women apparently became worse under treatment with clorothiazide.

If diuretic drugs do not prevent preeclampsia and do not have a favorable effect upon the course of the disorder, why use them?

Edema alone has almost always been the indication for which obstetricians have prescribed diuretic drugs. However, several studies have shown that generalized edema is physiologic and occurs in a high percentage of normal pregnancies. Moreover, in the absence of preeclampsia, infants born of women with edema of the hands and face weigh more at birth than do infants born of nonedematous women. It is not that the infants share in the edema, for they do not lose excessive weight following birth.

Robertson[12] studied 83 women prospectively from early pregnancy; 69, or 83 percent, developed visible edema and the others had occult edema as shown by progressive increases in the volumes of their legs and circumferences of their ankles and fingers. Two-thirds had edema of the hands or face at some time. Robertson could find no relation between the degree or distribution of the edema and the development of preeclampsia.

Edema of the hands or face has long been accepted as an early sign of preeclampsia, but the belief stems from retrospective studies of charts of women with preeclampsia. When one goes back over the medical record looking for premonitory signs, in about half of the cases one finds that the patient's wedding ring fitted tightly at perhaps the 30th week of gestation; thus edema of the fingers pointed to oncoming preeclampsia! But how many such studies have included reviews of the records of women with normal pregnancies? None that I know of. The edema at thirty weeks may have been physiologic and had nothing to do with preeclampsia. The prevalence of such edema is higher in preeclampsia than in normal pregnancy and the edema often is more severe in preeclampsia, but the overlap is so broad that differentiation of physiologic from early preeclamptic edema may not be possible. In the recent past, the obstetricians' indiscriminate use of diuretic drugs has not been effective in preventing or treating preeclampsia; in most cases it has been directed against a physiologic change. In general, tampering with physiologic processes is not likely to be beneficial. In addition, there are specific contraindications to the use of diuretic drugs in pregnant women, and especially in those with preeclampsia or chronic hypertension; I have listed ten in an earlier publication.[13]

It is generally assumed that placental function is impaired in the hypertensive disorders of pregnancy. Gant and co-workers[14] have proved it by finding an average reduction of about 50 percent in the placental conversion of dehydroisoandrosterone to estradiol. Moreover, they have shown that the administration of a thiazide or furosemide reduces placental function by another 50 percent.[14] Why aggravate a significant abnormality already present in preeclampsia? One of the first effects of any diuretic agent is to reduce the plasma volume, thus augmenting another abnormality already present in preeclampsia, which appears even before the onset of hypertension.

The use of diuretic drugs in pregnant women is justified only in the presence of such medical emergencies as cardiac failure, pulmonary edema, or imminent acute renal failure.

ANTIHYPERTENSIVE DRUGS

Uncontrolled chronic hypertension is associated with vascular damage and cardiac hypertrophy, and greatly increases the risks of cardiac failure, cerebral hemorrhage, and sometimes of renal failure. In long-term studies, reduction of blood pressure by antihypertensive drugs has proved to be beneficial in nonpregnant patients with chronic hypertension, but their use during pregnancy has been controversial.

Many physicians in the past have regarded hypertension as compensatory and necessary for an adequate flow of blood to vital organs. However, most hypertension depends upon arteriolar constriction, and if it is reduced specifically, the resistance to flow decreases and perfusion is maintained at lower pressures. The effect upon placental blood flow is an important consideration in deciding whether to reduce the blood pressures of pregnant women with hypertensive disorders; however, this effect is unknown. The maternal blood supply of the human placenta is delivered by the spiral arteries, rather than by arterioles. The distal portions of the spiral arteries have lost their elastic tissue and the muscle is greatly modified, so that they appear to be loose and perhaps passive channels.

Dixon, Brown, and Davey[15] measured the time to disappearance of half of the initial radioactivity (T $\frac{1}{2}$) of ^{24}Na injected transparietally into the placenta, as an index of placental blood flow. They found T$\frac{1}{2}$ to be prolonged in women with preeclampsia and chronic hypertension. Antihypertensive drugs may have decreased the blood flow, for the authors wrote " . . . the longest T½ both before and after term were obtained in patients who had become normotensive after receiving Veriloid or Rauwiloid." Gant and co-workers[14] observed that the placental conversion of dehydroisoandrosterone to estradiol is decreased when preeclamptic or normal pregnant women are given antihypertensive drugs; although that points to impairment of placental function, the effect on blood flow is uncertain.

The anatomic changes in the maternal arteries supplying the placental bed in women with chronic hypertension or preeclampsia pose a mechanical impediment to blood flow[16] and reduction of the arterial pressure might aggravate the situation. Thus, the scanty evidence available suggests a possibly adverse effect of reductions in blood pressure upon uterine blood flow.

Findings in laboratory animals may be relevant, although they are contradictory. The uterine blood flow of normal pregnant sheep varies in strict proportion with the mean arterial pressure.[17,18] In pregnant sheep with Goldblatt hypertension, the uterine blood flow is somewhat decreased during the first week of hypertension, but thereafter returns to normal. Reduction of the blood pressure with diazoxide (Hyperstat[R]) decreases uterine perfusion markedly,[19] as it does in normotensive sheep, [20] and monkeys.[21]

De Swiet and Hoffbrand[22] measured the uterine blood flow in unanesthetized pregnant rabbits by the injection of radioactive microspheres and found it to be dependent upon the perfusional pressure. Venuto et al.[23] using the same method in anesthetized pregnant rabbits, reported that the uterine blood flow was essentially constant over a wide range of arterial pressures; that is, the flow seemed to be autoregulated. Are the opposite findings explained by the use of anesthesia? If so, it seems strange that a presumably advantageous autoregulation of the uterine perfusion should be observed during anesthesia and not be present in the unmodified natural state.

Work with rabbits in Ferris' laboratory,[23] with dogs in the Terragnos' laboratory,[24] and with monkeys in Speroff's laboratory[21] indicates that the perfusion of the pregnant uterus may be modified or even regulated by the local effects of angiotensin and prostaglandin E (PGE). Infusions of angiotensin increase the uterine blood flow, even though the hormone is the most potent vasoconstrictive agent known, and the infusion greatly augments the amount of PGE in the uterine venous blood. PGE is a vasodilating agent which inhibits and possibly outweighs the constrictive effect of angiotensin. Infusion of inhibitors of prostaglandin synthetase, such as indomethacin or meclofenamate, reduces the output of PGE and results in a decrease in uterine blood flow, with an increase in systemic arterial pressure. Autoregulation of blood flow in the pregnant uterus of the rabbit may not depend entirely on the angiotensin-PGE system, for Venuto et al.[23] reported that the perfusion is essentially constant over a wide range of hypotension in animals given inhibitors of prostaglandin synthetase.

All of the above observations in rabbits, dogs and monkeys were made in anesthetized animals. Their significance, therefore, is questionable, because anesthesia modifies vascular responses. Assali, Brinkman, and Nuwayhid[25] reported that although angiotensin increases uterine blood flow in pregnant sheep anesthetized with various agents, it has the opposite effect in unanesthetized ewes, with rather marked reductions in uterine perfusion. Harbert, Cornell, and Thornton[26] found angiotensin to decrease the uterine blood flow significantly in conscious monkeys. Moreover, if PGE is produced in the human uterus, what can be the site of its vasodilating action? No arterioles are interposed between the spiral arteries and the intervillous space of the placenta.

Ramsey[27] has observed intermittent constriction of individual arteries in the innermost layer of the myometrium, sufficient to reduce or shut off the blood flow to the intervillous space. Inasmuch as the myometrium synthesizes renin, it is possible that angiotensin and PGE are produced and act locally on the myometrial arteries. Chorionic tissue also produces renin, and one could speculate that it uses the angiotensin-PGE system to ensure an adequate flow of blood to itself. But what would be the site of vasodilatation? The PGE probably does not recirculate to the myometrium, because most of it is removed from the blood on a single transit through the lungs. Bay, Greenspan, and Ferris[28] have found increased levels of PGE in the peripheral venous blood during late pregnancy, but its source is unknown.

Thus, we cannot rationalize with any certainty the use of antihypertensive drugs on the basis of their improving the life line to the fetus. The next step is to consider the effect of the drugs on fetal salvage. Several papers have reported no improvement, but no worsening either. More recently, control of hypertension by methyldopa (Aldomet[R]) has been said to have a favorable effect in women with chronic hypertension.

CHRONIC HYPERTENSION

Kincaid-Smith, Bullen and Mills[29] treated 32 pregnant hypertensive women with methyldopa for from 3 to 6 months, with an average reduction in blood pressure of 35/24 mm Hg. The incidence of superimposed preeclampsia (38%) was not decreased by the treatment, nor was its course modified favorably. The perinatal loss of 9.3 percent was lower than had been expected on the basis of earlier experience.

Leather and associates[30] administered methyldopa and a diuretic drug to 22 women with hypertension before the 20th week of gestation, and by random assignment, followed 24 others as controls. Three late abortions and two perinatal deaths occurred in the controls, with none in the treated groups. They added to their study almost equal numbers of women whose blood pressures had been normal in midpregnancy and who later developed hypertension. Overall, the perinatal loss was six cases in each of the control and treated groups.

Redman and co-workers[31] selected women whose blood pressures ranged between 140/90 and 170/110 before the end of the second trimester. They treated 101 with methyldopa, or hydralazine if the methyldopa was ineffective, and followed 107 as controls. They usually induced labor at 38 weeks of gestation. There were four late abortions in the control group, and none in the treated group. Among the controls there was one stillbirth and one neonatal death from an intracranial hemorrhage associated with a precipitous delivery. There was one stillbirth associated with superimposed preeclampsia in the treated group. The incidences of superimposed preeclampsia were about the same in the two groups and, as in the study by Leather et al.,[30] the slightly improved rate of fetal salvage is accounted for by fewer late abortions.

Although some authors advocate treatment of any blood pressure in excess of 140/90, we use antihypertensive drugs only if the diastolic pressure is maintained at 110 mm Hg or higher. We try to keep the diastolic pressure between 90 and 100 mm Hg. However, if the hypertension is severe, initially, we do not attempt to lower it quickly by more than 25 percent. We virtually never use diuretic drugs and that lessens the efficacy of the other antihypertensive agents. If the hypertensive woman is under treatment when she first comes to the obstetric clinic, we continue the medication, but stop the diuretic drug. In initiating treatment, we admit the patient to the hospital. If she is close to term, we usually start with hydralazine, 10 mg t.i.d., and increase the dose as needed. If the response is not satisfactory, or if she is far from term, we begin with methyldopa, again building up the divided doses, as needed, to as much as 2 g/day.

PREECLAMPTIC HYPERTENSION

Quite arbitrarily, we use antihypertensive agents only when the diastolic pressure exceeds 110 mm Hg. Preeclamptic hypertension seems to be more responsive than are renal and essential hypertension to hydralazine, and we use this drug almost exclusively. We start with 10 mg intravenously; if the diastolic pressure does not fall to between 90 and 100 mm Hg within 20 minutes, we repeat the dose. Usually the first dose, or the first and second doses are effective. If not, the doses are increased at intervals of 20 minutes. We seldom temporize with severe preeclampsia, but if the patient is far from term and if we do postpone delivery, we wean her from intravenous hydralazine while giving it orally.

Some now advocate the use of diazoxide and furosemide for the rapid reduction of hypertension in pregnancy. It is an unsatisfactory combination. Inasmuch as diazoxide is quickly bound by plasma proteins, it must be injected rapidly to be effective. In my opinion, the necessity for lowering blood pressure is seldom so urgent as to call for the irretrievable injection of an arbitrary dose of a potent agent that suddenly lowers the blood pressure, sometimes to shock levels. Diazoxide arrests labor and, as previously mentioned, reduces the uterine blood flow markedly.

Morishima et al.[32] observed that newborn guinea pigs were severely depressed and acidotic following administration of diazoxide to the mothers. They continued the study, using monkeys and baboons with spontaneous or induced labor. Diazoxide produced tachycardia, prolonged hypotension, and acidosis in the fetuses. Diazoxide has an antidiuretic effect, and furosemide is frequently administered with it. Speroff and coworkers[21] observed that a single injection of furosemide causes a progessive decrease in uterine blood flow of the pregnant monkey, with a fall of approximately 85 percent by 40 minutes.

THE MANAGEMENT OF SEVERE PREECLAMPSIA
AND ECLAMPSIA

The only rational management is one empirically proven to be effective. The objectives are to prevent convulsions in women with preeclampsia, to arrest them in women with eclampsia, and to deliver an undamaged, surviving infant.

Pritchard[33] has achieved a record unmatched in the history of eclampsia, using only magnesium sulfate, sometimes hydralazine, and delivery. He reported a series of 154 consecutive cases of eclampsia without a maternal death (which he extended to 179 before an accident befell the next patient). Excluding postpartum cases, in antenatal eclampsia the uncorrected perinatal loss was 15.4 percent, with more than half having had no detectable fetal heart beat when treatment was begun; excluding infants weighing less than 1,000 g, the perinatal loss was 9.9 percent. Every infant survived who weighed 1,800 g or more and whose fetal heart beat was heard at the beginning of treatment. For comparison, the maternal mortality in eclampsia has ranged up to 70 percent in the past and is now from 5 to 10 percent in leading clinics. The perinatal mortality in antenatal eclampsia varies greatly, but a common level is from 25 to 40 percent.

Pritchard's method sets a standard against which any other must be measured. In the past, misguided management and overtreatment probably have cost more lives than has the disease itself. Pritchard uses no diuretic drugs, no sedative agents (except in labor, as in any patient), no mannitol, no hypertonic dextrose, no albumin, and no heparin. Except in women with diastolic pressures exceeding 110 mm Hg, magnesium sulfate is the only agent used. Proof that any other method is better must entail testing in at least 200 cases of eclampsia and, despite the internists' enthusiasm for new drugs in preference to oldfashioned magnesium sulfate, the new drugs are potentially hazardous for both mother and fetus.

Recently there have been reports of the use of dazepam (Valium[R]) as an anticonvulsant agent in the management of preeclampsia-eclampsia. It seems to be less efficacious than magnesium sulfate in stopping eclamptic convulsions. Moreover, there are reports of adverse effects upon the infant. Cree, Meyer, and Hailey,[34] for instance, found that the newborn infant cannot metabolize diazepam and has significant circulating levels of the drug for eight days after birth. The Apgar scores often were depressed and some of the infants required endotracheal intubation. Many were hypotonic and even flaccid for up to two days, while some had to be fed by tube because of suppression of the sucking reflex. Thermogenesis was also impaired.

A generation ago, many obstetricians treated threatened abortion with "safe" diethylstilbestrol. We now know that many young women who were exposed to the drug as fetuses have developed abnormalities of the vaginal epithelium, with an occasional clear cell carcinoma. The internist forgets that the obstetrician is dealing with two patients with a combined life expectancy of more than a century.

Some observations contradict the hypothesis that PGE increases the uterine blood flow. Speroff and co-workers[35] found the inhibition of prostaglandin synthetase to increase, rather than to decrease, the uterine blood flow in three of four pregnant monkeys. Gerber et al.[36] observed that a large proportion of radioactive microspheres injected into the left cardiac ventricles of pregnant dogs are trapped in the pulmonary capillaries; that is, they had traversed a shunt. When the uterine circulation was excluded, few microspheres appeared in the lungs; that is, the shunt is in the pregnant uterus. Inasmuch as the hemochorial placenta has no capillaries (or even arterioles), the shunt appears to be the intervillous space. Gerber et al. estimated the placental blood flow from the radioactivity in the placenta plus that in the lungs in six dogs, and measured the uterine blood flow with an electromagnetic flow meter in 2; they found that indomethacin increased the flow by 37 percent, rather than decreasing it as Terragno et al.[24] had reported. The indomethacin almost completely blocked the release of PGE. PGE increases intrauterine pressure by augmenting myometrial tonus, which, in turn, compresses myometrial blood vessels. Gerber et al observed that the increase in uterine blood flow elicited by indomethacin is associated with a decrease in intrauterine pressure.

The only experiments indicating autoregulation of uterine blood flow are those in which radioactive microspheres of 15 micrometers in diameter were used in rabbits for the estimation of the flow. Gerber et al. point out that those experiments indicated that only about 5 percent of the cardiac output goes to the pregnant uterus, whereas other methods show the cardiac fraction to be 15 percent or more.

ACKNOWLEDGMENT

This chapter has been based, in parts, on a report in the December 1977 issue of *Resident and Staff Physician*. The permission of the Publisher to reproduce parts of the quoted article is gratefully acknowledged.

REFERENCES

1. Sellheim, H. Die mammäre Theorie über Entstehung des Eklampsiegiftes. *Zbl. Gynäkol.* **34:** 1609–1615, 1910.
2. Latzko, W. Naturforscherversammlung zu Cöln, 1908. Cited by Heinze, H. Ein Beitrag zur Therapie der Eklampsie. Arch, Gynäkol. **93:** 151–187, 1911.
3. Hunter, C A, Jr., Howard, W F et al. Amelioration of the hypertension of toxemia by postpartum curettage. *Amer. J. Obstet. Gynecol.* **81:** 884, 1961.
4. Edebohls, G M. Renal decapsulation for puerperal eclampsia. *N.Y. Med. J.* **77:** 1022, 1903.
5. Sitzenfrey, A. Die Nierenenthülsung mit besonderer Berücksichtigung ihre Anwendung bei Eklampsie. *Beitr. Klin. Chir.* **67:** 129, 1910.
6. Zangemeister, W. Beitrag zur Auffassung und Behandlung der Eklampsie. *Deutsche Med. Wchschr.* **37:** 1879, 1911.
7. Wieloch: Zur Behandlung des präeklamptischen und eklamptischen Stadiums durch Suboccipitalstich nebst Druckmessung. *Arch. Gynäkol.* **132:** 296, 1927.
8. Finnerty, F A, Jr., Buckholz, J H and Tuckman, J. Evaluation of chlorothiazide (Diuril) in the toxemias of pregnancy. *JAMA* **166:** 141, 1958.
9. Kraus, G W, Marchese, J R and Yen, SSC. Prophylactic use of hydrochlorothiazide in pregnancy. *JAMA* **198:** 1150, 1966.
10. MacGillivray, I, Hytten F E et al. The effect of a sodium diuretic on total exchangeable sodium and total body water in preeclamptic toxaemia. *J. Obstet Gynaecol. Br. Commonw.* **69:** 458, 1962.
11. Salerno, L J, Stone, M L and Ditchik, P. A clinical evaluation of chlorothiazide in prevention and treatment of toxemia of pregnancy. *Obstet. Gynecol.* **14:** 188, 1959.
12. Robertson, E G. The natural history of oedema during pregnancy. *J. Obstet. Gynaecol. Br. Commonw.* **78:** 520, 1971.
13. Chesley, L C. Hypertensive Disorders in Pregnancy. New York, Appleton-Century-Crofts, 1977.
14. Gant, N F, Madden, J D et al. The metabolic clearance rate of dehydroisoandrosterone

sulfate. IV. Acute effect of induced hypertension, hypotension, and natriuresis in normal and hypertensive pregnancies. *Amer. J. Obstet. Gynecol.* **124**: 143, 1976.

15. Dixon, H G, Browne, J C M et al. Choriodecidual and myometrial blood-flow *Lancet* **2**: 369, 1963.

16. Brosens, I A, Robertson, W B et al. The role of the spiral arteries in the pathogenesis of preeclampsia. *In* Wynn, R M. (Ed.) *Obstet. Gynecol. Ann* **1**: 177, 1972.

17. Griess, F. Pressure flow relationship in the gravid uterine vascular bed. *Amer. J. Obstet. Gynecol.* **96**: 41, 1966.

18. Ladner, C, Brinkman, C R, III, et al. Dynamics of uterine circulation in pregnant and nonpregnant sheep. *Amer. J. Physiol.* **218**: 257, 1970.

19. Brinkman, C R, III, and Assali, N S. Uteroplacental hemodynamic response to antihypertensive drugs in hypertensive pregnant sheep. *In* Lindheimer, MD, Katz, AI and Zuspan, FP. (Eds.) Hypertension in Pregnancy. New York, John Wiley & Sons, 1976, pp. 363–373.

20. Caritis, S, Morishima H O et al. The effect of diazoxide on uterine blood flow in pregnant sheep. *Obstet. Gynecol.* **48**: 464, 1976.

21. Speroff, L, Haning, R V, Jr. et al. Uterine artery blood flow studies in the pregnant monkey. *In* Lindheimer, MD. Katz, AI. and Zuspan, FP. (Eds.) Hypertension in Pregnancy. New York, John Wiley & Sons, 1976, pp. 315–326.

22. De Swiet, M. and Hoffbrand, B I. Effect of bethanidine on placental blood flow in conscious rabbits. *Amer. J. Obstet. Gynecol.* **111**: 374, 1971.

23. Venuto, R C, Cox, J W. et al. Effect of changes in perfusion pressure on uteroplacental blood flow in pregnant rabbits. *J. Clin. Invest.* **57**: 938, 1976.

24. Terragno, N A; Terragno, D A et al. Prostaglandins and the regulation of uterine blood flow in pregnancy. Nature **249**: 57, 1974.

25. Assali, N S; Brinkman C R, III, et al. Comparison of maternal and fetal cardiovascular functions in acute and chronic experiments in sheep. *Amer. J. Obstet. Gynecol.* **120**: 411, 1974.

26. Harbert, G M, Jr., Cornell, G W. et al. Effect of toxemia therapy on uterine dynamics. *Amer. J. Obstet. Gynecol.* **105**: 94, 1969.

27. Ramsey, E. M. Vascular anatomy. *In* Wynn, R M. (Ed.) Biology of the Uterus. New York, Plenum Press, 1977, pp. 59–76.

28. Bay, W H, Greenspan, R et al. Factors controlling plasma renin and aldosterone in pregnancy. *Circ. Res.* (In press).

29. Kincaid-Smith, P., Bullen, H. et al. Prolonged use of methyldopa in severe hypertension in pregnancy. *Brit. Med. J.* **1**: 274, 1966.

30. Leather, H M; Humphreys, D M. et al. A controlled trial of hypertensive agents in hypertension in pregnancy. *Lancet* **2**: 488, 1968.

31. Redman, C W G; Beilin, L J. et al. Fetal outcome in trial of antihypertensive treatment in pregnancy. *Lancet* **2**: 753, 1976.

32. Morishima, H O, Cohen, H. et al. The inhibitory action of diazoxide on uterine activity in the subhuman primate: Placental transfer and effect on the fetus. *J. Perinat. Med.* **1**: 13, 1973.

33. Pritchard, J A. Standardized treatment of 154 consecutive cases of eclampsia. *Amer. J. Obstet. Gynecol.* **123**: 543, 1975.

34. Cree, J E, Meyer, J. et al. Diazepam in labour: Its metabolism and effect on the clinical condition and thermogenesis of the newborn. *Brit. Med. J.* **4**: 251, 1973.

35. Speroff, L, Haning, R V, Jr. et al. Uterine artery blood flow studies in the pregnant monkey. *Perspect. Nephrol. Hyperten.* **5**: 315, 1976.

36. Gerber, J G, Branch, R A et al. Indomethacin is a placental vasodilator in the dog. *J. Clin. Invest.* **62**: 14, 1978.

20

Antepartum Heart Rate Monitoring

EDWARD GORDON, M.D.
AND
BARRY S. SCHIFRIN, M.D.

Of the many tests available for monitoring the fetus, the most longstanding and widely applied is ausculation. Heart tones were probably first described in 1650 by Marsak.[1] This technique of fetal surveillance was not generally applied, however, until the early 1800's with the publications of Meyer and DeKergaradec.[2] In the mid-1800's, Bodson described the signs of fetal distress as excessive frequency and great irregularity, while Kennedy emphasized that marked slowing of the fetal heart during contraction and slowness of return were signs of danger to the child.[3,4] Neither the technique of listening nor the criteria changed much over the ensuing century. As late as 1963, Cox stated that intermittent auscultation for a limited period of time would suffice to predict fetal distress and would provide enough time to prevent progression of fetal hypoxia.[5]

Despite its universal acceptance, the benefits of intermittent auscultation have never been documented. The technique has many obvious pitfalls: it is both intermittent and subjective. Counting errors may be considerable and listener bias may be extreme.[6] Subtle changes may be missed and obvious changes frequently do not correlate with disturbed fetal outcome. On the other hand, the disappearance of heart tones in a baby with a previously normal heart rate has been documented. These limitations were emphasized in a report from the collaborative project of the National Institute of Neurological Diseases and Stroke (NINDS) by Benson et al. In their report, based on over 25,000 deliveries, the authors concluded that auscultation of the fetal heart rate was of little value in the definition of early fetal distress.[7] While no comparable study of the value of auscultation during the antepartum period has been performed, it is reasonable to assume that in the absence of the stress of contractions, transient auscultation will be similarly unrewarding.

Increasingly, the stethoscope has been supplanted by electronic fetal monitors. In contrast to intermittent auscultation, such monitoring appears to provide reliable and reproducible information about fetal well-being during the antepartum period.[8] While these techniques have been applied to a large number of high-risk pregnancies, recent evidence suggests that they may ultimately play a role in routine antepartum surveillance.[9] The purpose of this chapter is to consider the role of antepartum fetal heart rate monitoring during pregnancy and to discuss in some detail the potential benefits and limitations of these techniques.

BASIS FOR TESTING

Electronic fetal monitoring during the antepartum period awaited the development of devices capable of counting fetal heart rate from the maternal abdominal wall. Also required was the availability of reliable and sensitive end points specific for asphyxial fetal compromise. The former was provided by the availability of ultrasound (Doppler) and microphonic techniques for counting the fetal heart rate from the maternal abdomen. One specific end point (late decelerations) was discovered in the course of the investigation of heart rate patterns during labor by Hon, Caldeyro-Barcia and others.[10,12] These authors, and others subsequently, showed that late decelerations in the heart rate pattern were indeed a reliable sign of fetal hypoxia. More recently, emphasis has been placed on the presence of variability and accelerations in the heart rate as signs of fetal well-being.[13] These developments have improved the sensitivity of testing, and even more importantly, have highlighted the limitations of intermittent auscultation. As has been shown, the more regular the fetal heart rate (i.e., the less the variability), the more ominous is the condition of the fetus. Out of these developments grew the two most widely used monitoring tests, the non-stress test (NST) and the contraction stress test (CST). While other tests have been proposed--such as the atropine transfer test and the exercise and hypoxemic stress tests--these have not achieved popular acceptance.[14]

EXTERNAL FHR MONITORING TECHNIQUES

Currently, there are three techniques for obtaining the FHR from the maternal abdominal wall. These include ultrasound, microphone, and the abdominal wall ECG. The basis for each technique, as well as the likelihood of satisfactory tracing and the potential quality of the tracing are elaborated in Table 1. It can be seen that ultrasound produces a satisfactory record most frequently and is the easiest to use. However, a number of influences restrict its accuracy. Ultrasound depends upon the detection of motion (Doppler effect). Optimally, only the fetal heart valve should be detected. But it is apparent that motion of the mother, maternal vessels, as well as movement of the fetus and the fetal heart may all be detected, confounding the signal. As a result, the ultrasound technique frequently introduces spurious amounts of beat to beat (short term) variability. For these reasons, we do not use variability (short term) as an end point in either the NST or the CST. Only long term changes, such as accelerations (NST) and decelerations (CST), are used.

External transducers frequently have a far more restricted range of counting than does the direct electrode applied to the fetal scalp during labor. With external techniques, heart rates above 160–180 bpm tend to be half-counted, while those below 60–70 bpm may in fact be double-counted.[15] Maternal obesity, excessive amniotic fluid or fetal/maternal movement can all compromise the quality of the tracing.

External Measurement of Uterine Activity

The relationship of changes in heart rate to the stress of uterine contraction is the cornerstone of the interpretation of fetal heart rate patterns. Contractions interfere with uterine blood flow in direct proportion to the amplitude and duration of the contraction.[16] Adequate registration of contractions is necessary if one is to appreciate the nature of the fetal response. In the past, the frequency and intensity of contractions were determined by

Table 1. Comparison of FHR Techniques.

TECHNIQUE	BASIS	POTENTIAL SATISFACTORY TRACINGS	POTENTIAL QUALITY
Ultrasound	Valve movement	1 (95%)	3
Phonocardiogram	Heart sounds	2 (80%)	2
FECG	ECG	3 (65%)	1

palpation of the maternal abdominal wall. This technique is highly subjective, not reproducible and requires the presence of an observer at all times. The electronic technique has supplanted manual palpation. Currently available tocotransducers allow continuous registration of uterine activity (and fetal movement) by responding to changes in the tension of the maternal abdominal wall overlying the uterus. If neither the belt holding the transducer nor the position of the mother is disturbed, such transducers can provide reliable information about the frequency and relative strength of uterine contractions. It is widely appreciated that the amplitude of the contraction on the recorder is in great measure determined by the tension of the encircling belt. It is apparent, therefore, that baseline uterine tone cannot be determined with this technique, although changes in tone can be appreciated if none of the variables mentioned above is changed. Similarly, the amplitude of the contraction under these circumstances is not absolute, and quantification of the amount of stress applied to the fetus is not determinable.

Indications For Testing[14]

Indications for antepartum testing include those conditions which carry the potential for utero-placental insufficiency. Among these the most common are hypertension, suspected post-maturity or intrauterine growth retardation (IUGR). Testing is similarly indicated in patients with abnormal findings on auscultation, or those in whom estriol values are abnormal. Recent studies by Schifrin and colleagues suggest that NST-CST testing may play a role in routine antepartum testing.[9]

Contraindications

There are no known contraindications to the NST. Contraindications to the CST include those conditions in which the induction of contractions with oxytocin might result in premature delivery (multiple gestation, threatened premature labor, etc.) or in suspected cases of placenta previa. Serious complications of testing are unusual. There are no known complications to NST. Uterine hypertonus has been seen in about 5 to 10 percent of CST patients infused with oxytocin, but serious fetal harm has not ben reported.[17] Nor has CST been implicated as a cause of premature delivery.[8]

Timing of Tests

In high risk pregnancies, testing is begun on clinical indication, but generally no earlier than 28 weeks of gestation. In the report by Schifrin et al.[9] testing was started on low risk patients beginning at about 32 to 34 weeks' gestation. Testing is usually repeated at weekly intervals. There has been an increasing tendency to test more frequently in diabetics and in those pregnancies longer than 44 weeks of gestational age.

Technique of Testing

Since both the non-stress test (NST) and the contraction stress test (CST) have many features in common, they will be described together. The patient is placed in a semi-recumbent position with moderate tilt in order to reduce the possibility of an aorto-caval compression. Testing is done in a quiet room free of distractions. While stretcher beds are used most commonly, testing is being carried out more often in recliner chairs with considerable increase in patient comfort. Blood pressure measurements should be obtained frequently, the first measurement being performed with the patient in either the lateral or the sitting position. Measurements are made every 10 to 15 minutes to provide early detection of supine hypotension. An FHR transducer, most commonly the ultrasound transducer, is applied to the maternal abdomen and adjusted for maximum signal quality. The tocotransducer is then applied over the fundus, or more satisfactorily, over a palpable fetal extremity. With the transducer in place, baseline heart rate and the frequency and intensity of contractions are determined, as are accelerations of decelerations in response to either contractions or fetal movement. While the tracing provides strong clues to the presence or absence of fetal movement, it is wise to have these confirmed by either manual palpation or by questioning the patient.

CLASSIFICATION OF ANTEPARTUM TESTS

The non-stress test (NST) attempts to define fetal well-being on the basis of the fetal heart rate response to fetal movement or contractions. A number of studies have demonstrated that when the fetal heart accelerates in response to fetal movement or uterine contractions, babies are invariably born in good condition. Those babies who fail to demonstrate this feature fare less well.[13]

The NST is poorly named. Although neither stress nor stimulus is applied externally, spontaneous fetal movement (FM) or uterine contractions (UC) represent provocative stimuli. Accelerations represent a highly complex response involving reflex CNS pathways and myocardial performance. The pathologic response of the NST, that is, the absence of accelerations, does not provide specific information about the type of fetal problem, if any. Both the FHR fluctuations and the transient accelerations with FM are reduced or absent when the fetal CNS is depressed by chronic drug usage (tranquilizers, narcotics, barbiturates), and in normal fetuses during periods of quiet sleep. The response of the CST is more specific. Late decelerations, in response to either spontaneous or induced UC, define compromise of placental respiratory function. This response is apparently far more primitive than the accelerations noted with movement. Late decelerations will develop in virtually all fetuses, anomalous or not, if sufficient hypoxia is present.[18]

Interpretation of NST

Successful NST tracings are classified as reactive, non-reactive, or sinusoidal according to Schifrin.[14] Although this classification includes rate and variability criteria, these have minimal impact on the interpretation of the NST. Decreased baseline variability tachycardia or bradycardia are not relevant end points of either the NST or the CST. The reactive test requires two accelerations of at least 15 bpm in amplitude and 15 seconds in duration usually associated with FM or UC. Table 2

The recording is carried out until two accelerations are observed within any 10-minute period. There is no minimal time limit. If a reactive pattern has not been recorded within 40 minutes, the test is deemed non-reactive. This time limit has been chosen because normal fetuses undergo rest/activity cycles of about 40 minutes in duration. The range of these cycles is quite variable, however. Within this 40 minutes stimulation of the baby and/or mother with sound or glucose may induce a reactive pattern. Irrespective of the duration of monitoring or the stimulus used, if accelerations are evoked, the test is regarded as reactive.

In the sinusoidal pattern, accelerations are absent and the baseline contains repetitive oscillations. This pattern has been observed in pathological

Table 2. Classification of NST.

PATTERN	DESCRIPTION			
	FHR	ACCELERATIONS		
		NUMBER IN 10 MIN.	AMPLITUDE BPM	DURATION SEC.
Reactive	110–150 bpm	≥ 2	≥ 15 bpm	≥ 15 sec.
Nonreactive	110–150 bpm	< 2	< 15 bpm	< 15 sec.
Sinusoidal	110–150 bpm	Absent	Oscillations superimposed on baseline freq. 2–5 cpm, amplitude 5–15 bpm.	

cases of Rhesus isoimmunization, fetal anemia, and maternal hypertension, but have also been seen in normal and anomalous fetuses and following narcotic administration to the mother.[19] In some instances, the sinusoidal pattern is short-lived and followed by reactive NST. In this setting the pattern should be regarded as reactive. At present it appears that a sinusoidal pattern should not be used as an indication for delivery by itself.

The reactive NST appears to be the most reliable sign of fetal well-being yet devised. On the other hand, the non-reactive NST is a poor predictor of unfavorable outcome. While this group contains a much higher incidence of abnormal babies than does the reactive group, the majority of those with non-reactive NST do well.[9]

CST Interpretation

The initial 15 minutes of recording are evaluated for uterine contractions (UC). If UC are less than 3 per 10 minutes and if late decelerations do not accompany UC, oxytocin is infused via a constant infusion pump into an existing intravenous line. The initial rate of infusion is about 0.5–1.0 milliunits (mU) per minute. Thereafter, the rate of infusion should be doubled every 20 minutes. Oxytocin should be discontinued as soon as a satisfactory test is obtained. Monitoring is continued until the UC have returned to baseline levels. Oxytocin is discontinued if contractions last longer than 90 seconds or if they are more frequent than 4 per 10 minutes. With this schedule, the incidence of hypertonus is about 7 percent. About half of these episodes of hypertonus are accompanied by fetal bradycardia.[20] We do not continue an oxytocin infusion longer than 1 hour after sufficient UC have been induced. Successful tests are classified as negative, positive, and equivocal

This scheme rests upon finding a "10 minutes window" which satisfies the criteria of a positive or negative test. Diagnosis of equivocal CST is made only in the absence of either a positive or negative window. According to this scheme, occasional decelerations or decelerations associated with hypertonus are disregarded in the presence of a subsequently negative window. On occasion, a positive window will develop as a result of uterine hypertonus. In this circumstance, the test should be regarded as equivocal rather than positive. The benefits of this scheme include a high incidence of negative tests (greater than 90%) and a very low incidence of both positive (3%) and equivocal (1%) test results[14] compared to those reported previously.[8]

Results of Testing

As can be seen, the majority of CST and NST test results reveal no fetal compromise. About 90 percent of tests are normal. Positive CST tests are found in about 3 percent of tests in recent series, but are higher in older reports. Variable decelerations are found more often than late decelerations, their incidence increasing with advancing gestation. They are usually seen in association with a reactive pattern. While they are frequently unexplained, they should stimulate a search for oligohydramnios.[21] Variable decelerations associated with non-reactive NST may be much more ominous than non-reactive NST alone, especially if the variable decelerations are repetitive and contain rebound accelerations.[22]

The frequency of unsatisfactory tests depends upon the technique of monitoring and other factors (see above).

False Results

The confidence in test results which predict normal is far greater than the confidence of the test results which suggest fetal compromise. False non-reactive NST are four times more common than are true non-reactive NST results.[17] The false-positive CST ranges from 25 to 65 percent.[8,9] False normals, on the other hand, are quite infrequent and usually the result of accidents or other conditions not predictable at the time of testing. The only exception to this is the terminal infant who may have a negative CST. This phenomenon has been observed in both anomalous and nonanomalous fetuses dying during labor.[23] Characteristically, variability and accelerations will be absent.

Combined NST-CST Testing

The limitations of CST are obvious. The test is time-consuming, costly, cumbersome, and yields infrequent positive tests. The ease and speed of the NST make it an ideal screening test. Numerous studies attest that there is little loss of sensitivity in accepting a reactive NST as the equivalent of a negative CST. Considering the limitations of the non-reactive NST, we currently use a combined program for testing. We begin with the NST; if the pattern is reactive, we presume there is no fetal indication for intervention. If the NST is nonreactive, we consider it non-diagnostic and proceed to the CST. The benefit of this combined test procedure has been illustrated in a number of high-risk pregnancies and in a recent study of low-risk pregnancies.[8,9,20] Perinatal mortality has been improved and the duration of high-risk pregnancies increased. By inference, the incidence of iatrogenic prematurity has been minimized. These results, however, are valid only when this scheme is make part of an organized program of perinatal care. The importance of the program is illustrated by comparing the results of studies in which test results were blinded to those in which abnormal results are used as an indication for intervention. In blinded studies those with positive tests suffered a perinatal mortality of about 25 percent.[20,24] In studies in which results of testing guided intervention, the perinatal mortality in a high-risk group of patients was about 10 per 1,000.[9,25,25] These data suggest that electonic fetal monitoring reliably predicts fetal wellbeing and provides a clue to timely intervention in the potentially compromised fetus. Such monitoring may have a role in universal antepartum fetal surveillance.

REFERENCES

1. Marsac, P. Cited by Le Goust, P.: Limousin Ode, Niort, 1650.
2. DeKergaradec, L. H. S. A. Memoire sur lauscultation applique a letude de la grossesse, Paris, 1822.
3. Kennedy, E. Observations on Obstetric Auscultation. New York, J. H. G. Lansley, 1843.
4. Bodson, M. Quoted by Kennedy.[3]
5. Cox, L. W. Fetal anoxia, *Lancet* 1: 841, 1963.
6. Hon, E. H. An Atlas of Fetal Heart Rate Patterns. New Haven, Harty Press, 1968.
7. Benson, R. C. et al. Fetal heart rate as a predictor of distress. *Obstet. Gynecol.* 32: 259, 1968.
8. Freeman, R. K. The use of the oxytocin challenge test for antepartum evaluation of uteroplacental respiratory function. *Am. J. Obstet. Gynecol.* 121: 481, 1975.
9. Schifrin, B., Foye, G. et al. Routine fetal heart rate monitoring in the antepartum period. (In press)
10. Hon, E. H. Observations on "pathologic" fetal bradycardia. *Am. J. Obstet. Gynecol.* 77: 1084, 1959.
11. Caldeyro-Barcia, R., Mendez-Bauer, C., Posiero, J. J. et al. Fetal monitoring in labor. *In* Maternal and Child Health Practices, Problems Resources Methods of Delivery (Gold, E. M., Wallace, H. M., Lis, E. F., Eds.) Springfield, Ill., Charles C Thomas, 1973, pp. 332–394.
12. Kubli, F. W., Hon, E. H., Khazin, A. F., et al. Observations on heart rate and pH in the human fetus during labor. *Amer. J. Obstet. Gynec.* 104: 1190–1206, 1969.
13. Rochard, F., Schifrin, B. S. and Sureau, C. Non-stressed fetal heart rate monitoring in the antepartum period. *Am. J. Obstet. Gynecol.* 126: 699, 1976.
14. Schifrin, S. Antepartum fetal heart rate monitoring. (Edited by L. Gluck) Chicago, Year Book, 1977, pp. 205–224.
15. Afriat, C. and Schifrin, B. Sources of error in fetal heart rate monitoring. *J. Obstet. Gynec. Neonat. Nurs.* 12: 11–15, 1976.
16. Martin, C. B. Uterine blood flow and uterine contractions in monkeys. *Clin. Res.* 20: 282, 1972.
17. Martin, C. B. and Schifrin, B. Prenatal fetal monitoring, perinatal intensive care. (Edited by Aladjem, S. and Brown, A. K.) St. Louis, C. V. Mosby, 1977, pp. 155–173.
18. Schifrin, B. S. Fetal heart rate patterns following epidural anesthesia and oxytocin infusion during labor. *J. Obstet. Gynaec. Brit. Comm.* 79: 332, 1972.
19. Gray, J. H., Cudmore, D. W., Luther, E. R. et al. Sinusoidal fetal heart rate pattern associated with alphaprodine administration. *Obstet. Gynec.* 52: 678–681, 1978.
20. Schifrin, B. S., Lapidus, M. and Doctor, G. Contraction stress test for antepartum fetal evaluation. *Obstet. Gynec.* 45: 433–438, 1975.
21. Gabbe, S., Ettinser, B. et al. Umbilical cord compression associated with amniotomy: laboratory observations. *Am. J. Obstet. Gynecol.* 126: 353–355, 1976.

22. Freeman, R. K. and James, J. Clinical experience with the oxytocin challenge test. II. An ominous atypical pattern. *Obstet. Gynecol.* **46:** 255, 1977.
23. Cetrulo, C. L. and Freeman, R. K. Problems and Risks of Fetal Monitoring, Chap. 4. *In* Risks in the Practice of Modern Obstetrics (Aladjem, S., Ed.) 1975, pp. 82–103.
24. Pose, S. V., Castillo, J. B., Mora-Rojas, E. O. et al. Test of fetal tolerance to induced uterine contractions for the diagnosis of chronic distress. *In* Perinatal Factors Affecting Human Development. Pan-Am. Health Org. Scientific Publication, No. 185, 1969.
25. Visser, G. H. A. and Huisies, H. J. Diagnostic value of the unstressed antepartum cardiotocogram. *Brit. J. Obstet. Gynaecol.* **54:** 321, 1977.
26. Nochimson, D. J., Turbeville, J. S., Terry, J. E. et al. The nonstress test. *Obstet. Gynec.* **51:** 419–421, 1978.

21

Cesarean Section in Perspective

R. CLAY BURCHELL, M.D., F.A.C.O.G.

The sudden increase in cesarean births concerns everyone—women, physicians, and all those concerned with health care. For many years the incidence of section remained stable at approximately 3 or 4 percent, including both primary and repeat sections.[1] In fact, 5 percent was considered an absolute top limit for good obstetric practice. Recently there has been an upsurge in incidence.[2,3]

Experience at Hartford Hospital illustrates this trend (Fig. 1). In 1960, the rate was almost 9 percent, which was considered high at the time.[4] Upon analysis, however, the operation was quite safe at this hospital and the results were good, so there appeared no reason to modify the procedure on medical grounds. The incidence remained fairly stable until 1968 and then increased slowly so that by 1972 it was about 11 percent.[5,6] From 1972 through 1976, the rate increased about 2 percent per year, since indications changed in three major categories.[7]

1. In 1972, patients with a *breech presentation* had a vaginal birth unless there was another obstetric indication for section. By 1976, these patients were delivered by cesarean section in most instances unless the course of labor demonstrated that there was little possibility of any complication.

266

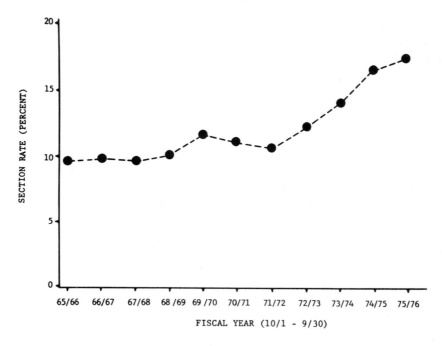

Fig. 1. Note that section rate was fairly stable from 1960 to 1972 with a marked increase after that year.

2. *Cephalopelvic disproportion,* another indication, was modified during this period. Patients and obstetricians became less tolerant of long labors; what was considered a normal labor was modified so that most patients were delivered in less than 12 to 14 hours and virtually no labor was allowed to continue beyond 20 hours.

3. *Fetal distress,* the third indication showing significant increase, included a number of indications. Attitudes toward premature rupture of the membranes had changed, and more patients were induced on this account than previously. There was some concern about post-date pregnancy, and if this was an indication for section it was included in this category. Finally, some sections resulted from the increased use of fetal monitoring.

The increase in cesarean sections has upset obstetricians and raised two primary questions: Is the rate too high, and is this liberal use of the operation in the best interests of mother and baby? Classical indications for cesarean section have been extended, contributing to the increase. The cause of this trend is not readily apparent, but new technology and malpractice conditions are commonly thought to have had an influence. Moreover, there seems to be an underlying pressure upon physicians to utilize section as an answer for most obstetric problems. In order to provide background and perspective, the history of cesarean section over the last century will be reviewed.

HISTORICAL PERSPECTIVE

What is termed the modern era of cesarean section was ushered in by Max Sänger's epic monograph in 1882.[8] In retrospect, the impact of this single manuscript was to revolutionize obstetrics over the next century! Basically Sänger said that treatment of the uterine wound was crucial and that buried sutures should be utilized to close the uterus in all patients. Astonishingly, Sänger reported only one case, and many of his ideas came from frontier medicine practiced in the United States.[9]

What Sänger did was to promote basic technique that made a fatal operation relatively safe and thus paved the way for the increasing use of cesarean section to solve obstetric problems over the ensuing years. Previously section had been the most fatal of surgical operations. Maternal mortality was nearly 100 percent. For example, it was 85 percent in Great Britain and Ireland in 1885,[10] 92 percent in New York City in 1887[11] and 100 percent in greater Paris for an entire period from 1786 to 1876.[12] In 90 years not a single woman in Paris survived cesarean section! No wonder it was termed "sacrificial obstetrics."

Conditions were such that the "radical operation" of Porro was considered a tremendous improvement when it was introduced in 1876.[13] This operation (a section with supracervical hysterectomy) had a maternal mortality of only 50 percent and hence was much less dangerous than the "classical operation" (removal of fetus with unsutured uterus left in situ). Termination of childbearing ability seemed a small price to pay for improved maternal mortality. Six years later, Sänger reversed the trend toward hysterectomy by modifying the classical operation so that it was as safe or safer than the Porro operation.

Sänger was influenced by reports from the United States.[14,15] Subsequently Harris compiled statistics for many years in the United States and emphasized in his reports of results that a "timely operation" was critical.[16,17] Harris showed that the maternal mortality during the 1880's was 92 percent in New York and 75 percent in New Orleans when the operation was done by physicians as a last resort. At the same time, the mortality was only 12.5 percent when the operation was performed on slaves in Louisiana; here it was performed early in labor because there was little concern about the mother. The mortality was 7 to 15 percent for early repeat sections, and only 10 percent when the operation was performed in early labor. An astonishing fact was that in the collected cases, mortality was about 44 percent when women did sections on themselves or were gored by cattle (less than half the mortality of having it done by a physician in late labor)!

Thus, two simple but significant steps made a universally fatal operation relatively safe and reduced maternal mortality by 80 to 90 percent: perform the procedure before or early in labor and suture the uterus. The "timely operation" was again emphasized by Witredge Williams in 1930.[18] Maternal mortalities were less than 2 percent in early labor, 10 percent in late labor, 15 percent after induction of labor, and 27 percent after failed forceps in the second stage of labor. It is interesting to note that many of the fetal indications for section at the present time fall into the last three categories where the mortality had ranged from 10 to nearly 30 percent.

During the next thirty years cesarean section mortality was steadily reduced with the introduction into obstetric practice of antibiotics, blood transfusions and safe anesthesia. Infection and hemorrhage had been leading causes of maternal death; antibiotics treated infection directly, and blood transfusions prevented direct death from hemorrhage as well as prevented severe anemia, a contributing factor in mortality from infection.

From the beginning of time, there had been no perfect solution for difficult or impossible vaginal birth. The introduction of forceps solved the problem to some extent. Cesarean section seemed to be the answer, but the high maternal mortality prohibited its use. By 1960, however, section had gradually become safe enough so that it could be utilized without restraint for most obstetric problems, and physicians could focus their attention on the fetus. As a result of obstetric progress, "the age of the fetus" began.

AGE OF THE FETUS

The rate at which discoveries in fetal medicine have been applied into practice since 1960 has been astonishing. The pregnant uterus has always been an emotional as well as physiologic barrier for fetal investigation. After discoveries were made that held therapeutic promise, there was cogent reason to invade the uterus, and the emotional restraint was broken. The pregnant uterus was no longer considered sacred! One discovery led to another with a true renaissance in fetal medicine.

Early advances in fetal medicine were concerned with the hostility of the intrauterine development. In 1961, Liley[19] utilized *amniocentesis* in rhesus-sensitized pregnancies to determine the optimal time for delivery. Previously amniocentesis had been used as a research technique to study amniotic fluid or to measure intrauterine pressures, but this was the first time that a widespread diagnostic utility had been demonstrated which paved the way for its subsequent generalized use.

In 1963, Greene[20] reported experience with *urinary estriol excretion* as a measure of placental function. This was another assessment of the intra-uterine environment, although the determinations did not require that the uterus be invaded. Originally it was known that low or falling urinary estriol levels were associated with abnormal pregnancies, and it was thought that the determination measured placental function. Then in 1964,[21] Diczfalusy showed that the fetus and the placenta were members of an integrated team in elaborating estrogens so that the test measured both placental and fetal function. Thus the concept of the "fetoplacental unit" was established.[22,23]

Electronic fetal monitoring was another significant step forward. There had been interest in fetal electrocardiograms for some time and then in the early sixties, fetal heart rate was correlated with uterine contractions to monitor a kind of natural stress test.[24,25] Uterine contractions impede blood flow and reduce the area of exchange within the intervillous space. Normally, there is sufficient reserve so that this stress is not reflected clinically in the fetal heart rate. If there is less reserve, the rate is modified by increased uterine tonus, and specific patterns of change are predictive of fetal distress.[26-28]

Stress testing for patients not in labor was an extension of the use of ex-ternal noninvasive electronic monitoring.[29] Oxytocin was employed to pro-duce contractions which were then correlated with fetal heart rate changes. It was discovered that a negative stress test was predictive of fetal well-being and that repeated weekly negative stress tests would theoretically pre-vent stillbirths. Subsequently the same results were found with non-stress tests in which fetal movement was correlated with fetal heart rate.[30-32] Loss of fetal movement in itself is a hazardous sign. When fetal movement was not sufficient for the test, a regular oxytocin challenge test could be per-formed.

Chemical monitoring of the fetal pH was also useful in some situations. Saling demonstrated a way to obtain blood from the fetal scalp in 1962 after the membranes had been ruptured.[33] This has recently been correlated with electronic monitoring to determine more precisely the fetal status. Serial determinations demonstrate whether or not continued labor would be harmful.

Although medical *ultrasound* has been available for some years, its use has been much more extensive since 1970.[34] Fetal size and hence growth patterns can be determined by this technique.[35,36] As other measures of fetal status become more sophisticated, it becomes increasingly important to diagnose intrauterine growth retardation and to determine ac-curately when the pregnancy is at term. Ultrasound has enabled obstetri-cians to do this.

The safety of the intrauterine environment has been the focus of our discussion to this point. The tests described helped obstetricians to determine when the fetus was in danger and whether or not the mother was near term. Then in 1971 Gluck described a test done on amniotic fluid which would predict the chances of fetal survival outside the uterus.[37] This was a milestone! For the first time there was an intrauterine test that would allow the physician to balance the risks of intra and extra-uterine environments and choose the best one for the fetus.[38-40]

Prematurity had always been a serious threat to the newborn, and in most cases neonatal deaths resulted from the respiratory distress syndrome (RDS). The lungs were simply not developed sufficiently to function normally.[41,42] Investigators found that surfactant was not present in the lungs of stillbirths and infants who had RDS. Then Gluck discovered that the *lecithin/sphingomyelin ratio in amniotic fluid* would predict whether or not there was sufficient surfactant for normal respiration. At about the same time, progress was made in treating infants with RDS.[43]

There was progress in fetal medicine on other fronts. One of the most dramatic areas involved the concept of treating the fetus therapeutically while it was still in the uterus. Soon after Liley's discovery that the severity of rhesus sensitization could be determined from amniotic fluid, he began to correct the fetal anemia with an intrauterine transfusion of blood into the abdominal cavity of the fetus![44] As a result, pregnancy could be maintained until the severely affected fetus was mature enough to survive after birth. *Intrauterine transfusion* was a significant and dramatic step which emphasized that fetal therapy was in fact possible and thus encouraged other investigators.[45-47]

Currently studies are progressing on large numbers of patients to determine whether or not Liggins' observations that steroids given to the mother before birth would enhance lung maturity.[48] After some testing on sheep, Liggins gave women who were between 28 and 32 weeks of gestation steroid preparations before delivery, and demonstrated that fetal survival was improved.[49,50] The incidence and severity of RDS was reduced. Evidence is increasing that these results are reproducible in large series of patients.[51-53] If this proves true, it will mean that physicians can not only determine which fetuses will develop RDS if delivered, but can actually prevent the complication when early birth is mandatory or inevitable.

Another longstanding problem has been idiopathic prematurity stemming from the mother simply going into labor before term. In this situation, there is insufficient time for steroids to have an effect (48 hours) so that these infants may still die from the respiratory distress syndrome. A number of drugs including alcohol[54-56] and sympathomimetic agents have shown promise in preventing premature labor.[57-61]

Considered from a broad perspective, the problem during pregnancy is to insure a receptive intrauterine environment until the fetus is fully mature at term. Sometimes the environment is so hostile that it will not support life and the fetus will die if not delivered early. On the other hand, if birth occurs before the newborn infant is able to function in an extra-uterine environment, death also results.

Normally there are more than six weeks between the time when the fetus is mature enough to survive after birth and when the uterus is no longer nurturing. This "safe interval" may be shortened in a complicated pregnancy so that there are only a few days or a week of safety. At times the uterine environment is hostile before fetal maturity, in which case there is no "safe interval."

As recently as twenty years ago, the obstetrician's ability to modify care in a therapeutic way was limited to delivering the fetus when it was suspected that the intrauterine environment was hostile. Knowledge of what was or was not a hostile environment was based on empirical evidence alone. In many instances, the best judgment was incorrect and the fetus was stillborn because delivery was too late or the infant died neonatally because delivery was too early.

It is a measure of real progress in the last two decades that today the obstetrician is able to assess the hostility of the intrauterine environment, determine whether or not the fetus will survive if delivered, prevent premature labor in many instances and help to insure survival if the uterus will support the fetus for as long as 48 hours. The new tests are so valuable because they enable the obstetrician to determine the boundaries or absence of a "safe interval." From the fetal viewpoint, the development of fetal medicine is as significant as the increasing safety of cesarean section with respect to the mother.

The reciprocal action between the safety of section and the ability to determine and modify fetal well-being has initiated a true socio-medical revolution! Today cesarean section is safer than vaginal birth in many obstetrical situations such as breech presentation, multiple gestation, wherever midforceps operations are indicated and probably, for the delivery of all premature infants. Although section is not safer than vaginal birth for the mother, it is safe enough, so that most mothers, fathers and obstetricians feel the additional risk is counterbalanced by the benefit to the fetus.

Actually, the dangers for the fetus in some of these situations have been known for years. The perinatal mortality with a breech presentation delivered vaginally has always been high; about five times that with a normal cephalic presentation. Section was little utilized in the past because it was unsafe and bad results were tolerated as inevitable. Today, most breeches are delivered by section as a means of reducing perinatal morbidity and mortality.

However, controversy still surrounds the role of cesarean section in twin gestations. We have always known that the perinatal mortality is greater for the second twin than for the first. Now the only question is whether parents and society want the second twin to have the same chance as the first; the price is slightly more risk for the mother. If each fetus is to have the same chance, then all twin gestations will be delivered by cesarean section.

The same argument applies to premature infants. At one time pregnancies were terminated early to prevent cephalopelvic disproportion in patients with contracted pelves. This proved to be a disaster because premature infants did not withstand the trauma of birth well enough even though they were small. Today, many infants born between 28 and 32 weeks of gestation are saved. Evidence is accumulating that section is indicated for these births because labor is stressful, the head of the premature infant being fragile and particularly susceptible to intracranial hemorrhage. Increasingly, cesarean section will replace vaginal birth for most obstetric complications on strictly medical indications.

There are other pressures for section when there is a problem with pregnancy. As a response to technological advances, society has adopted the concept of the "perfect baby" and has become intolerant of anything less. Irreducible fetal mortality and morbidity are national goals. Couples are having smaller families, but more than ever want the one, two or three children they have to be perfect. There is little tolerance for the concept that in some situations nature has not been kind and, for example, has presented parents and obstetrician with a breech presentation. It is expected that modern medicine can overcome the problem. One has the impression that few individuals are comfortable today with anything less than supreme effort to have a perfect baby, even though there are some troublesome side effects such as high cost and increased risk for the mother. In some cases the pregnant woman almost becomes a laboratory animal with respect to all the tests that are required. Once entrenched, a trend toward perfection like this one is very difficult to reverse or even modify.

High societal expectations and an intolerance for less than perfect results have also contributed to the number of malpractice suits in obstetrics, and secondarily to the number of cesarean sections. The effect of legal liability has been indirect rather than direct. Malpractice punishes for what patients and society dislike rather than rewards for what is desired. Recent suits make it very clear that patients dislike and do not expect less than perfect results. Time after time the allegation in a suit is that a cesarean section should have been performed sooner.

Malpractice also tends to make medical practice rigid and "cements" new concepts into general usage. Fetal monitoring is perhaps an example of this. Ten years ago electronic fetal monitoring was in the experimental and research stage. Application to practice really began about five years ago and now it is almost universal. No one really knows whether or not all patients should be monitored, but malpractice suits have been lost because patients were not monitored. Thus, practice has totally changed in five years—more because it was indefensible not to monitor, than because there was evidence that monitoring was desirable in all patients.

Another factor in increasing the section rate beside societal expectation and legal liability is the number of advocates for the fetus that have developed within recent years. Traditionally one person, the obstetrician or family physician, had two patients during pregnancy, the mother and the fetus. The goal was to end the pregnancy with two healthy patients, one of which would sometimes be transferred to a pediatrician. Now the mother still has one physician but the fetus has additional advocates. Some, such as the obstetric specialist in maternal fetal medicine and the pediatric neonatologist, are physicians. Other fetal advocates are really new concepts such as the "perinatal unit" and national planning efforts which have classified obstetric units into "levels" depending upon their ability to care for the sick newborn.[62]

The net result of this advocacy is to focus attention upon the fetus rather than the mother, and lead everyone to the conclusion that birth should be as safe and easy as possible for this particular baby at this time. When this movement began no one considered that cesarean section might well be the safest possible birth for "this particular baby."

It would appear that this trend is leading obstetrics to the time when cesarean section will be legitimately utilized to solve virtually all obstetric birth problems. The result will be two types of births: cesarean section for the complicated and simple vaginal birth for the uncomplicated. Vaginal birth will be confined either to spontaneous delivery or elective low forceps. It is difficult to fault this concept because, given today's hard evidence, it is certainly the best thing for the baby—and if real thought is given to selection, probably the best thing for mother and baby.

The fascinating thing to consider is that this whole revolution, high societal expectations, the ability to determine and control when an individual fetus should be delivered, and the concept that parents can plan for the number of children they desire, would either never have taken place or be of no avail if cesarean section had not become increasingly safe over the last century; safe enough so that it could be utilized as the foundation for this revolution in obstetrics.

Viewed in this light, a section rate of 15 to 20 percent does not imply an irresponsible number of operations performed by irresponsible physicians, but the culmination and logical end-point of a trend that began 96 years ago when Sänger demonstrated to the world that cesarean section was safe enough to be considered as an option for birth.

In view of what has happened, some of the editorial comments of George Kosmak in the *American Journal of Obstetrics and Gynecology* celebrating the 50th anniversary of Sänger's monograph have a haunting quality[63]:

"Perhaps the occasion should call forth a word of comment on the acceptance of this obstetric operation, no longer as a procedure solely of necessity, but rather as one of choice.

" . . . we must continue to seek, as Sänger did, the means to place it on a firmer basis, with due regard to the indications for its performance and the qualifications of the operator. Perhaps the success of such efforts will show a lowered mortality and morbidity rate during the next half century, with consequent greater safety to the mother that such progress may be recorded with justified pride in a future issue of this Journal, should it survive to commemorate the hundredth anniversary of the Sänger operation."

REFERENCES

1. Jones, O. H. Trends in the incidence of and indications for cesarean section at Charlotte Memorial Hospital during the last ten years. *Am. J. Obstet. Gynec.* **87:** 306–319, 1963.
2. Hibbard, L. Changing trends in cesarean section. *Am. J. Obstet. Gynec.* **125:** 798–804, 1976.
3. Hughey, M. J., LaPata, R. E. et al. The effect of fetal monitoring on the incidence of cesarean section. *Obstet. Gynecol.* **49:** 513–518, 1977.
4. Klein, J. Perinatal morbidity and mortality associated with cesarean section. I. A study of cases in which stress is not a factor. *Obstet. Gynecol.* **16:** 527–534, 1960.
5. Klein, J. Perinatal morbidity and mortality associated with cesarean section. II. Fetal salvage in the presence of stress factors. *Obstet. Gynecol.* **20:** 160–173, 1962.
6. Klein, J. Cesarean section in twin pregnancies. *Obstet. Gynecol.* **25:** 105–111, 1965.
7. Rink, K. Changing indications for cesarean section. Summer Student Fellowship Report. Hartford Hospital, 1977.
8. Sänger, J. Der Kaiserschnitt bei Uterusfibromen nebst Vergleichender Methodik der Sectio Caesarea und de Porro Operation. Leipzig, W. Engelmann, 1882.
9. Eastman, N. J. The role of frontier America in the development of cesarean section. *Am. J. Obstet. Gynec.* **24:** 919–929, 1932.
10. Radford, T. Observations on the caesarean section and other obstetric operations. Manchester, 1865.
11. Harris, R. P. Lessons from a study of the cesarean operation in the city and state of New York, and their bearing upon the true position of gastroelytrotomy. *Am. J. Obstet.* **12:** 82–91, 1879.
12. Budin, *in* Tarnier et Budin: Traité de l'art des accouchements. IV, 495, 1901.

13. Porro, E. Della amputazione utero-ovarica come complemento de Taglio cesareo. *Ann. Univ. med. e cher.* **237:** 289–351, 1876.
14. Harris, R. P. The operation of gastro-hysterotomy (true caesarean section), viewed in the light of American experience and success; with the history and results of sewing up the uterine wound; and a full tabular record of the caesarean operations performed in the United States, many of them not hitherto reported. *Am. J. Med. Sci.* **75:** 313–342, 1878.
15. Lungren, S. S. A case of cesarean section twice successfully performed on the same patient. *Am. J. Obstet.* **14:** 78–94, 1881.
16. Harris, R. P. Special statistics of the caesarean operation in the United States, showing the successes and failures in each state. *Am. J. Obstet.* **14:** 341–361, 1881.
17. Harris, R. P. Cattle-horn lacerations of the abdomen and uterus in pregnant women. *Am. J. Obstet.* **20:** 673–685, 1887.
18. Williams, J. W. Obstetrics: A textbook for the use of students and practitioners. New York, D. Appleton and Co. 6th Ed., 1930.
19. Liley, A. W. Liquor amnii analysis in the management of the pregnancy complicated by rhesus sensitization. *Am. J. Obstet. Gynecol.* **82:** 1359, 1961.
20. Greene, J. W., Jr. and Touchstone, J. C. Urinary estriol as an index of placental function. *Am. J. Obstet. Gynecol.* **85:** 1, 1963.
21. Diczfalusy, E. Endocrine functions of the human fetoplacental unit. *Fed. Proc.* **23:** 791, 1964.
22. Diczfalusy, E. Steroid metabolism in the foeto-placental unit. *In* The Foeto Placental Unit. Proceedings of an international symposium held in Milan, Italy, Sept. 4–6, 1968. Amsterdam, Excerpta Medica Foundation, 1969.
23. Merkatz, I. and Solomon, S. The fetoplacental unit. *Clin. Obstet. Gynaec.* **13:** 665–687, 1970.
24. Hon, E. H. Observations on pathologic fetal bradycardia. *Am. J. Obstet. Gynec.* **77:** 1084, 1959.
25. Mendez-Bauer, C., Poseiro, J. L. et al. Effects of atropine on the heart rate of the human fetus during labor. *Am. J. Obstet. Gynec.* **85:** 1033, 1963.
26. Caldeyro-Barcia, R., Mendez-Bauer, C. et al. Control of human fetal heart rate during labor. *In* Donald E. Cassels (Ed.) The Heart and Circulation in the Newborn and Infant. Chicago, 1965. New York, Grune and Stratton, 1966.
27. Hon, E. H. The human fetal circulation in normal labor. *In* Donald E. Cassels (Ed.) The Heart and Circulation in the Newborn and Infant. International Symposium on the Heart and Circulation in the Newborn and Infant. Chicago, 1965. New York, Grune and Stratton, 1966.
28. Kubli, F. W., Kaeser, O. and Hinselmann, M. Diagnostic management of chronic placental insufficiency. *In* Pecile, A. and Finzi, C. (Eds.) The Feto-Placental Unit. Amsterdam, Excepta Medica Foundation, 1969.
29. Ray, M., Freeman, R. K. et al. Clinical experience with the oxytocin challenge test. *Am. J. Obstet. Gynec.* **114:** 1, 1972.
30. Sadovski, E. and Yaffee, H. Daily fetal movement recording and fetal prognosis. *Obstet. Gynecol.* **41:** 845, 1973.
31. Sadovsky, E., Mahler, Y. et al. Correlation between electromagnetic recording and maternal assessment of fetal movement. *Lancet* **1:** 1141, 1973.
32. Sadovsky, E., Yaffee, H. and Polishuk, W. Fetal movement monitoring in normal and pathologic pregnancy. *Int. J. Gynaec. Obstet.* **12:** 75, 1974.
33. Saling, E. Neues Vorgehen zur Untersuchung des Kindes unter Gebrut. *Arch Gynäk.* **197:** 108, 1962.
34. Thompson, H. E., Holmes, J. H. et al. Fetal development as determined by ultrasonic pulse echo techniques. *Am. J. Obstet. Gynecol.* **92:** 44, 1965.

35. Hellman, L. M., Kobayashi, M. et al. Growth and development of the human fetus prior to the twentieth week of gestation. *Am. J. Obstet. Gynecol.* **103**: 789, 1969.
36. Campbell, S. The prediction of fetal maturity by ultrasonic measurement of the biparietal diameter. *J. Obstet. Gynaecol. Br. Commonwlth.* **76**: 603, 1969.
37. Gluck, L., Kulovich, M. et al. Diagnosis of the respiratory distress syndrome by amniocentesis. *Am. J. Obstet. Gynecol.* **109**: 440, 1971.
38. Gluck, L. Biochemical development of the lung: Clinical aspects of surfactant development, R.D.S. and the intrauterine assessment of lung maturity. *Clin. Obstet. Gynec.* **14**: 710, 1971.
39. Gluck, L. and Kulovich, M. Lecithin/sphingomyelin ratios in amniotic fluid in normal and abnormal pregnancy. *Am. J. Obstet. Gynecol.* **115**: 539, 1973.
40. Gluck, L., Kulovich, M. et al. The interpretation and significance of the lecithin/sphingomyelin ratio in amniotic fluid. *Am. J. Obstet. Gynecol.* **120**: 142, 1974.
41. Pattle, R. E. Properties, function and origin of the alveolar lining layer. *Nature* **175**: 1125, 1955.
42. Avery, M. E. and Mead, J. Surface properties in relation to atelectasis and hyaline membrane disease. *Am. J. Dis. Child.* **97**: 517, 1959.
43. Gregory, G. P., Kitterman, J. A. et al. Treatment of idopathic respiratory distress syndrome with continuous positive airway pressure. *New Eng. J. Med.* **284**: 1333, 1971.
44. Liley, A. W. Intrauterine transfusion of the foetus in hemolytic disease. *Brit. Med. J.* **2**: 1107, 1963.
45. Bowman, J. M., Friesen, R. F. et al. Fetal transfusion in severe Rh isoimmunization. *JAMA* **207**: 1101, 1969.
46. Stern, K., Goodman, H. S. and Berger, M. Experimental isoimmunization to hemoantigens in man. *J. Immunol.* **87**: 189, 1961.
47. Freda, V. J., Gorman, J. G. and Pollock, W. Successful prevention of experimental Rh sensitization in man with an anti Rh gamma 2 globulin antibody preparation; a preliminary report. *Transfusion* **4**: 26, 1964.
48. Liggins, G. C. and Howie, R. N. A controlled trial of antepartum glucocorticoid treatment of prevention of the respiratory distress syndrome in premature infants. *Pediatrics* **50**: 515, 1972.
49. Liggins, G. D. Premature delivery of foetal lambs infused with glucocorticoids. *J. Endocr.* **45**: 515–523, 1969.
50. Liggins, G. C. and Howie, R. N. Prevention of RDS by maternal steroid therapy. Modern Perinatal Medicine, L. Gluck (Ed.) Chicago, Yearbook Medical Publishers, 1974, p. 415.
51. Baden, M., Bauer, C. R. et al. A controlled trial of hydrocortisone therapy in infants with respiratory distress. *Syndrome Pediat.* **50**: 526, 1972.
52. Ballard, P. L., Ballard, R. A. and Granberg, P. Serum glucocorticoid levels following beta methasone therapy to prevent respiratory distress. *Pediat. Res.* **9**: 393, 1975 (Abstract).
53. Granberg, P., Ballard, R. A. et al. Effect of antenatal betamethasone in preterm infants. *Pediat. Res.* **9**: 396, 1975 (Abstract).
54. Fuchs, F. Treatment of threatened premature labor with alcohol. *J. Obstet. Gynaec. Brit. Commonwlth.* **72**: 1011–1013, 1965.
55. Fuchs, R., Fuchs, A. R. et al. Effect of alcohol on threatened premature labor. *Am. J. Obstet. Gynec.* **99**: 627, 1967.
56. Zlatnik, F. and Fuchs, F. A controlled study of ethanol in threatened premature labor. *Am. J. Obstet. Gynecol.* **112**: 610–612, 1972.
57. Ahlquist, R. P. A study of the adrenotropic receptors. *Am. J. Physiol.* **153**: 586–600, 1948.

58. Hendricks, C. H., Cibils, L. A. et al. The pharmacologic control of excessive uterine activity with isoxsuprine. *Am. J. Obstet. Gynec.* **82:** 1064–1075, 1961.
59. Landesman, R., Wilson, K. et al. The relaxant action of ritodrine, a sympathomimetic amine, on the uterus during term labor. *Am. J. Obstet. Gynecol.* **110:** 111–114, 1971.
60. Barden, T. P. Effect of ritodrine on human uterine motility and cardiovascular responses in term labor and the early post partum state. *Am. J. Obstet. Gynec.* **112:** 645–652, 1972.
61. Bieniarz, J., Moteu, M. and Scommegna, A. Uterine and cardiovascular effects of ritodrine in premature labor. *Obstet. Gynecol.* **40:** 65–73, 1972.
62. Towards Improving the Outcome of Pregnancy. Recommendations for the Regional Development of Maternal and Perinatal Health Services. The National Foundation - March of Dimes. White Plains, New York, 1976.
63. Kosmak, G. W. The modern cesarean operation (Editorial comments) *Am. J. Obstet. Gynecol.* **24:** 930, 1932.

22

Ovarian Tumors
Complicating Pregnancy

PAUL PEDOWITZ, M.D., F.A.C.O.G.

Much confusion exists regarding the management of ovarian tumors complicating pregnancy. The minimal exposure to this complication during training—and subsequently in practice—contributes in large measure to this confusion. The prevailing opinions of many colleagues are based upon either limited experience or gut reactions as to the efficacy of the various therapeutic regimens. Frequently their opinions are based upon data that either antedate modern anesthesia and surgical technique, or are anecdotal in nature.

To clarify the situation, a review of the literature during the past ten years (1968–1977) was made to determine:

1. The optimum time for surgical intervention;
2. The risk of abortion following surgery;
3. Postoperative management.

It quickly became apparent that the majority of reports during the past ten years were simply case reports.[1-7] These were reported because of either the rarity or hormonal activity of the neoplasms, or the complications associated with them. However, there were seven reports of institutional experiences, and this presentation is an analysis of these 626 cases.[8-14]

The incidence of ovarian tumors complicating pregnancy, as reported in the literature, varies from a low of 1:2552 deliveries to a high of 1:512 deliveries (Table 1). In this collective series, there were 626 cases in 574,717 deliveries, an incidence of 1:919. Six hundred-and-six of the cases were benign - an incidence of 1:948 deliveries. There were 20 malignant tumors for an incidence of 1:28,736 deliveries. Any ovarian tumor seen during the reproductive years can be found to complicate pregnancy.

As expected, benign cystic teratomas and simple serous cysts were the most common tumors complicating pregnancy (Table 2). These accounted for more than one-third of all the tumors reported. Only five of the benign tumors were solid in nature. Approximately one-sixth of all of the tumors were not neoplasms but functional cysts of the ovary, and more than 90 percent of these were related to pregnancy. Only 3.2 percent of the tumors were malignant. The most common malignant tumor complicating pregnancy in women under 30 was dysgerminoma, and in women over 30, cystadenocarcinoma. All of the malignant tumors were either solid or semi-solid. Despite the patient's age there should be a high index of suspicion that the ovarian neoplasm is malignant if it is solid or semi-solid.

Ovarian tumors complicating pregnancy are, as a rule, asymptomatic. They are symptomatic only if they become hormonally active or if a complication ensues. It is obvious that only functioning virilizing tumors will produce characteristic symptoms. The author had a personal case who developed hirsutism, male voice, enlarged clitoris, male escutcheon, hypertension and an abnormal glucose tolerance curve during the third trimester of pregnancy. The patient had an uneventful vaginal delivery and a solid adnexal mass was discovered at the six weeks post-partum examination. Following removal of the virilizing thecoma, there was a reversion of

Table 1. Incidence of Ovarian Tumors Complicating Pregnancy

AUTHOR	CASES	TOTAL DELIVERIES	INCIDENCE
Chowdhury[8]	30	54,000	1:1820
Ruckhaberle et al.[9]	150	108,150	1:721
Saunders & Milton[10]	19	48,482	1:2552
Chung & Birnbaum[11]	199	160,889	1:803
White[12]	37	35,461	1:958
Buttery et al.[13]	164	153,890	1:938
Siuanesaratnam & Sinnathuray[14]	27	13,845	1:512
TOTAL	626	574,717	1:919

Table 2. Histopathology of 626 Ovarian Tumors Removed During Pregnancy

		NO.	%
Benign Tumors			
Cystic Teratomas		131	
Simple Serous Cyst		130	
Mucinous Cystadenoma		77	
Serous Cystadenoma		72	
Paraovarian Cyst		22	
Endometrioma		20	
Fibroma		4	
Cyst Adenofibroma		4	
Thecoma		1	
	Sub Total	461	73.6
Type Not Stated		39	5.8
Functional Tumors			
Corpus Luteum Cyst		92	
Follicle Cyst		10	
Lutein Cyst		4	
	Sub Total	106	17.4
Malignant Tumors			
Serous Cystadenocarcinoma		6	
Dysgerminoma		5	
Mucinous Cystadenocarcinoma		4	
Granulosa Cell Tumor		2	
Anaplastic Carcinoma		1	
Choriocarcinoma		1	
Solid Adenocarcinoma		1	
	Sub Total	20	3.2
	TOTAL	626	100.0

the abnormal glucose tolerance curve and of the hypertension to normal status and a gradual resolution of the virilization. The most common complication was torsion of the ovarian tumor (Table 3). The two tumors most likely to undergo torsion were benign cystic teratoma and corpus luteum cyst. The incidence of this complication, however, did not differ significantly from that of the non-pregnant state. Hemorrhage into or rupture of a tumor can occur during pregnancy, labor or the puerperium. However, infection in a cyst, with abscess formation, characteristically occurs during the puerperium.

The majority of cases are diagnosed during the first trimester, before the uterus fills the pelvis (Table 4). As pregnancy progresses beyond the first trimester, a decreased number of cases are diagnosed until the puerperium. At this point, because the uterus no longer fills the abdomen, cases overlooked during pregnancy become apparent.

The operation of choice in the management of benign ovarian tumors complicating pregnancy is ovarian cystectomy. Unilateral salpingo-oophorectomy or oophorectomy should be reserved for Stage 1A ovarian malignancies, adnexa that have undergone torsion with resultant necrosis, or ovarian tumors that contain no salvageable ovarian tissue. As noted in Table 5, the majority of cases were treated in this fashion. Hysterectomy was reserved for cases of advanced ovarian malignancy.

An important question that needs clarification is the effect of the surgery upon fetal outcome. From Table 6, taken from Buttery et al.[13] it would appear that surgery performed during the first 13 weeks of pregnancy is associated with an increased risk of abortion. Of the 47 cases operated on in the first trimester, the fetal outcome was known in 26. Of these, 9 terminated in abortion, an abortion rate of 34.6 percent. This far exceeds

Table 3. Complications in 626 Ovarian Tumors During Pregnancy

COMPLICATION	NO.	%
Torsion	96	15.4
Hemorrhage into Tumor	27	4.4
Rupture	19	3.0
Infection	19	3.0
Not Stated	199	31.8
No Complications	266	42.4
	626	100.0

Table 4. Duration of Pregnancy When Ovarian Tumor was Diagnosed

DURATION	NO.	%
First Trimester	227	36.2
Second Trimester	109	17.4
Third Trimester	53	8.4
Intrapartum	12	1.9
Puerperium	26	4.1
Not Stated	199	32.0
TOTAL	626	100.0

Table 5. Type of Operation Performed in 626 Cases of Ovarian Tumors Complicating Pregnancy

OPERATION	NO.	%
Cystectomy	216	34.3
Unilateral Salpingo-oophorectomy	48	7.7
Oophorectomy	28	4.4
Total Abdominal Hysterectomy with Bilateral Salpingo-oophorectomy	10	1.6
Laparotomy with Biopsy	1	0.2
Not Stated	323	51.8
TOTAL	626	100.0

Table 6. Fetal Outcome in Relation to the Period of Gestation at Operation[13]

Fetal Outcome

GESTATION (WEEKS)	ALIVE	STILL-BIRTH	NEONATAL DEATH	ABORTION	UNKNOWN	TOTAL CASES
0 to 13	16(+1)[1]	1	---	9	21	47
14 to 27	45(+1)[1]	---	2(+2)[1]	1	12	60
28 to delivery	17	3	1	---	---	21
Puerperium	19(+1)[1]	2	3(+1)[1]	---	---	24
Postabortal	---	---	---	12	---	12
TOTAL	97(+3)[1]	6	6(+3)[1]	22	33	164

[1] Second twin

the risk of spontaneous abortion during the first trimester. There were 175 cases from the collective data who had surgery performed in the first trimester and in whom the fetal outcome was known (Table 7). Twenty-eight percent (40 cases) terminated in abortion, a rate significantly greater than the expected spontaneous abortion rate. Further analysis of these abortions (Table 8) reveals that in 7 cases the pregnancy was terminated in the course of treatment for either malignancy or tubal pregnancy and that 2 patients were aborting at the time of the laparotomy. In addition, 5 aborted following surgery for an acute abdomen. It has been shown that elective laparotomy per se does not, but that laparotomy for acute abdomen does increase the risk of abortion.[15] In addition, an inadequate incision as well as excessive uterine manipulation during surgery also increase the risk of

Table 7. Pregnancy Outcome in 175 Cases when Surgery Performed in the First Trimester

	NO.	%
Abortions	49	28.0
Pregnancy Continued	126	72.0
TOTAL	175	100.0

Table 8. Analysis of 49 Abortions Occurring in the 175 Operations Performed During the First Trimester

ETIOLOGICAL FACTORS IN THE 16 ABORTIONS
HAVING KNOWN DETAILS

Acute Abdomen due to Torsion of, Hemorrhage into, or Rupture of Cyst	5
Hysterectomy for Malignancy	5
Associated with Tubal Pregnancy	2
Aborting at Time of Laparotomy	2
None of the Above	2

The remaining 33 abortions occurred from among 123 cases in which exact details were not given. The only detail given was that torsion occurred in 99 of the 123 cases.

abortion. Although I advocate Pfannenstiel incisions for routine gynecological laparotomies, it is not the incision of choice when performing a laparotomy for ovarian tumors complicating pregnancy. Therefore, critical analysis of the collective data does not support the concept that elective laparotomy in the first trimester carries an increased risk of abortion.

As stated previously, the finding of a solid or semi-solid mass requires prompt surgical intervention regardless of the period of gestation. However, many gynecologists feel more comfortable waiting until the 14th to 16th week to remove the cyst. In women past 35, wherein the risk of ovarian malignancy is greater, it would be more judicious to perform the laparotomy as soon as diagnosed, even though the tumor may feel cystic. Ovarian cysts diagnosed in the third trimester are best treated following delivery unless they are incarcerated in the pelvis, are solid or semi-solid to touch, or undergo a complication demanding prompt surgical intervention.

Asymptomatic cysts less than 6 cm in diameter discovered during the first trimester can be treated either conservatively or aggressively. Since these are corpus luteum cysts of pregnancy, they will regress by the 14th to 16th week of pregnancy. If they persist until the beginning of the second trimester, laparotomy is indicated. During the first trimester, aggressive management consists of laparoscopic examination to exclude corpus luteum cyst of pregnancy followed by immediate cystectomy.

Through the years it has been my feeling that the postoperative management of the pregnant patient should be identical to that of the non-pregnant one. In 1968, I performed a unilateral salpingo-oophorectomy for torsion of a corpus luteum cyst in a women who was 6 weeks pregnant. Although progestational agents were not administered postoperatively, she had an uneventful antenatal course and delivered a 4000 gram infant. Despite this, my belief that progestational agents were not needed was still not based on scientific fact. In 1972, Csapo[16] demonstrated that the luteo-placental shift of progesterone formation occurs early and is well advanced by the seventh week of pregnancy. Clinical substantiation of the scientific fact that administration of progestational agents was unnecessary following laparotomy was not long in coming. White in 1973[12] removed the corpus luteum of pregnancy in 5 cases between 7-1/2 and 12 weeks of gestation. Only two of these patients received supplemental progesterone therapy, yet all 5 went to term and delivered live infants. In 1975, Hill et al.[15] found no difference in abortion rates between patients treated actively with high doses of progestational agents and sedatives to prevent uterine motility and those treated as if no pregnancy existed. Between the two groups, there was no difference in the incidence of premature labor and no significant difference in the fetal mortality. Therefore, it does not appear that progestational therapy is indicated following laparotomy.

The conclusions thus reached are that:

1. Surgical intervention for ovarian cysts can be performed safely during the first trimester without increasing fetal risk.
2. The finding of semi-solid or solid ovarian tumors, regardless of the period of gestation, warrants prompt surgical intervention to rule out ovarian malignancy.
3. Surgical intervention in the third trimester is best delayed until the puerperium unless there are circumstances that demand prompt treatment.
4. Postoperative supplemental progestational therapy does not appear to be warranted.

REFERENCES

1. Creasman, W. T., Rutledge, F. and Smith, J. F. Carcinoma of the ovary associated with pregnancy. *Obstet. Gynecol.* **38:** 111, 1971.

2. Wolff, E., Glasser, M. et al. Virilizing luteoma of pregnancy. Am. J. Med. **54:** 229, 1973.
3. Thomas, E., Mestmann, J. et al. Bilateral luteomas of pregnancy with virilization. A case report. *Obstet. Gynecol.* **39:** 577, 1972.
4. Wildemeersch, D. A. A. Primary ovarian carcinoma in pregnancy. A case report. *Z. Geburtsh. Perinat.* **179:** 471, 1975.
5. Magré, J., Leroux, P. et al. A cellular Leydig cell tumor of the ovary and pregnancy. *J. Bull. Fed. Soc. Gynecol. Obstet. Lang. Fr.* **23:** 107, 1971.
6. Cislo, M. and Wieczorek, E. A rare case of term pregnancy with co-existing ovarian teratomata. *Ginekol. Pol.* **46:** 985, 1975.
7. Wiesiolek, J. and Strzalkowski, J. A case of bilateral ovarian dysgerminoma in a woman in labour. *Pol. Tyg. Lek.* **27:** 430, 1972.
8. Chowdhury, N. N. R.. Ovarian tumors complicating pregnancy. *J. Obstet. Gynecol., India* **18:** 439, 1968.
9. Ruckhaberle, B., Bilek, K. and Ruckhaberle, K. E. Ovarian tumors and pregnancy. *Zentralbl. Gynaekol.* **94:** 1729, 1972.
10. Saunders, P. and Milton, P. J. Laparotomy during pregnancy: An assessment of diagnostic accuracy and fetal wastage. *Br. Med. J.* **3:** 165, 1973.
11. Chung, A. and Birnbaum, S. Ovarian cancer associated with pregnancy. *Obstet. Gynecol.* **41:** 211, 1973.
12. White, K. C. Ovarian tumors in pregnancy. Am. J. Obstet. Gynecol. **116:** 544, 1973.
13. Buttery, B. W., Beischer, D. W., Fortrine, D. W. and Macafee, J. Ovarian tumors in pregnancy. *Med. J. Aust.* **1: 345, 1973.**
14. Siuanesaratnam, V. and Sinnathuray, T. A. Ovarian tumors complicating pregnancy in a Malaysian study. Med. J. Malaysia **30:** 291, 1976.
15. Hill, L. M., Johnson, C. E. and Lee, R. A. Ovarian surgery in pregnancy. *Am. J. Obstet. Gynecol.* **122:** 564, 1975.
16. Csapo A., Pulkkinen, M. O. M. et al. The significance of the human corpus luteum in pregnancy maintenance. *Am. J. Obstet. Gynecol.* **112:** 1061, 1972.

23

Family Planning as an Integral Part of Maternity Care

HOWARD C. TAYLOR, JR., M.D.

Until a few years ago, it was thought in this country that there were three common causes of maternal death, *sepsis, hemorrhage,* and *eclampsia.* The history of the control of sepsis begin with recognition of the contagiousness of the worst and commonest forms, and continues with the application of the principles of asepsis, discovery of the streptococcus and finally, the antibiotics. The first step toward the elimination of hemorrhage as a cause of death may be dated from the work of Landsteiner[3] in Vienna in 1901 on substances causing agglutination and hemolysis of blood when samples from two individuals are mixed together, and of Jan Jansky of Prague in 1907 who classified blood into four main groups. Thereafter many years had to elapse before simple, safe methods of blood transfusion could be evolved to make possible its present general use. Eclampsia too now produces only a rare fatality in developed countries, reduction in these deaths not being attributable to the discovery of a specific cause, but to conscientious antepartum supervision to recognize the earliest signs of pre-eclamptic toxemia.

Thus in the United States and elsewhere with similar medical services, the three great killers of pregnant, parturient and puerperal women have nearly disappeared. At the very least, the means for their elimination are clearly in sight. What then are the tasks of medicine today? For the child, there is certainly much to be done through applied genetics, and a developed science of intra-uterine environment and perinatal management. For the welfare of the mother, I consider the chief problems to be faced are in the social and economic rather than in what has traditionally been regarded as the medical field. Yet the solution, to many of these problems defined as "social" rest heavily on our profession.

In many ways these problems are more difficult than some the physician has struggled with in the past. In the first place, they are harder to define. There is no social streptococcus such as characterizes puerperal fever. The equivalent of the hemorrhagic shock syndrome cannot be visualized among the social ills. No convulsions give dramatic warning of approaching social disaster. Women do not die, at least in the hospital, from persistent mistakes in lifestyle or from hard luck in their personal relationships or in their choice of companions.

The area of social aspects surrounding obstetrics is almost limitless. To mention just a few of the special problems, there are abortion, teenage pregnancy, the consequences of promiscuous sexual activity, high reproduction rates among potentially incompetent parents, and many others. The search for a solution, or at least mitigation of some of these problems, meets with economics at one extreme and with psychology at the other, with, in many situations, a necessary mixture of both.

Among these many diffuse and often controversial situations is one where there is substantial agreement among thoughtful people. This is what we call "family planning." Leaving aside general advantages relating to life patterns, I would like to review briefly the direct relationship of family planning to maternal and infant mortality. This subject readily divides itself into two parts, 1) the effect on the individual of poorly adapted family patterns and, 2) the health effect on nations or regions of excessive rates of population growth.

DIRECT INDIVIDUAL EFFECTS OF POOR FAMILY PLANNING

The pattern of childbearing within a given family, of course, has its effects on each member. With regard to the mother alone, there is the well-known effect of age, the increasing mortality after 35 and a more disputed higher risk before the age of 20 years. High parity tends to be related to increasing age, but seems to be an independent factor also in increasing risk. The direct effect on mortality of short spacing between pregnancies is harder to demonstrate, but its relation to chronic ill health is often apparent.

For the child, figures have shown increased infant or neonatal mortality in infants born to women under 20 and over 40 and to those conceived shortly after termination of a previous pregnancy. The available statistics on these points were compiled in the U.S. some years ago; the special care provided under situations of increased risk in our modern institutions may substantially reduce the differentials. In a modern society, it is only the risk of reproduction at an advanced age that seems, for the present, beyond remedy. No such improving security is available in the immediate future for much of the developing world, where ill health and malnutrition add greatly to the risk of death when births occur at short intervals and at unfavorable ages.

INDIRECT EFFECTS ON MATERNAL AND CHILD HEALTH OF EXCESSIVE POPULATION GROWTH

The indirect effect of unduly rapid population growth on the general health provides an even more far-reaching influence, although somewhat controversial as to what is cause and what is effect. This is particularly a problem of the countries of Africa, Asia and Latin America. Underdevelopment, with its low standards of living and education, undoubtedly favors uncontrolled reproducing. Conversely, the high birth rate limits improvements in sanitation, in nutritional resources and in the development of adequate health services.

It seems to me appropriate at this conference on "New Techniques and Concepts in Maternal and Fetal Medicine" to remind ourselves of the enormous work to be done, not only in the devising and testing of what is new, but in spreading what is already known to the majority of the women of the world.

First, in regard to maternal mortality, I would like to discuss the recent records of two university hospitals. In one such hospital in the United States (Table 1) among 22,499 deliveries from 1968–1973, there were eight maternal deaths, only one due to any of the classical triad of causes.[5] In one West African University Hospital (Table 2) among approximately the same number of deliveries in about the same period of time, there were 183 deaths. Of these, 69 were due to anemia or hemorrhage, 13 to sepsis and 7 to eclampsia. These figures are probably not far from typical for much of the developing world.[4]

Attempts have been made to calculate the number of children's lives that could be saved annually if the best conditions now available prevailed in the developing countries.[11] Total deaths of children under one year of age and from one to four years have been estimated for India, Pakistan, the Arab Republic of Egypt and Brazil (Table 3). These have been compared with the theoretical figures that would prevail if current rates for Sweden

Table 1. Causes of Maternal Deaths among 22,499 Deliveries at a University Hospital in a Developed Country.

		NUMBER OF CASES
Obstetric Causes	Eclampsia	1
	Pulmonary embolus	1
	Abortion (tetanus)	1
Associated Causes	Suicide	1
	Ruptured cerebral aneurysm	1
	Cancer	3
Total		8

Table 2. Causes of Maternal Deaths among 22,280 Deliveries at a University Hospital in a Developing Country.

CAUSE	NUMBER OF CASES
Severe anemia	34
Acute hepatic failure	28
Postpartum hemorrhage	22
Septicemia	13
Hemoglobinopathies	8
Ruptured uterus caused by obstructed labor	7
Antepartum hemorrhage	7
Severe preeclampsia and eclampsia	7
Anesthetic deaths	7
Total	133
Deaths caused by abortions	12
Deaths caused by ectopic pregnancy, including one advanced extrauterine pregnancy	6
Total	18
Deaths from associated causes	32
Grand total	183

were applied. The difference indicates the number of lives that might be saved if the conditions of health and medical services enjoyed here were available; the total for India amounted to nearly six million annually.

It should be emphasized that the social and economic factors which are the immediate cause of these excess deaths are by no means exclusively the result of high birth rates. Nevertheless, a population growth rate that is disproportionately large in comparison with the rate of economic expansion surely bears a major responsibility.

Experimental programs are under way in the U.S. to provide so-called "sex education," often with fairly detailed instruction in the use of con-

Table 3. Estimates of Preventable Deaths among Infants and Preschool Children.

	NUMBER OF CHILDREN			
AGE GROUP	INDIA	PAKISTAN	EGYPT	BRAZIL
Under 1 year				
Deaths at current rate	3,238,000	927,000	171,000	617,000
Deaths if Swedish rates applied	57,000	43,000	19,000	47,000
Lives to be saved	3,181,000	884,000	152,000	570,000
1 to 4 years				
Deaths at current rates	2,928,000	1,059,000	173,000	193,000
Deaths if Swedish rates applied	47,000	14,000	3,000	6,000
Lives to be saved	2,881,000	1,045,000	170,000	187,000

traceptives to all school children. This may be, I think, a risky innovation with unpredictable results. Premarital instruction in contraceptives, however, seems justified and indeed desirable for those who wish it. Yet many women in this country come to their first delivery with no practical knowledge or intelligent motivation. If this is a rather common situation in America, it is little short of universal in the developing world.

EARLY HISTORY OF POSTPARTUM FAMILY PLANNING

For many years contraceptive advice was often given by the obstetrician at a postpartum visit, but only to his personal private patients. This practice expanded in the 1930's although in New York at least, some obstetricians preferred to refer their patients to one of the super-specialists of the day, one who was proficient in fitting of the diaphragm.

In spite of their probable greater need, the poorer patient delivered in the hospital wards received no such advice for many years. A so-called "birth control clinic" was established at The Sloane Hospital in New York in 1926, but the indications for supplying information were about as strict as for therapeutic abortion. A relaxation of the rules occurred gradually over the next several decades. At first patients who requested it were admitted to the clinic, and only in recent years were puerperal women, more or less routinely, advised to go there. The principal indication was at first based on the belief that the best interest of the woman's own health required a two-year interval between births.

Only in recent years has the general apprehension about over-population led to a change in emphasis. It is no longer thought enough to offer contraceptive advice or perhaps recommend it for individual health reasons, but rather to persuade families to limit the number of their children for the collective good. The techniques to be used, and the means to motivate families to employ them, have been numerous and varied and have given rise to at least ill-defined divisions of medical and public health practice. Among these many programs is the so-called "Postpartum" approach or, as I prefer to call it, "Maternity Centered Family Planning."

Of fairly recent origin is the utilization of the maternity experience to achieve a high percentage of so-called "acceptors" of contraception as a social or demographic objective. Such postpartum programs are generally fairly common even in many of the less developed countries now, although first trials with this approach were begun only a few years ago.

The early 1960's was a period of high enthusiasm for the once condemned, but by then rehabilitated, intrauterine device. To test its safety and efficacy, Dr. Christopher Tietze set up a number of programs, one of which was at the Presbyterian Hospital with Dr. Robert Hall.[2] Under his direction, essentially every woman delivered on the ward service was visited at the bedside by a social worker, with relevant explanations and reference to the birth control clinic. The percentage of so-called acceptors was very high. This was essentially a postpartum family planning program and so far as I knew, the first to attempt to reach all delivered women. Thereafter the problem was to see how successful such a approach would be in different institutions and how the principle could be adapted to a variety of conditions of delivery.

PREDICTABLE ADVANTAGES OF THE POSTPARTUM APPROACH

In August of 1965, there was a conference in Geneva sponsored by the Rockefeller and Ford Foundations and by the Population Council in relation to forms of family planning programs. Impressed with the success of our own small program at home, I read a paper on The Theoretical Advantages of the Postpartum Approach.[6]

These basic advantages have been referred to repeatedly and are listed in Table 4.

1. The postpartum period is critical, for the woman has demonstrated her fertility and will soon conceive again without contraception. Statistics indicate that two-thirds will be pregnant five months after the first menstrual period, four-fifths after a year, if no contraception is used.

2. The organization of an obstetrical service provides personnel, space and equipment and thus avoids the expense of duplication in setting up an independent clinic.

3. The relevance of the subject of child-spacing is apparent to the preg-

Table 4. Special Advantages of a Maternity-Based Family Planning Program.

1. *Physiologic*
   Identification of the fertile woman: concentration of effort on the "high-risk" group
   Lactation providing time and continuing contacts through child health clinics
2. *Educational*
   The alternative to a lacking school system
   An acutely favorable situation with respect to motivation
   Susceptibility to advice from those to whom trust has been given for safe deliverance
3. *Accessibility*
   Universality of contact after first pregnancy
   Birth registration and dissemination of information
   The special opportunity for beginning with women of low parity
   Special means of reaching the indifferent or apathetic
4. *Acceptability*
   Virtue by association
   Effects of a lowered perinatal mortality
   Development of a medical intrastructure
   Availability of foreign aid

nant or puerperal woman, and she is receiving instruction from doctors, nurses or social workers whom she has learned to trust for her own safe deliverance.

4. Where maternity services are well organized and all women receive regulated private care, it would be possible to universalize information and instruction in contraceptive techniques.

5. Finally, in some countries where birth control programs for demographic purposes are disapproved of, hospital clinics for individual maternal and child welfare are acceptable.

In this Geneva paper, it was, however, pointed out that as a world program, the postpartum approach would face the problems of varying excellence in available obstetrical care. It was suggested that four grades of service, with respect to the ease of setting up and probable effectiveness of a postpartum program, might be recognized:

1. Hospital deliveries by physician or qualified midwife.
2. Home deliveries by physician or qualified midwife.
3. Home deliveries by relatively unqualified persons such as the village midwife (for instance, the "dai" of India), but with some government supervision.
4. Home deliveries with no qualified supervision during pregnancy, labor or the puerperium.

It is under the conditions of the last two categories that the majority of women in the rural areas of the developing world are delivered.

THE INTERNATIONAL POSTPARTUM PROGRAM

A so-called International Postpartum Study was initiated by The Population Council in 1966 and was continued over a nine-year period. It served to demonstrate the effectiveness of the approach, at least so far as hospital-delivered patients were concerned.

The Program began with 26 participating hospitals but the number had increased to 138 by 1974. Through 1973, the total of deliveries and abortions managed in the participating hospitals amounted to over three million (3.2).

In evaluating the success of the program, two categories of acceptors, the direct and indirect, were recognized. The Direct Acceptors were those adopting family planning practices within the first three months after delivery. The Indirect Acceptors were those who adopted family planning practices more than three months after delivery and those, who though not delivered in a particular hospital, heard about the services through intermediate sources and applied at the clinic for advice and prescriptions.

The general results, as shown in Table 5, indicate that on the average about a fifth of all delivered women were direct acceptors. Including the indirect acceptors increased the rate to a third of the women delivered.[1]

These overall figures conceal an enormous variation between the results in individual institutional programs. The direct acceptor rate ranged from a low of 2 percent to a high of 67 percent. These variations depended in part on the regions of the world where the program was situated, but also upon the organization of preparatory educational classes for the antepartum

Table 5. International Postpartum Program Acceptance Rates by Year, 1966 1973.

YEAR	OBSTETRICAL AND ABORTION CASELOAD (THOUSANDS)	TOTAL ACCEPTOR RATE	DIRECT ACCEPTOR RATE
1966	198	36	19
1967	289	42	24
1968	297	33	18
1969	470	27	15
1970	589	28	16
1971	690	34	21
1972	622	36	22
1973	340	31	19
Total program	3,496	33	19

period, and upon the conviction and energy of the local program director and his staff.

A STUDY OF THE POSSIBILITIES FOR A WORLD POSTPARTUM PROGRAM

The theoretical listing of the advantages of the postpartum approach, coupled with growing evidence of the practical success of the International Program for hospital-delivered patients, produced a temporary period of optimism in the early 1970's. Indeed some of us thought a formula had been discovered which, if widely applied, might solve the problem of uncontrolled world population increase.

Major difficulties obviously would have to be overcome, chief of which was the generally low standard of maternity care which prevails throughout much of the so-called developing world. In the less developed countries, about four-fifths of the people live in rural areas, where hospitals in our sense of the word do not exist. Even in the cities, large numbers of women are delivered at home and in the country areas, this practice is almost universal. Here physicians are not available. Many countries have midwife training programs, but the majority of women are still delivered by the so-called traditional birth attendent, the village midwife, who under various names (the "dai" of India or the "dukon" of Indonesia), is depended upon by the village women of the developing world.

The qualifications of these women differ widely. At one extreme are women with an elementary school education, who have had a number of hours of formal instruction and who are more of less integrated into the government maternity services. At the other extreme are totally illiterate women, with little sense of cleanliness or asepsis, who ply their trade unsupervised and unknown to any existent medical or health organization.

With a dim understanding of these conditions, Dr. Bernard Berelson, then President of the Population Council, and I set out to determine "what would it take in everything required—in personnel, physical facilities, transport, supplies and equipment, and funding—to bring some minimal professional and paraprofessional attention to every pregnant woman in a number of developing countries before, during and after delivery for the double purpose of promoting maternal/child health and family planning."[8]

We knew that we were undertaking a difficult job and hoped at least we would get some approximate figures. We did not realize how difficult, nor how approximate our figures might be. Let me describe briefly the steps in our investigation and note the results obtained:

1. First we set up a model (Fig. 1) for a rural maternal-child service that

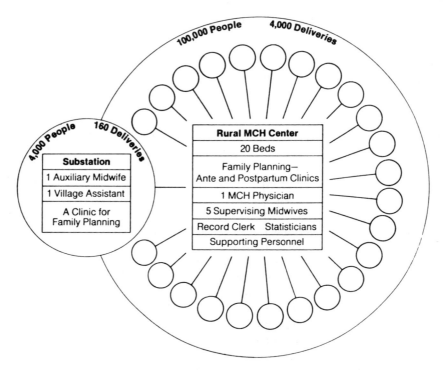

Fig. 1.   Rural model for an MCH Center with 25 substations to serve a population of 100,000 with an estimated 4000 annual deliveries.

we believed would do the job. There were in fact two models, one for the country and one for the cities, but since the former was to serve 80 percent of our projected patient load, I shall discuss only this.

The rural model was devised for 100,000 people or 4,000 annual deliveries in a country with a birth rate of 40 per Thousand. It was to be directed from a central maternity, with family planning and maternity clinics, a 20-bed ward for complicated cases and a staff including one maternity and one chid health physician and five supervisory midwives. Dependent upon this central structure and personnel would be 25 substations, one for each 4,000 people, each staffed by an assistant midwife and a village woman associate.

2. The next step was to try to determine how much of this model, particularly in terms of physical structures and various categories of personnel, was already available in a number of sample countries. To determine this, knowledgeable collaborators with access to official figures were sought and obtained in ten countries: Columbia, Ghana, the states of Orissa and the

Punjab in India, Indonesia, Iran, Kenya, The Philippines, Thailand and Turkey.

With this basic information the study attempted to determine what additional structures must be supplied and what additional personnel would be needed to make programs possible based on the postulated model. The work was completed over a two-year period (Table 6).

The annual cost of the program was expressed as sums that must be added to the national health budget for each man, woman or child in the population. The figures arrived at ranged from 32 cents to $1.65 for various countries. The general average for all countries studied amounted to 60 cents per capita. These figures involved for most countries a substantial but not exorbitant increase in the national budget for health.

Reference to suitable sources showed that the average per capita gross national product of the ten countries studied was about the same as for the developing world as a whole. Using figures on population, it was thus possible to arrive at an approximate, although somewhat hypothetical figure, for the total annual cost of upgrading maternity care in the world to give reasonable security for mother and child and the opportunity to provide universal motivation and instruction in family planning. The annual cost for the entire developing world, with unknown China excluded, would be about one billion dollars.

It should be remembered that at the time when this work was finished the

Table 6. Comparative Costs of Proposed Program and of Health Budgets in Various Countries expressed in U.S. Dollars.

REGION AND COUNTRY	ANNUAL PER CAPITA COSTS	
	PROPOSED PROGRAM	HEALTH BUDGET
Asia		
Philippines	0.06	0.53
Thailand	0.38	1.10
Indonesia	0.41	0.06
Punjab, India	0.32	1.07
Orissa, India	0.36	0.87
Middle East		
Iran	0.92	4.83
Turkey	0.55	2.80
Africa		
Kenya	1.65	1.68
Ghana	0.93	3.66
Latin America		
Colombia	0.36	1.20

two principal authors believed the postpartum, i.e., the "maternity centered" idea was a most promising approach to family planning and perhaps the best way to a solution of the population problem. In addition to the ultimate goal of population control, there were the statistics on maternal and infant deaths which cried out for world attention. A billion dollars a year seemed a low and easily attainable amount. The paper with these conclusions was published seven years ago.

THE FIRST FIELD TRIALS

We did not expect the United Nations, the U.S. Congress and various governments of the world to suspend all other activities to undertake our program. We did expect it to receive a little attention. A press conference, poorly attended, was held and there was a small article on an inside page of *The New York Times*. But that was all! It was evident that some sort of practical demonstration must be mounted if the proposed system was to be widely accepted.

Organizing the field trials has proven even more difficult than had been anticipated. National governments were generally less eager to provide opportunities, even if funds were brought from outside sources, than we had expected. Eight countries were visited and tentative plans drawn up for each, but in the end only four projects were actually instituted. These were in Indonesia, the Philippines, Turkey and (somewhat belatedly) in Nigeria. Several years were spent in getting projects approved and necessary money raised, the latter chiefly from the United Nations Fund for Population Activities. Since each project, when started, was to run for five years, final statistical results are not yet available.[9]

In selecting areas for the projects, we felt that relatively large populations were essential, because small groups would be subjected to such intense propaganda and given such excellent treatment that results would be irrelevant to what might become, we hoped, a world program. Our study areas have therefore had populations ranging from 300,000 to 600,000 people (Table 7).

The program (Fig. 2) required first detecting the pregnant woman in the village and persuading her to attend the maternal child health clinic. Thereafter there were to be at least two antepartum visits teaching the idea of family planning, delivery by a trained midwife or by a traditional birth attendant under midwife supervision, and two postpartum visits—at the second of which a decision on contraception, usually the pill or the IUD, was to be made. In addition, we attempted to provide two years of infant care, with attention to nutrition and immunization, each visit of the child with her mother being the occasion for strengthening the woman's commitment to continuation of family planning.

Table 7. Location and General Characteristics of Three Projects.

COUNTRY	REGION	AREA (SQ KM)	NO. OF INHABITANTS	POPULATION PER SQ KM
Indonesia	Modjokerto	640	622,000	972
Philippines	Bohol	2,000	430,000	215
Turkey	Yozgat	14,123	513,000	36

	DETECTION	ANTEPARTUM	PARTURITION	POSTPARTUM	INFANCY
M.C.H.		Maternity Care		P.P. Care	Immunization Nutrition
F.P.		Education Motivation		Motivation Initiaton	Continuation

Fig. 2. Schedule of maternal child health and family planning care.

From the beginning it was evident that conditions varied so widely in the different countries that we could not possibly apply the standard model for physical structures and for staffing that we had used in our original theoretical calculations. The term "less developed country" covers an enormous range of living standards, notably in available government health services.

Let us consider some of these specific differences with particular reference to the means available for the improvement of maternal and child health.[10]

Indonesia was the location of the first project to get underway (Table 8). The area assigned to us was the regency of Modjokerto, about 50 miles from the city of Surabaya, at the opposite end of the island of Java from the capital city of Jakarta. The project area is relatively small, about 800 square kilometers, the population very large (perhaps 700,000) and the density consequently very high, about 750 people per square kilometer. Although the project called for some additional centers, 99 percent of the women will be delivered at home, 90 percent by untrained or partly trained indigenous midwives.

The project in Indonesia has run its five years. As an experiment in the effectiveness of "Maternity Centered" family planning, simultaneous results have been confused by the development of a national plan for the provision of contraceptive materials, especially pills, at various clinics and designated stations.

Table 8. Expected Conditions of Delivery in Percentages for Each Project.

	HEALTH CENTERS OR HOSPITALS	HOME BY TRAINED AUXILIARY	HOME BY INDIGENOUS MIDWIFE
Indonesia	5	15	80
Philippines	10	30	60
Turkey	30	50	20

The Turkish project is situated in the Province of Yozgat, east of the capital of Ankara, in the Central Anatolian plateau (Table 8). In a geographical sense, it is the largest, spread over 14,000 square kilometers, thus providing an opportunity to study the problems of giving services at considerable distances. Even with a total population of over half a million people, the density is only 36 people per square kilometer. There are 25 hospitals or maternity centers in the province. A large number of midwives have been trained in Turkey and the majority of deliveries take place at home with this type of worker in attendance.

The project in Turkey seems to have gone well, but is complicated by the fact that the process of "socialization" of medical services by the government, undertaken step-wise province-by-province, has just reached Yozgat province.

The Philippine project, which has perhaps ran the smoothest, is situated in the island of Bohol, several hundred miles South of Manila, just North of the Mindanao Sea. Half of the island, consisting of 2,000 square kilometers and containing 430,000 people, is devoted to the project. The area is already equipped with 17 Maternal Child Health Centers, each staffed by one trained midwife (Table 8). Although a majority of rural Philippine women must be delivered at home by the uncertified indigenous midwife, this woman called the "hilot" has usually had some instruction and tends to work well in association with the government midwife.

The fourth project, in Nigeria, was instituted after I had ceased to be active in developing these overseas projects. It is situated near Calabar in the Eastern Region of the country. Early reports indicate a considerable interest but a concern which is chiefly for maternal and child health rather than for family planning.

The Maternity Centered Field Program of the Council in Java, the Philippines and Turkey is nearing completion. Statistics are not yet all in, but much experience has been gained. It is not possible to claim that the results projected from the hypothetical study have been achieved, but it has been shown that such projects can be set up and made to operate even in the most remote areas.

The cost will be greater for the world than the billion dollars a year

Taylor and Berelson had predicted. Perhaps it will be ten times as high but is 10 billion a year too much to provide for the security of the mothers and children of the developing world and for their introduction to family planning?

Besides a probable cost much above our estimates, far more time will be needed to get such a project fully underway than we had hoped for. Government officials, though in favor of health and often of birth control, are not necessarily disturbed by conditions which to us seem so pathetic, but which they find more or less acceptable because they have always existed. Bureaucratic red tape is a robber of time in Jakarta, Ankara and Manila as it is in Washington. Beyond these governmental problems, there is the shortage of needed personnel, which may involve the devising and setting up of appropriate training programs. Finally, there are the cultural attitudes of the people themselves, who again are somewhat reconciled to loss of life in relation to reproduction and unconvinced that the individual should restrict his reproductive activities for some future, collective benefits.

The annual defense budget for the United States amounts to many billions, with similar sums being spent by the U.S.S.R. Let us suppose, fancifully perhaps, that the U.S. decided to cut its arms budget by 5 billion, the money saved to be devoted to a maternity program for the developing world. Russia could then be challenged to do likewise. Inconceivable perhaps, but I do not think our influence in the world or our security would be diminished appreciably even if Russia refused to go along.

CONCLUSIONS

In spite of all of these difficulties, the plan seems sound and—with adequate support—practicable. As a population control device it has the enormous advantage of being coupled with a program for maternal and child health. A coordinated world plan, deployed on a single guiding principle, should have a force not apparent in the heterogeneous projects scattered about the world today.

A final question may be asked about the role of the physician in solving the dual problems of maternal-child health and over-population. There has been, in the last few years, a growing opinion that the medical component of the program for population has been overestimated. Economic development has been stressed as the means to reduce birth rates, rather than the motivation supplied by workers in family planning clinics. The demographers, who in a sense, discovered the fact of the population explosion, often seem to think that the cure must also be found within their field. Part of the diminished faith in what has been characterized as the "family planning approach" to population control is doubtless due to the slowness with which the world is responding to the threat of a population catastrophe.

Yet we as a profession can do more than we have. In particular, I believe that every maternity service should have a contraception clinic and that all delivered women should be told of the importance at least of spacing. The offering of clinic services should be as routine and as carefully checked as the taking of antepartum blood for serology testing.

It is true that the birth rate in the United States is now very low and, as long as our borders are intact, we need have no fear of overpopulation. But what we and other similarly advanced nations do is observed and gradually accepted by other nations. A universal acceptance of the idea of routine "maternity centered" or postpartum family planning would be a long step toward a stable world population and result in a vast improvement in maternal and child health.

It is clear that the geographic area we are working in is becoming a part of "one world." What happens in Africa, Asia and Latin America will deeply affect, if not ourselves, certainly our children. In vast areas of this developing world, it is not new techniques and concepts that are needed, but the will and the means to apply principles already tried and proven in our Northern and Western World.

REFERENCES

1. Castadot, R. G. et al. The International Postpartum Family Planning Program: Eight Years of Experience. Reports on Population/Family Planning. No. 18: 15, 1975.
2. Hall, R. E. Continuation and pregnancy rates with four contraceptive methods. *Am. J. Obstet. Gynecol.* **116:** 671, 1973.
3. Landsteiner, K. Ueber Agglutinations-Erscheinungen normalen menschlichen Blutes Wien. Klin. *Wochenschrift* **14:** 1132, 1901.
4. Ojo, O. A. and Savage, V. Y. A ten-year review of maternal mortality rates in the University College Hospital, Ibadan, Nigeria. *Am. J. Obstet. Gynecol.* **118:** 520, 1974.
5. The Sloane Hospital Data on Maternal Mortality from 1968–1973. (Analyzed 1974.)
6. Taylor, H. C., Jr. A family planning program related to maternity service. *Am. J. Obstet. Gynecol.* **95:** 726, 1966.
7. Taylor, H. C., Jr. and Berelson, B. Maternity care and family planning as a world program. *Am. J. Obstet. Gynecol.* **100:** 885, 1968.
8. Taylor, H. C., Jr. and Berelson, B. Comprehensive family planning based on maternal/ child health services: A feasibility study for a world program. *Studies in Family Planning,* **2:** 22–54, 1971.
9. Taylor, H. C., Jr. and Lapham, R. J. A program for family planning based on maternal/ child health services. *Studies in Family Planning,* **5:** 71, 1974.
10. Taylor, H. C., Jr. and Rosenfield, A. G. A family planning program based on maternal and child health services. *Am. J. Obstet. Gynecol.* **120:** 733, 1974.
11. Wray, J. D. Table adapted from "Will Better Nutrition Decrease Fertility?" Ninth Congress of Nutrition, Symposium on Nutrition, Fertility and Reproduction. Mexico City, 1972. Based on data from A. Berg and R. J. Muscat. The Nutrition Factor, Its Role in national Development, Washington, D.C. The Brookings Institution, 1973.

24

Physiologic Approaches to the Resuscitation and Management of the Asphyxiated Newborn

LEO STERN, M.D.

The need to resuscitate a newborn infant is the end result of a variety of causes which lead to peripartum asphyxia. Whether expected or unanticipated, the importance of this condition for perinatal survival and health is enormous. Approximately 25 percent of the total perinatal mortality in North America can be related directly or indirectly to asphyxia.[1] Its toll in subsequent morbidity and permanent central nervous system (CNS) damage among survivors, with resultant cerebral palsy and motor and developmental retardation, further adds to the critical role of birth asphyxia, and thereby its correct management, with respect to both initial survival and future functional integrity of the newborn.

Classically, the assessment of the degree of asphyxia has rested on the Apgar score, a rating from 0 to 10 being assigned based on a 0 to 2 score for heart rate, respiratory rate, muscle tone, reflex irritability and color. The scoring system is valid only if accurately assessed, with close attention being given to the exact time at which the score is recorded. There is a crucial difference in prognosis between a 1 minute, 5 minute and 10 minute Apgar rating. Whereas the initial score at 1 minute may be misleading in either direction, an *accurate* 5 minute score appears to correlate very well with the degree of asphyxia as assessed by excess lactate accumulation and acid-base studies. A very low 10 minute score indicates severe asphyxia and a considerably less optimistic prognosis. There appears to be an inverse relationship between the serum lactate level and the cumulative 1, 5 and 10 minute Apgar score in that the lower the latter, the higher the former will be. When this relationship is dissected out, however, it would appear that the key figure is the 5 minute Apgar score, hence the objective basis behind the reasoning that a 5 minute Apgar score is a better predictor of both immediate asphyxia and future outcome than are the other two. Recent reassessment of the usefulness of such a clinical scoring system would indicate that either heart rate with time-to-first-cry, or time-to-first-cry alone, may be simpler, more efficient, and at least as accurate a predictor as the classical total score itself.[2] In the final analysis, PaO_2 as an index of hypoxemia, $PaCO_2$ as an index of hypercarbia, and pH as the indicator of the resultant combined metabolic and respiratory acidosis are the most accurate methods of assessment. Unfortunately, clinical necessity demands that resuscitative measures be initiated without awaiting these results, although further measures beyond the initial stages should clearly be guided by these parameters.

PRINCIPLES OF RESUSCITATION

Adequate oxygenation with moist, warm oxygen must be assured immediately. If assisted ventilation is indicated because of inadequate or absent respiratory efforts, this can be effected initially with a bag and well-fitting mask equipped with a small circuit blow-off valve near the mouth. More permanent ventilatory assistance will require the use of a mechanical respirator with or without intratracheal intubation (see below).

Correction of the accompanying acidosis may be accomplished by adequate oxygenation (the major component of the acidosis is metabolic due to tissue hypoxia), together with ventilatory increase in pH as a result of correction of the respiratory acidosis as the accumulated CO_2 is blown off. If the acidosis is severe, however, the period before such correction may permit severe acidemia to persist for several hours with resultant deleterious systemic effects (pulmonary and peripheral vasoconstriction, reduced surfactant synthesis, bilirubin-albumin dissociation). Rapid correction of acidosis can be achieved with intravenous sodium bicarbonate. Although the irritative potential makes it preferable to administer this via a peripheral vein, the immediate necessity for such therapy in a badly asphyxiated infant often necessitates using the umbilical vein for this purpose.

An initial dose of 3 to 5 mEq/kg given over a 1 to 2-minute period should then be followed with slower intravenous correction based on a measured low pH and calculated base deficit (negative base excess). An acceptable formula for calculation of amounts to be used is: $-\text{BE} \times 0.6 \times$ body weight (kg) with half of the correction administered initially over a 30-minute period and the remainder within the next 2 to 4 hours. Although hyperalkalemia is difficult to produce, the dangers of both hyperosmolarity and hypernatremia are present with such therapy, and it should therefore not only be judiciously used but carefully monitored.[3]

Temperature

The importance of adequate thermoregulation and maintenance of an optimal thermal environment cannot be overemphasized. Too often in the drama and haste of the above procedures, poor temperature control is allowed to result in hypothermia. Moreover, the infant's metabolic response to inadequate thermal ambient conditions may invalidate much of the success of the other measures.

It is a common misconception that "cooling" lowers oxygen consumption in the newborn. Quite the opposite is true. The maximal thermal comfort zone (neutral zone of environmental temperature), where oxygen consumption is minimal yet sufficient to maintain the body temperature for a newborn, is 32 to 34°C. Below this zone even minimal changes in environmental temperature result in an obligatory increase in oxygen consumption,[4] a demand which the already stressed newborn would be unable to meet. The obligatory increase is lessened under conditions of hypoxia, as a result of which, however, the body temperature itself will tend to fall more readily. The proper thermal microenvironment should also minimize heat losses via conduction (do not leave the baby naked on a cold surface), evaporation (dry skin surface, avoid dry O_2), convection (keep away from air conditioners), and radiation (do not carry out procedures near the cold outside wall of the nursery or delivery room).

The directive to keep oxygen moist stems from the consequent reduction of evaporative heat loss via the lung. That it must be kept warm arises from the fact that cold oxygen (it is always cold directly from a tank or wall source) delivered via a face mask will cause an increase of O_2 consumption even if the rest of the body is kept warm. This phenomenon results from the fact that the forehead and trigeminal areas are the most sensitive peripheral thermoreceptors in the systemic metabolic response to "cold" exposure.[5]

For all of these reasons, an area either in or adjacent to the delivery room, adequately heated, with sufficiently warmed, moist oxygen available, should be set aside for optimal effectiveness of these maneuvers. A variety of commercially purchased or self-constructed types of radiant heating equipment can be so utilized, with their precise nature and location best adapted to local conditions.

Intubation

Tracheal intubation has long held a hallowed place in the routine of neonatal resuscitation. Although obstructed respiration is rare as a cause of asphyxia, intubation may indeed be lifesaving if true obstruction exists. Moreover, in choanal atresia, the infant may die if some form of oral airway is not established (a small mouthpiece is usually sufficient), since infants are obligatory nose breathers at the time of birth. Intubation by itself, however, by preventing closure of the glottis, blocks the grunting reflex and will thereby lower PaO_2 as a result of reduced expansion of the smaller alveoli in the periphery of the lung. This changes the ventilation perfusion ratio and enhances the physiologic right-to-left shunt which occurs as a result of the continued perfusion of nonventilated alveoli. Moreover, since the tube is longer and narrower than the trachea, it will increase dead space and resistance in the airway. The end result is a fall in PO_2 and a rise in PCO_2 which can be reversed when the tube is removed.[6] Thus, unless there is a clear obstruction to be relieved or surmounted or unless either a manually operated bag or mechanical ventilator is to be attached to the tube, *intubation by itself is of no advantage.* Not only may it clearly be physiologically harmful, but time and energy expended may also detract from other more effective resuscitative measures.

Cerebral Edema

With severe asphyxia, cerebral edema secondary to anoxic swelling of the central nervous system may occur. The edema, which usually takes 24 to 36 hours to manifest itself, may be responsible for the symptoms of increased intracranial pressure, CNS depression, and convulsions. Therapy with intravenous mannitol, 1 to 2 gm/kg given over a 4-hour period, has proven effective in reducing the edema, although reaccumulation may necessitate repeat courses of therapy. The efficacy of the osmotic diuresis induced should be followed by serial determinations of serum osmolality as a reflection of changes in the CNS. Postanoxic seizures should be treated with anticonvulsant medication.

Anesthetic and Sedative Depression

Asphyxia due to depression secondary to maternal anesthesia and sedative administration should be treated with resuscitation and supportive measures as above. While there are specific antidotes for morphine, it must be remembered that when these are given in excess, their action will mimic that of morphine itself. Neonatal depression from morphine and pethidine (Demerol, Meperidine) given to the mother just prior to delivery should be distinguished from the "Neonatal withdrawal syndrome" occurring in chronic maternal heroin, morphine, and methadone usage. Here the infant is in a state of hyperactivity, and therapy with either phenobarbital, chlorpromazine, or diazepam will be required.

Magnesium sulfate intoxication either as a result of therapy for maternal pre-eclampsia or through its unwarranted use as a rectal enema for the supposed management of hyaline membrane disease should be recognized by history.[7] This condition may result in profound depression and death of the infant. Exchange transfusion, preferably with citrated blood, will not only remove circulating Mg^{++}, but its complexing with the citrate in the exchange mixture will further inactivate the excess magnesium ion still present after the exchange procedure.[8]

Intoxication with local anesthetic agents either accidentally following caudal or pudendal injection, or via enhanced reversed-gradient fetal-maternal absorption following paracervical block, will result in asphyxia which may be both profound and difficult to recognize. In the case of accidental injection of the fetus, a puncture site on the scalp (in a vertex presentation) affords a clue as to the underlying cause: the infants show convulsions at birth with intermittent bouts of bradycardia and apnea. In the case of misdirected paracervical blocks with mepivacaine (Carbocaine), high levels of the drugs have been recovered from blood, urine and cerebrospinal fluid (CSF) of an intoxicated infant.[9] If suspected in time, immediate exchange transfusion may be life-saving. Unlike the situation with magnesium intoxication, there is no added effect of citrate binding, and either citrated or heparinized blood can be used for the procedure.

While the above principles are generally applicable to resuscitation of the asphyxiated newborn, a number of them require a clearer understanding of pathophysiology and of their own ultimate importance in the final outcome for any such infant, whether or not the principles inherent in the resuscitation procedure are adhered to. It is clear that the more attention paid to the pathophysiology and understanding of events the greater the likelihood for success with the undertaking. Consequently, some of these areas will now be explored in detail.

Temperature Regulation

The principles of thermocontrol already referred to indicate the penalty the organism must pay in response to an improper environmental temperature. The mandatory increase in oxygen consumption can only be met by increasing minute ventilation. Since minute ventilation is a direct multiple of tidal volume × respiratory rate, and since the tidal volume in the newborn infant tends to be a relatively fixed phenomenon, the only response the infant is capable of making to meet this requirement is to increase his or her respiratory rate. While such increases are possible up to a point, the infant already suffering from respiratory distress is clearly incapable of going much above an already elevated rate—which may approach 60 or 80 or even more respirations per minute, and exposure to the cold stimulus may be sufficient to cause total respiratory collapse.

The metabolic response to cold involves an increase in norepinephrine excretion and with it a rise in free fatty acids.[10] The rise in free fatty acids is accompanied by an inverse decline in the blood glucose level with resultant hypoglycemia.[11] Moreover, the free fatty acids themselves are powerful displacers of bilirubin from their albumin binding sites since they appear to be competitive for at least one of the sites at which bilirubin may be bound. The resultant competition for bilirubin binding sites may predispose (as will the accompanying acidosis) to development of kernicterus at lower levels of serum bilirubin.

The increase in norepinephrine is also assumed to be the responsible agent for the demonstrated fall in PO_2 under conditions of cold exposure, a fall which has been attributed to an increase in peripheral right-to-left shunting in the lung resulting from norepinephrine-induced pulmonary vasoconstriction.

Finally, it should be pointed out that if the cold stimulus exposure is severe enough or protracted enough, it will ultimately result in peripheral vasoconstriction and acidosis which in turn will lead to an entirely new and self-perpetuating series of adverse consequences. As noted below, there is the additional phenomenon that a fall in pH is one of the simplest ways of separating bilirubin from its albumin bond, thereby—as in the case of the free fatty acid elevation—also predisposing toward easier and earlier development of CNS toxicity from bilirubin.[12]

Acidosis

Acidosis occurring from asphyxia is a combination of both hypercapnia and hypoxemia thereby resulting in a mixed respiratory and metabolic acidosis with a resultant fall in pH. In assessing the severity of the acidosis, however, it must be remembered that the pH index can be misleading if one simply considers changes in pH as an arithmetic progression. The pH is the inverse logarithm of the hydrogen ion concentration and thus there is far greater significance to the degree of fall between 7.20 and 7.10 than there would be in the fall from 7.30 to 7.20. The use of hydrogen ion concentration as a direct index of acidemia will somewhat obviate this difference by providing at least a linear progression in terms of the severity of the acidosis itself.

While bicarbonate correction has been advocated for acute combatting of the immediate effects of acidosis, we must remember that it is not lack of bicarbonate that is responsible for the acidosis, but that all efforts must be directed at correcting both the hypercapnia and hypoxemia that have brought about the acidosis if other than transient relief is to be anticipated. The rationale for immediate correction of a low pH (particularly one below 7.20) stems from the fact that acidosis is a powerful pulmonary as well as peripheral vasoconstrictor. The pulmonary vasoconstriction results in pulmonary hypertension and in a reduction in pulmonary blood flow which has been shown to be a crucial factor in surfactant production and turnover. Thus, the infant with respiratory embarrassment at birth, who is allowed to become acidotic, may well perpetuate the pulmonary insufficiency with secondary alveolar collapse as a result of reduced surfactant synthesis and its attendant hypoxemic and hypercapnic changes. This will result in more acidosis, thereby perpetuating a vicious cycle which can only be interrupted if the acidosis is immediately and promptly corrected.

In addition, there is a generalized enzymatic depression that occurs under acidotic conditions, and a number of immediate life-supporting reactions are thereby endangered. The fact that all enzyme systems do work at an optimal pH affords a ready explanation for the increase in hyperbilirubinemia that occurs under acidotic conditions, an increase which is even more dangerous because of the tendency of the acidosis to dissociate bilirubin from its albumin bond (see above).

Hypoxemia

The assessment of hypoxemia presents a major problem in the newborn. The clinical ability to equate cyanosis or color with the state of plasma and tissue oxygen delivery is at best a rather risky and generally inaccurate affair. This arises from two major differences in the newborn as opposed to the adult. The physiologic polycythemia and plethora make assessment of color in an already suffused infant a difficult matter. Moreover, the oxygen dissociation curve is shifted to the left because of the content of fetal hemoglobin, so that by the time cyanosis is clinically apparent there has already been a fall in arterial oxygen tension to levels as low as 50 percent of their normal value in the newborn.[13] Furthermore, we know that it is not saturation but arterial oxygen tension which determines the driving force between plasma and tissue oxygen and thereby the rate and amount of oxygen delivery to the tissues. Because of this, a more physiologic measurement would be the use—either directly or derived of the P_{50}—which represents the arterial oxygen tension at which hemoglobin is 50 percent dissociated. It is differences in the P_{50} which would explain why some infants show tissue acidosis at a given PO_2 while others will not. The variation in their condition is a direct result of tissue oxygen delivery which combines all of these factors rather than the arterial oxygen tension alone.

Like acidosis, hypoxia also influences a number of oxygen-dependent enzymatic reactions, in addition to controlling the level of aerobic glucose metabolism to the central nervous system. Hypoxia appears as well to be a powerful stimulus to calcitonin release with resultant secondary hypocalcemia, a phenomenon which may appear with any form of induced hypoglycemia. The hypoglycemia-hypocalcemia relationship is apparently mediated by the glucagon response to the hypoglycemia and secondary calcium loss due to the ability of glucagon to promote calcium loss in the renal tubule.

MECONIUM ASPIRATION

Even though the aspiration of meconium may present primarily as a pulmonary problem, it is inseparable from the birth asphyxia now generally believed to be associated invariably with its occurrence. The majority of perinatal mortality classifications have shifted away from allowing meconium aspiration to be classified with the other pulmonary causes of perinatal mortality and morbidity, and have requested that they be classified together with the other causes of birth asphyxia. Such a change in the positioning of the disease is likely to become universal by 1980 with the adoption of the new World Health Organization classification by sufficient member states.

The asphyxia may be either intrapartum or may occur at the time of birth. Forewarning is often given by the appearance of meconium (especially in a vertex presentation) in the amniotic fluid either on amnioscopy or at rupture of the membranes just prior to delivery. It is assumed that under asphyxiating conditions, increased gastrointestinal movements result in the expulsion of meconium into the amniotic fluid. It is not known for certain whether the breathing movements made by the fetus can actually inhale meconium into the lungs prior to birth, but there is clear evidence that swallowing movements permit large amounts of meconium to be present in the upper pharynx and airways, which can subsequently be inhaled with the first respiratory efforts of the newborn.

The aspiration of meconium into the smaller bronchi and alveoli results in both alveolar and bronchiolar obstruction, although the major brunt of such obstruction mechanically is probably at the level of the smaller bronchioles, giving rise to an obstructive bronchitis which may produce enormous elevations of $PaCO_2$. Moreover, the tendency of meconium to stick to the bronchial walls yields a partially fixed type of obstruction with alveolar overdistention as the alveoli tend to over-expand in expiration. Pathophysiologically there is also a loss of effective ventilating surface and continued perfusion of underventilated areas of the lung, resulting in reduction in arterial oxygen tension and in the extreme elevation of PCO_2 in the blood.

Treatment consists primarily of the avoidance of peripartum asphyxia and minimization where it can be detected either clinically or through intrapartum fetal monitoring. An infant born with meconium in the amniotic fluid or suspected of being asphyxiated should be removed from the delivery table immediately, since there may be further expulsion of meconium directly onto the infant's face and mouth if he is left lying in the vicinity. Attempts at aspiration of the meconium from the upper pharynx and airways seem profitable, although it is not possible to reach areas lower down. Bronchoscopy is contraindicated because of the difficulty in performing it in the newborn and the sticky nature of the meconium which is extremely difficult to remove from the bronchial passages by such means.

Although meconium has been reported experimentally to favor the growth of bacteria, there is no evidence that the meconium itself is unsterile, and antibiotics are probably not indicated solely for the meconium. However, many of these cases occur after prolonged rupture of the membranes, and under those circumstances, antibiotic coverage has been advocated in view of the high incidence of infection which increases as the time of membrane rupture begins to exceed 24 to 48 hours.

The use of corticosteroids is extremely controversial, but there is no real evidence that it is helpful. If corticosteroids are being used, they will not "break up" the meconium or hasten its disappearance. They are utilized solely for their anti-inflammatory propensity, since meconium is highly irritating and causes secondary edema and swelling of the bronchial walls around it. The doses used should be high, given preferably within the first 3 hours and certainly no later than 6 hours after birth, and sharply tapered and discontinued by 48 to 72 hours of age.

Severe respiratory failure has been known to occur and may require management with oxygen and a ventilator. If assisted ventilation is necessary, continuous distending pressure either in the form of continuous positive airway pressure or continuous negative pressure is *contraindicated* since the alveoli are already overdistended and any further pressure will tend to increase an already high $PaCO_2$. The underlying CNS injury may often predominate either as clinical respiratory difficulty or as convulsions and cerebral edema. The seizures should be managed with anticonvulsant therapy, and the cerebral edema may require mannitol for its treatment and control.

Complications include alveolar collapse and pneumothorax. Pneumothorax is far more common, and a variety of extrapulmonary air complications ranging from interstitial emphysema to pneumomediastinum with or without pneumothorax commonly occur. On occasion, subcutaneous emphysema, pneumopericardium, and pneumoperitoneum have been reported as well.

The major cause of extrapulmonary air collection is the partially fixed obstructive nature of meconium in the smaller bronchi with resultant over-distention in expiration as the bronchi narrow during the expiratory phase of the respiratory cycle. Unlike hyaline membrane disease, where reduced compliance of the lung makes it relatively resistant to large shifts when collapse occurs, no protective mechanism exists in the meconium aspiration syndrome, and there is a greater tendency toward large tension pneumothoraces. These need to be treated rapidly and aggressively by either needle aspiration or tube drainage of the air. If continued air collection occurs in the form of a bronchopleural fistula, constant pressure applied to the draining tube may help.

In the long term, no residua are to be expected from meconium aspiration. Because the disease is associated with birth asphyxia, the prognosis for intellectual and developmental outcome represents the major problem. Thus the outcome can be predicted easily for the lung irrespective of how bad the situation may look radiographically, since the meconium will invariably be removed from the lung without any apparent permanent damage. It is for the central nervous system, which has sustained a greater or lesser degree of injury at the same time, that the prognosis must for obvious reasons be more guarded.

PREDICTION OF OUTCOME

In assessing the efficacy of any approach toward so acute and critical a problem as the asphyxiated newborn infant, attention must be paid not only to the maneuvers taken and the principles on which they are based but to the nature of the individual or individuals being assigned the task. It is unfortunate that there is a natural tendency to utilize the most junior and inexperienced personnel for what may indeed be the most critical and difficult task associated with the entire birth process. We therefore require not only a better understanding of the principles upon which our efforts at resuscitation and subsequent management of the asphyxiated newborn are to be based, but more careful attention as to who should be assigned the priority task of implementation. Even attention to the best principles will fail if those who are obliged to carry out the procedures are inexperienced in how the principles are to be applied. This period of life is so critical for not only survival, but future outcome, that it clearly merits the attention of the best personnel available in any institution or locale.

REFERENCES

1. Quebec Perinatal Mortality Committee Annual Reports, 1967–1969. Ministry of Health, Province of Quebec, Canada.
2. Chamberlain, G. and Banks, J. Assessment of the Apgar score. *Lancet* **2**: 1225, 1974.
3. Finberg, L. Dangers to infants caused by changes in osmolal concentration. *Pediatrics* **40**: 1031, 1967.
4. Bruck, K. Temperature regulation in the newborn infant. *Biol. Neonate* **3**: 65, 1961.
5. Mestyan, J., Jarai, I., Bata, G. and Fekete, M. The significance of facial skin temperature in the chemical heat regulation of premature infants. *Biol. Neonate* **7**: 243, 1964.
6. Harrison, V. C., Heese, H. and Klein, M. The significance of grunting in hyaline membrane disease. *Pediatrics* **41**: 549, 1968.
7. Outerbridge, E. W., Papageorgiou, A. and Stern, L. Magnesium sulphate enemas in a newborn: Fatal systemic magnesium absorption. *J. A. M. A.* **224**: 1392, 1973.
8. Bajpai, P. C., Denton, R. L., Stern, L. and Sugden, D. The effect on serum ionic magnesium of exchange transfusion with citrated as opposed to heparinized blood. *Canad. Med. Assoc. J.* **96**: 148, 1967.
9. Stern, L., Outerbridge, E. W. and Fawcett, J. Paracervical block in obstetrics. *Lancet* **2**: 322, 1969.
10. Schiff, D., Stern, L. and Leduc, J. Chemical thermogenesis in newborn infants: Catecholamine excretion and the plasma non-esterified fatty acid response to cold exposure. *Pediatrics* **37**: 577, 1966.
11. Dole, V. P. A relation between non-esterified fatty acids in plasma and the metabolism of glucose. *J. Clin. Invest.* **35**: 50, 1957.
12. Stern, L. and Denton, R. L.: Kernicterus in small premature infants. *Pediatrics* **35**: 484, 1965.
13. Stern, L. The use and misuse of oxygen in the newborn infant. *In* Symposium on Respiratory Disorders in the Newborn, Pediat. Clin. N. A. (Gluck, L., Ed.) Philadelphia, W. B. Saunders Co., **20**: 477, 1973.

25

Group B Streptococcal Infections in the Newly Born

FRANKLIN C. BEHRLE, M.D.

Although streptococcal infections have long been recognized as a significant cause of infection in the pediatric population, until recently the Group A streptococcus has held a virtual monopoly as the principal causative agent. Within the past decade, however, the emergence of Group B streptococcal infections limited largely to neonates has presented a fascinating new dimension to streptococcal disease which has raised many perplexing questions. Not the least of these is why this organism, known as a pathogen for many years in the dairy cattle industry, has rather suddenly appeared as the commonest cause of bacterial infections in many newborn nurseries both in this country and abroad. Furthermore, the ubiquity of the organism among pregnant and non-pregnant adult females[1] remains unexplained and poses serious problems in relation to the epidemiology of neonatal infections.

CHARACTERISTICS OF THE ORGANISM (FIG. 1)

Man and cattle constitute the principal hosts for this organism which appears to have a predilection for the urogenital tract, rectum, breast, and

HEMOLYSIS ——————— β (80%); α (3%); γ (17%)

HOST ————————— MAN, CATTLE

SITE ————————— RESPIRATORY, UROGENITAL, RECTAL, BREAST

PATHOGENICITY —— SEPSIS, MENINGITIS, PNEUMONIA, SUPPURATIVE
ARTHRITIS, MASTITIS (CATTLE, (?) HUMAN)

TYPES ————————— I (a,b,c); II; III

Fig. 1.   Group B streptococcus (Agalactiae).

occasionally, the respiratory tract. Most organisms produce a zone of beta-hemolysis on culture media and are commonly reported as "non-Group A beta-hemolytic streptococci." Nevertheless, beta-hemolysis is present in only 80 percent, the remainder showing a weak zone of hemolysis (14–17%) or none at all (3–6%). Those strains producing beta-hemolysis are usually distinguishable from Group A strains by their lack of inhibition by bacitracin discs; however, this distinction is not totally reliable, since approximately 10 percent of Group B strains are bacitracin-sensitive. Precise serological identification can be made in only a few laboratories at present, but further presumptive identification is possible by the CAMP reaction[2] and the hippuricase-broth assay.[3]

Human strains have been classified into three major types (I, II, III) with

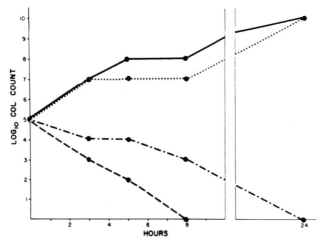

Fig. 2.   Growth of group B streptococci without antibiotics (—) and with 10 μg/ml gentamicin (••••). Reference strain III with 10 μg/ml ampicillin (— – —) and with 10 μg/ml ampicillin and 2 μg/ml gentamicin (----).

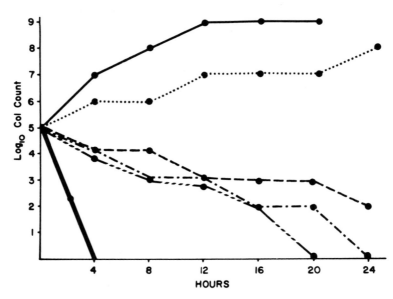

Fig. 3.   Growth of group A (●●●●) and group B (— streptococci without antibiotic. Killing of group A streptococcus by 1 μg/ml ampicillin (—). Killing of group B streptococcus strains Ja and Tr with ampicillin: Ja 1 μg/ml (----), Ja 10 μg/ml (— · — -), Tr 1 μg/ml (— ---- —).

additional sub-typing of I into Ia, Ib, Ic. All five have been implicated in neonatal disease, with one or another predominating depending on the geographic location and/or timing of a specific outbreak of disease. Currently type III appears to be the most virulent of the group in this country, particularly in relation to the "late-onset" form of disease.

While the Group B streptococcus (GBS) demonstrates sensitivity to penicillin G and a variety of other antibiotics, including the amino-glycosides, there are significant differences in sensitivity when compared to Group A organisms. These differences are of practical importance in the management of clinical infections. Schauf et al.[4] have demonstrated that higher blood levels (i.e., higher dosages) of penicillin G are required to achieve bactericidal action with Group B streptococci when compared with Group A strains (Fig. 2). In addition, the combination of penicillin G with an aminoglycoside provided a better bactericidal activity than with either antibiotic used alone (Fig. 3). Comparable *in vivo* studies have not yet appeared.

CLINICAL FEATURES

GBS infections in neonates have demonstrated a high degree of variability with respect to the organ system(s) attacked, the severity of the infection, the onset, and the type of organism involved. Undoubtedly this variability occurs for multiple reasons, among which are the source of the organism (maternal vs. nosocomial), the degree of resistance of the newborn, and the virulence of the agent.

Two very distinct clinical pictures have been described—an "early onset" form characterized by onset within the first few hours to days of life, a fulminant course, and a high mortality rate, and a "late onset" type seen after the second week of life and commonly presenting with the clinical signs of meningitis. However, further experience has shown that such clear-cut distinctions are arbitrary and that no true temporal hiatus exists between the two types. Rather, the majority of cases occur within the first week followed by sharp drop-off and then a steady but gradual decline over the next several months.[5] For unexplained reasons, GBS infections are rarely encountered in later life.

Whereas the early form tends to involve the lungs and produce septicemia and shock and the late form the meninges, there are numerous exceptions to this (e.g., meningitis has been encountered in the first few days of life and septicemia in the later period).

One very troublesome feature of early-occurring disease in premature infants is the great difficulty in differentiating it from idiopathic respiratory distress syndrome (RDS). Several reports [6,7] have indicated that GBS infections in premature infants may be indistinguishable from classical RDS. This appears to be true for both the clinical and X-ray features of the latter disease. Furthermore, postmortem histological examination of the lungs of some premature infants has revealed the presence of both hyaline membranes and polymorphonuclear exudate, and lung cultures have grown GBS organisms. Therefore, it is evident that both RDS and GBS infection can exist simultaneously. On the other hand, in term infants, early GBS infections are often manifested by respiratory distress of a nonspecific nature, and in conjunction with signs of shock suggesting sepsis. Roentgenograms of the chest in these infants usually show diffuse, infiltrative lesions characteristic of pneumonia. A highly consistent and helpful additional finding in the author's experience has been the combination of a low total white cell count with a low polymorphonuclear ratio in association with early fulminant infections.

The difficulties in diagnosing GBS infections in premature infants make it imperative to consider this entity in any infant presenting with findings of idiopathic RDS, and serious thought should be given to early administration and continuation of appropriate antibiotics until the results of cultures are available. Term infants who appear septic should be suspected of infection with this organism and given immediate combined antibiotic treatment in doses sufficient to exert a bactericidal effect. In addition to blood cultures, cultures should be obtained from the skin, throat, urine, and cerebrospinal fluid of the infant, and the vagina and rectum of the mother. Positive cultures from multiple sites are the rule in early infections, and a high correlation exists between the type of organism isolated from the infant and that obtained from the mother.

The incidence of disease caused by the various serotypes varies considerably. Whereas early reports suggested a predominance of types Ia, Ib, Ic in conjunction with the early form of the disease and type III with "late onset" disease, more recently types II and III have been seen commonly in the early and type III in the late form.[8-10]

Mortality rates remain high for this entity despite more widespread knowledge of its prevalence and the availability of effective antibiotics. Early disease carries a 50 to 70 percent mortality, and later onset 20 to 30 percent. Unusual manifestations of infection have been the cause for myriad reports and have included descriptions of osteomyelitis, omphalitis, mastitis, pericarditis, otitis media, endocarditis, ethmoiditis, empyema purulent arthritis, and septic shock accompanied by disseminated intravascular coagulation. Infants surviving meningitis are prone to develop the same types of sequelae encountered with other bacterial agents.

Several reports[11-13] have appeared to warn of recurrence of seemingly adequately treated GBS disease. Whether these represent a true relapse or a re-infection is not clear. Either mechanism may be responsible in a given case. The comparative resistance of GBS organisms to blood levels of penicillin which are bactericidal to Group A organisms has been previously mentioned. Thus, the usual recommended dosage of penicillin G (100,000 u/kg/day) may be insufficient to eliminate all bacteria and result in sequestration of organisms and subsequent relapse of incompletely treated disease. Alternatively, recurrence may represent an entirely new infection. There is some evidence to show that following treatment eliminating all signs and symptoms of disease a carrier state may ensue in which the organisms continue to colonize the throat, anal region, and skin.[14] In such cases prompt intervention with antibiotics may have precluded adequate antibody formation and offered further opportunity for bacterial re-invasion. Furthermore, the widespread prevalence of these organisms in the environment of neonates also allows for nosocomial spread with subsequent invasion of a susceptible host.

EPIDEMIOLOGY

The epidemiology of GBS infections is still imperfectly understood, in spite of the wealth of information that has accrued within the past decade. Unquestionably, there is a very high colonization rate of the organism in the vagina and rectum of both pregnant and non-pregnant women.[1] In those reports in which care has been taken to obtain specimens from the lower vaginal tract and perianal region, to use selective culture media, and in which sampling has occurred at intervals throughout pregnancy, the incidence of positive cultures is at least 40 percent. Positive throat cultures are obtained with far less frequency. Many women appear to harbor the organisms for long periods of time, whereas others show only transient colonization. There is suggestive evidence that black women may carry a higher incidence of positive vaginal cultures than whites. Interestingly, the incidence of overt infections in black infants may be less than that of white infants.[5]

It is difficult to ascertain if the high prevalence rate of GBS colonization in women is a recent phenomenon or merely reflects a heightened interest in detection and the use of better techniques for growing the organism. Reported differences from various centers throughout the world may also involve other factors which have as yet not been systematically explored, e.g., geographic location, socioeconomic differences, parity, hygiene, race, birth control practices. An additional aspect, the identification of GBS colonization of the male urethra,[15] also needs further study. There is a good possibility that venereal transmittal plays an important role in spread of the organism, which may in part explain the failure to eradicate GBS from women treated with penicillin.

Infants may become colonized in a variety of ways. Those who demonstrate overt infection at or immediately following birth show a high

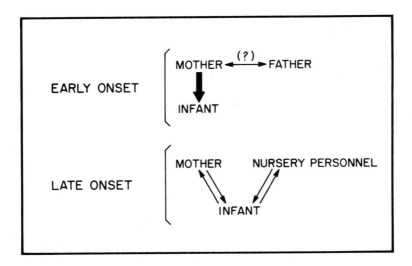

Fig. 4.   Mode of transmission Group B Streptococcus.

correlation between the serotype of the invading agent and that cultured from the mother. In instances where prolonged rupture of the membranes has existed, the infant may become infected prior to the onset of labor. Most often, however, it is believed the organism is acquired during passage through the birth canal. Asymptomatic infants may also show colonization in the face of negative maternal cultures, or colonization with a different serotype from that of the mother, implying nosocomial transmission. The high incidence of positive cultures reported in nursery personnel allows opportunity for this form of spread. Acquisition of GBS beyond the first few days of life may occur in several ways—from the mother, from other infants through hand contact by nursery personnel, or directly from nursery personnel who harbor the organism. The following scheme depicts various possibilities which exist during the early and late periods (Fig. 4).

IMMUNE DEFENSES

Although maternal carrier and infant colonization rates are high, overt infection in infants is infrequent, occurring in only 1 to 3 percent of infants colonized. Animal studies have shown a protective effect of type-specific antibodies, but human studies to date have been too few and limited in scope to provide a clear picture of the role of maternal antibody in conveying immunity to the neonate. Baker et al.[16] showed a higher incidence of antibodies to type III purified polysaccharide antigen in healthy infants as opposed to those with meningitis or sepsis caused by this type. There was also failure to detect specific antibody upon recovery from infection in 10 infants contrasted with 4 adults who had recovered. Klesius and co-workers[17] have investigated three factors: a heat-labile plasma factor, the phagocytic capacity of polymorphonuclear cells, and type-specific agglutinins. Their findings suggest that some newborns are deficient in one or more of these factors, implying that passive transfer of immunity is less than complete and that the inherent capability of some neonates to defend against the organism is relatively weak. Further studies to elucidate the role of the immunologic and other defenses of newborn infants are obviously needed, and could provide a rational approach to the prevention of disease.

TREATMENT

In light of the available evidence, any reduction in morbidity and mortality from GBS infections must depend on (1) strong suspicion and prompt administration of adequate penicillin and an aminoglycoside in any infant showing evidence of septic shock shortly after birth, and (2) a similar antibiotic regimen for any premature infant with signs of respiratory distress simulating idiopathic RDS. Penicillin should be administered in doses of 150,000–250,000 u/kg/24 hrs. intravenously, or if ampicillin is used the dosage should be 100–200 mgm/kg/24 hrs., either of these divided into 2 or 3 equal doses. Gentamycin, 5 mgm/kg or kanamycin 10–20 mgm/kg in divided doses every 12 hours should be added to penicillin on the basis of the *in vitro* studies showing potentiation by the combination. Treatment should be continued for a minimum of 10 days.

PROPHYLAXIS

Early reports offered hope that treatment of colonized pregnant women would eradicate the organism and remove the threat of infection from their offspring. Further evidence has failed to confirm this and at present the principal merit of detecting the pregnant carrier is to identify the infant who may be at risk in order to begin specific treatment at the earliest sign of illness following birth.

THE FUTURE OF GBS INFECTIONS

The major drawback to curbing GBS infections rests with our poor understanding of the nature of resistance to this organism by neonates. Accordingly, it is currently impossible to identify those infants at high risk prior to the onset of disease following birth. What is badly needed is a marker which will identify such infants prior to the time of their birth. It is hoped that efforts will be intensified to elucidate the factors related to neonatal immunity in order to focus on methods of prevention or early treatment for those infants at high risk, while sparing infants not in jeopardy from unnecessary therapeutics.

REFERENCES

1. Baker, C. J. and Barrett, F. F. Transmission of Group B streptococci among parturient women and their neonates. *J. Ped.* **83:** 919, 1973.
2. Christie, R., Atkins, N. E. and Munch-Petersen, E. A note on a lytic phenomenon shown by Group B streptococci. *Aust. J. Exp. Biol. Med. Sci.* **22:** 197, 1944.
3. Facklam, R. R., Padula, J. F. et al. Presumptive identification of Group A, B, and D streptococci. *Appl. Microbiol.* **27:** 107, 1974.
4. Schauf, V., Deveikis, A., Riff, L. and Serota, A. Antibiotic-killing kinetics of Group B streptococci. *J. Ped.* **89:** 194, 1976.
5. Anthony, B. F. and Okada, D. M. The emergence of Group B streptococci in infections of the newborn infant. *Ann. Rev. Med.* **28:** 355, 1977.
6. Ablow, R. C., Driscoll, S. G. et al. A comparison of early-onset Group B streptococcal

neonatal infection and the respiratory distress syndrome of the newborn. *N. Eng. J. Med.* **294:** 65, 1976.

7. Vollman, J. H., Smith, W. L., Ballard, E. T. and Light, I. J. Early onset Group B streptococcal disease: Clinical, roentgenographic, and pathologic features. *J. Ped.* **89:** 199, 1976.

8. Anthony, B. F. and Concepcion, N. F. Group B streptococcus in a general hospital. *J. Infect. Dis.* **132:** 561, 1975.

9. Baker, C. J. and Barrett, F. F. Group B streptococcal infections in infants. *J.A.M.A.* **230:** 1158, 1974.

10. Wilkinson, H. W., Facklam, R. R. and Wortham, E. C. Distribution by serological type of Group B streptococci isolated from a variety of clinical material over a five-year period (with special reference to neonatal sepsis and meningitis). *Infect. Immun.* **8:** 228, 1973.

11. Broughton, D. B., Mitchell, W. G. et al. Recurrence of Group B streptococcal infection. *J. Ped.* **89:** 183, 1976.

12. Dorand, R. D. and Adams, G. Relapse during penicillin treatment of Group B streptococcal meningitis. *J. Ped.* **89:** 188, 1976.

13. Truog, W. E., Davis, R. F. and Ray, C. G. Recurrence of Group B streptococcal infection. *J. Ped.* **89:** 185, 1976.

14. Paredes, A., Wong, P. and Yow, M. D. Failure of penicillin to eradicate the carrier state of Group B streptococcus in infants. *J. Ped.* **89:** 191, 1976.

15. Franciosi, R. A., Knostman, J. D. and Zimmerman, R. A. Group B streptococcal neonatal and infant infections. *J. Ped.* **82:** 707, 1973.

16. Baker, C. J., Kasper, D. L., Paredes, A. and McCormack, W. C. *Ped. Res.* **10:** 399, 1976 (Abstr.)

17. Klesius, P. H., Zimmerman, R. A. et al. Cellular and humoral immune response to Group B streptococci. *J. Ped.* **83:** 926, 1973.

26

Health Care Planning: Cost, Utilization and Regulation

MARTIN B. WINGATE, M. D.

HEALTH CARE PLANNING: COST, UTILIZATION AND REGULATION

The obstetrician who is not a member of one or more committees, the head of a section or department, or who is not committed to making administrative decisions is becoming increasingly rare. Probably he or she will become even more extensively involved in the future as a result of political pressure for cost containment, regionalization, medical/legal decisions, and the like. Many chiefs of service are being included in institutional decision-making and must become familiar with the budgeting process, program planning, and regulatory activities at local, state and federal levels. These responsibilities call for clinical as well as administrative management skills. The impact of these decisions upon his own department, his colleagues in practice and his patients must be considered.

COSTS

Health Care Expenditure

There is widespread recognition of the rising cost of health care in the United States both in terms of total dollars expended and as a percentage of the gross national product. The Health Care Financing Administration reported that in the fiscal year ending September 30, 1977 total health care spending reached $163 billion or $737. for each man, woman and child; this represents 8.8 percent of the gross national product. The total health care bill was 12 percent above the previous financial year, although the gross national product rose only 10 percent. Hospital care, both inpatient and outpatient, accounted for 40 percent of the cost and reached $65.6 billion, an increase of 14 percent over the previous year. Third parties financed more than 94 percent of hospital care costs. The cost of physician services constituted 20 percent of the total or $145.84 per capita, representing an increase of 13 percent above the previous year (Table 1). Over $38 billion was expended for Medicare and Medicaid, more than twice the amount spent five years ago. The physician cost here remained proportionately the same (Fig. 1).

This considerable increase in health care expenditure is related to a large number of factors, including the growth of sophisticated technology, changing characteristics of the populations served, social and welfare programs such as Medicare and Medicaid, the increasing spread of health insurance as a fringe benefit of employment contracts, administrative costs, and inflation.

Table 1.   Health Care Expenditures For Fiscal Year Ending September 30, 1977*

SOURCE	TOTAL DOLLARS (millions)	%
Direct payments	$12,502	38.8
Third-party payments	19,682	61.2
Private health insurance	11,817	36.7
Philanthropy and industrial inplant	42	0.1
Government	7,823	24.3
Federal	5,807	18.0
Medicare	4,431	13.8
Medicaid	1,032	3.2
Other	344	1.1
State and Local	2,016	6.3
Medicaid	795	2.5
Other	1,220	3.8
Total	$32,184	100.0

* Preliminary Report from Health Care Financing Administration.

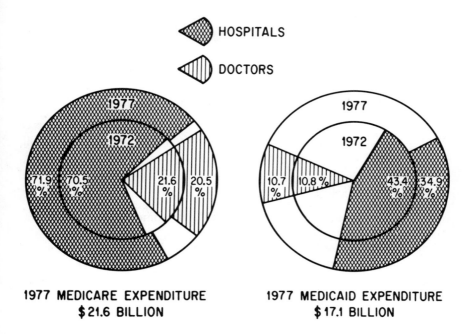

HOSPITALS

DOCTORS

1977

1972

71.9 %   70.5 %   21.6 %   20.5 %

1977

1972

10.7 %   10.8 %   43.4 %   34.9 %

1977 MEDICARE EXPENDITURE
$21.6 BILLION

1977 MEDICAID EXPENDITURE
$17.1 BILLION

Fig. 1.   Medicare and medicaid expenditures, 1972 and 1977 (H.E.W.).

Some of these factors have resulted in increased utilization of services. However the largest cost rise has involved hospitals. The cost of a semi-private hospital room increased 229 percent between 1967 and mid-1975, and operating room charges rose 235 percent during the same period.[1]

There has been a reduction in the daily census in hospitals as patients have been moved out of longterm facilities, but the daily census in short-term hospitals increased by 28 percent between 1963 and 1973. Con-comitantly, there was a doubling of the use of outpatient facilities during the same period.[2]

Hospital Costs

The steep rise in hospital costs has produced pressure for cost contain-ment by all levels of government. Hospital administrators, however, are ex-periencing escalating expenses, some of which are not readily controllable.

Inflation

Most of the cost escalation in acute care institutions can be attributed to inflation. In the years 1966 to 1975 acute care per diem rates increased from

$41 to $136. Over 50 percent of this increase was due to an increase in wages and prices of other resource costs and somewhat less than 50 percent to the increased use of traditional services or the introduction of new services.[3]

Population Growth and Increasing Insurance Coverage

In addition to the population growth and the expanded number covered by insurance, a growing proportion of the population served is elderly. This group requires more health services than does the population as a whole.

Increased Utilization

Increased utilization of short-term beds in some specialties such as psychiatry has occurred because of the closure of long-term facilities. The phenomenal growth of new medical technology has resulted in increased capital and equipment costs. New treatment methods requiring elaborate equipment are available only in hospitals and require multiple short-term stays for the patient.

Higher Personnel Costs

As a result of the new technology, more highly trained, highly paid personnel are required to operate the equipment often on a 24-hour basis. In addition, wages in the general labor force have risen over 100 percent in the last 15 years. Hospital wages, traditionally low, have risen even more rapidly as a "catch-up" period has occurred.[4]

Hospital Utilization Review Procedures

Review procedures and other efforts to curb increasing use have paradoxically increased per diem hospital costs. The effect of decreased hospitalization has produced an increase in the number of unoccupied beds. There are, however, fixed costs, in some cases estimated to be as high as $36,000 a year. The low occupancy rates, therefore, increase the cost per patient day as the cost is spread over the occupied bed/occupancy cost. Patients admitted to a hospital are more likely to have complex diseases which are expensive to manage because there is a trend to investigate and treat patients with less serious illnesses on an ambulatory basis. The first few days of inpatient care are the most expensive since most investigations and treatment are initiated at this time. Thus, shortening the average length of stay tends to increase cost per patient day.

Malpractice Insurance

Rates have risen as much as 400 percent in a year. The increasing malpractice suits and the increasing number of personnel covered by hospital malpractice insurance policies have produced a proportionate increase in patient per diem cost.

Financing of Capital Expenditure

There has been a significant reduction in the amount of money available for capital expenditure in hospitals from philanthropic and federal funds. By 1973, non-profit short-term hospitals were covering 62 percent, and for profit short-term hospitals 80 percent, of their construction costs with commercial loans. The use of commercial loans has raised hospital costs, for interest rates have risen significantly in the last few years.[5]

Regulatory Activity

The cost of compliance with the demands of the growing number of regulatory agencies concerned with health care delivery is discussed in a succeeding section.

SOME SHORT-TERM ACTIVITIES INITIATED OR PROPOSED TO CONTROL ACUTE CARE COSTS

Rate Regulation

Rate regulation for Blue Cross and Medicaid hospital per diem reimbursement has been used in many states in an attempt to slow the escalation in hospital rates. Rate regulation is an attempt to limit total expenditures for acute care rather than to reimburse hospitals for actual costs.

Cost "Caps"

Legislation has been proposed and is in effect in some states (New York) to limit hospital reimbursement to a fixed percentage per annum increase.

"Jawboning"

Federal and state agencies are intensifying their appeals to hospitals to voluntarily control costs.

SOME LONG-TERM ACTIVITIES INITIATED OR PROPOSED TO CONTROL ACUTE CARE COSTS

Reorganization

Reorganization of acute care facilities and services by regionalization, consortium formation, shared services and mergers.

Hospital Construction

Control of new hospital construction and renovation by Health Systems Agencies and State Health Planning Commissions is in effect in many areas.

Residencies

Altering the distribution of residents by specialty and sub-specialty in order to reduce the number and, thus, the proportion of secondary and tertiary residencies as compared to primary care resident positions.

National Health Service

Legislating a National Health Service so as to exercise cost control of utilization and reimbursement rates in all sections of the health care system.

UTILIZATION

The population entering the United States health care system is growing at a slower rate but by virtue of its changing characteristics, there is an increasing demand for health care. The well-publicized decline in the birth rate and the fertility rate (which has fallen even more abruptly than birth rate) is one of the reasons for a larger percentage of the elderly in the population. Compounding "the problem" is the greater life expectancy of both males and females.[6] This population group has a greater need for health care than do the younger age groups (Fig. 2).

Among the many reasons for the falling fertility rate are:
1. Extensive use of contraception.
2. Less restrictive abortion laws.
3. Increased availability of family planning services for the poor as well as for higher economic groups. The fertility rate has fallen more quickly among the poor than it has among other groups.

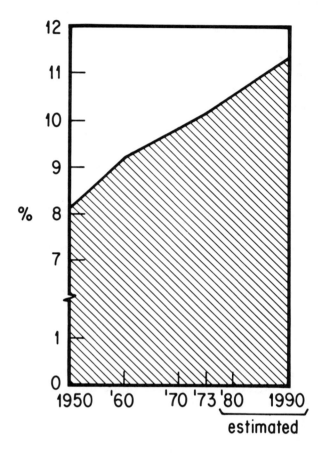

Fig. 2.   U.S. population by percentage. Age 65 and older (1950–1990). U.S. Department of Commerce, Bureau of the Census. Statistical Abstract of the United States, Washington, D.C. U.S. Gov't Printing Office, 1974, Table 3.35.

4. The ever rising cost of raising and educating children has encouraged the restriction of family size.
5. More women are working and wish to reduce the number of children to be cared for.
6. Large families are no longer "in fashion."
7. Religious restraint on utilization of family planning is less effective. Thus the birth expectation of Catholic women aged 20 to 24 has declined twice as fast as that of non-Catholics.[7]

It is already apparent that a large number of obstetric units have an increasingly low occupancy rate and some indeed have closed. There will be less demand for pediatric beds which are already less intensively utilized because of advances in pediatric care which have in turn reduced the need for hospitalization. Smaller family size may reduce the "flight" from the inner cities to the suburbs, and the population served by inner city health facilities may no longer decrease and may in some instances even increase.

The Medicaid program has permitted a significant proportion of poorer people to enter the health care system. Rising educational levels and increasing affluence has stimulated the demand for the most sophisticated medical care available.

Acute Care Bed Utilization

It has been estimated that 38 percent of all health care spending involves acute care. The exponential growth in biomedical sciences research in the past thirty years, stimulated by generous federal financial support, has increased the amount and complexity of medical knowledge. As a result, an increasing number of specialty and sub-specialty disciplines were developed requiring the introduction of highly technical investigation and management in the hospital setting. During the same time period considerable sums of money were made available through the Hill-Burton program to support new hospital construction. The combined effect of these factors led to increased dependence upon and utilization of these facilities by physicians. Criticism has been leveled at physicians because provision of this high technology to treat a relatively small proportion of the population has been financed at the expense of simpler and possibly more cost-effective methods of preventive medical care which can be applied to a large proportion of the population. Acute care bed utilization is also related to methods of financing health care. Most hospitalization financing is based upon a retrospective reimbursement of costs which allows for an almost automatic reimbursement of higher resource costs; this encourages growth in acute care capacity because of the near certainty of continually increasing reimbursement.

Accountability For Acute Bed Care Utilization

The variety of institutional and non-institutional health care services, most of which function on an autonomous or semi-autonomous basis, causes systems-oriented decision-making to become an almost impossible task. There is little chance that a community will be allowed to determine and to control its health care resources in an acceptable manner. The restrictions imposed by third-party insurers and public programs on reimbursement for other than hospitalization costs has created a dis-incentive to utilize ambulatory services most efficiently. In the name of accountability, a multitude of agencies at a local, state and federal level impose regulatory control over almost all aspects of acute care services. Little if any coordination of regulatory activity appears to exist, and problem-solving under such circumstances is extremely difficult.

Finally, account must be taken of the self-interest of the trustees, board of governors, administrators and medical staff and of the communities the hospital serves. Hospital management commonly make decisions within the narrow terms of their institution and its patient population rather than as part of a regional of national health care system. The community may also significantly influence utilization because of fears of reduced access to care. The closure of small hospital units may well mean that patients may have to travel many miles to have access to the health care that was formerly available locally.

REGULATORY ACTIVITY

An increasing proportion of the money spent on health care comes from federal sources. Congress has demanded a strict accounting of the use of federal funds. The taxpayer must be assured that his tax money will be spent efficiently and effectively. "There has been a deep-seated fear that federal money will be misused and misdirected if it is given to lower levels of government, state and local, without guidelines stating the accountability in terms of input through detailed guidelines and controls on objects of expenditures. However, these methods of accountability have sponsored red tape and rigidity without introducing incentives to more outputs".[8]

It is the contention of hospital administrators that hospitals are greatly over-regulated and that regulatory activity is increasing to a level which is detrimental to efficiency. In 1976, the Hospital Association of the State of New York set up a task force to inquire into the nature and extent of regulatory activity and to develop a program "for forcefully advising government and the public of the consequences of curtailment of services resulting from regulatory mandates imposed by the Health Department of New York State and other regulatory agencies."[9]

The collection of information has proven to be a major task. Almost every department in a hospital is subject to regulations but the variety of agencies involved make it impossible for any single administrator to keep track of all the regulatory inspections and reports required from his or her institution. Furthermore, no source or authority exists with an inventory of all the different regulations or regulators. One hundred and sixty-four different regulatory agencies have some jurisdiction over hospitals in New

York State; 96 are state operated, 40 federal, 18 city and county, and 10 are voluntary or quasi-public agencies. Sixty-seven agencies regulate policy procedures and administration; 59 scrutinize performance standards, 53 oversee professional standards; 51 investigate accounting recording procedures; and 51 are concerned with financial and statistical reporting.

The task force noted that 33 agencies were concerned with the protection of patient rights; 31 with patient safety and 25 with controlling hospital admission procedures. The task force concluded that "these procedures are wastefully expensive to a degree beyond the awareness of the general public who in the long run pay the extra costs in one way or the other."[9]

Bureaucratic rulings were often incomprehensible. A State Supreme Court Justice in a commentary on a State Health Department reimbursement regulation noted "the wording of the rules is of such a general and vague nature that they would be susceptible to many and varied interpretation as to their exact meaning. . . after reading the rules through in an effort to understand their meaning at least ten times, I did not feel that it is possible to state with any certainty in what manner many of the separately numbered sections should or could be interpreted."

There is frequent duplication of regulatory activity. The State Health Department team surveyed an institution for compliance with federal and state codes and wrote six separate reports on non-compliance that overlapped in the majority of the areas under review. Lack of a dietary inservice training program was cited six times, six different plans for correction were demanded, separate plans were requested by state and federal governments for each of the three units involved. Since there was only one dietary unit in the institution, the corrected plan had to be submitted six times so as to comply with demands!

In August, 1975 a State Health Department official informed the hospital that its "Pap" smear program did not meet standards. The official cited a regulation in support of the statement which did not in fact come into effect until six weeks after the inspection had taken place. The hospital remedied the deficiency and in May of 1976 it was informed by the department's Cancer Control Bureau that it was in 100 percent compliance. However, six weeks later, another unit of the State Health Department informed the State Hospital Review and Planning Council that there was no "Pap" smear program of any sort in the hospital concerned and therefore, since the hospital was not in compliance, it was subject to a 10 percent reduction in Medicaid and Blue Cross reimbursement. There was apparently no mechanism available to the hospital to appeal this erroneous administrative decision.

The task force noted that the State Health Department had changed its focus from one of epidemiologic surveillance to the regulation of health care facilities and services and was concerned not with serving patients but with saving dollars for the State. In the last ten years, the number of physicians employed by the State Health Department had declined, but its accounting staff had risen 8,500 percent, its attorney staff 1,000 percent, and its non-institutional employees, 75 percent. Most positions in the Health Department now were found to be regulatory.

In a statement published in 1973, the State Health Department described its mission. "The Department sets standards and exercises the right of regular inspection, audit and review over every aspect of health facility planning, construction and operation. In effect without Health Department approval new facilities may not be established and existing facilities may not continue to operate in New York State."

The task force made recommendations for coordination and reduction of regulatory activity to reduce the time and money on completing the regulatory procedures required for public accountability. But the health system is by no means the only segment of the community subject to over-regulation. Many businesses are concerned over bureaucratic regulatory activity. The government spent over $3.5 billion for its regulatory program in 1977, a 20 percent increase over 1976. Federal departments and agencies sent out over 9,800 forms and received 556 million responses. It was estimated that the cost to business was $20 billion. Colleges and schools estimate that it costs 50 cents to administer every dollar received from government. At the University of North Carolina, the computer center was totally involved for six months trying to handle the rules laid down by the Department of Health, Education and Welfare. Among the plethora of suggestions for improving the methods of public accountability and effectiveness, Rivlin[10] has suggested:

1. *Decentralization* - Breaking down central administration into more manageable units.
2. *Community Control* - Control of social services should be placed in the hands of the community being served.
3. *The Market Model* - Reliance should be placed on effective competition to spur the development of more efficient social service methods.

The success of these three methods depends upon development and use of better measures of effectiveness for social services and on vigorous and systematic attempts to find and test more effective methods, and then to *publicize* the results.[10]

REFERENCES

1. Medical Care. Rising Costs in a Peculiar Market Place. Federal Reserve Bank of Richmond Economic Review, March/April, 1975, p. 11.

2. American Hospital Association Statistics. Chicago, 1974, p. 7.
3. Forward Plan for Health FY 1978–1982. U.S. Dept. of Health, Education and Welfare.
4. The Effect of Changing Technology on Hospital Costs. Research and Statistics, Note 4. Washington, D.C., Social Security Administration, 1972.
5. Trends Affecting the U.S. Health Care System. DHEW Publication No. HRA 76–14503, 1975.
6. U.S. Department of Commerce Bureau of Census. Statistical Abstract of the United States, 1974. Washington, D.C., U.S. Government Printing Office, 1974.
7. Gold, E. Public Health Aspects of Future Obstetric and Gynecologic Services. Obstet. Gynecol. 462, 1973.
8. Rivlin, A.M. Systematic Thinking for Social Action. Washington, D.C., The Brooking Institute, 1971, pp. 125–126.
9. Hospital Association of New York. Report of the Task Force and Regulation HSANY, Albany, New York, 1977.
10. Rivlin, A.M. Systematic Thinking for Social Action. Washington, D.C., The Brooking Institute, 1971, p. 122.

27

Induced Abortion and Perinatal Statistics: Experience in Hungary

ANTAL JAKOBOVITS, M.D.,
HAROLD A. KAMINETZKY, M.D.,
LESLIE IFFY, M.D.,
AND
GARRY FRISOLI, M.D.

During the last three decades a considerable body of information has emerged from Europe concerning the effect of induced abortion upon subsequent reproductive performance. The most extensive investigations were undertaken in Hungary where abortion during the first 12 weeks of gestation became freely available to all women beginning in 1953. Much of the information referred to in this review results from an analysis of the material from the Central Bureau of Statistics in Budapest. Other data have been collected in major regional teaching centers.

Four separate abortion laws were introduced in Hungary between 1953 and 1974. The first three, introduced during the 1950's, represented a gradually increasing liberalization amounting ultimately to "abortion on demand" by the close of that decade. Implemented in 1974, the law restricted abortion to women who had borne 2 or 3 children and thus presumably had completely satisfied their childbearing desires.

Before liberalization, the law was stringent and the penalties for criminal abortion were severe. Nevertheless, it was estimated that of the 100,000 abortions induced annually during the early 1950's, all but 6,000 were illegal and resulted in a 5 percent decline in the national birth rate between

Table 1. Live Birth Rates in Countries with Legalized Abortion Systems, 1955–1968*

Year	BULGARIA	CZECHO-SLOVAKIA	HUNGARY	POLAND	RUMANIA	U.S.S.R.	YUGO-SLAVIA
			NO. PER 1000 POPULATION				
1955	20.1	20.3	21.4	29.1	25.6	25.7	26.8
1956	19.5	19.8	19.5	28.0	24.2	25.2	25.9
1957	18.4	18.9	17.0	27.6	22.9	25.4	23.7
1958	17.9	17.4	16.0	26.3	21.6	25.3	24.0
1959	17.6	16.0	15.2	24.7	20.2	25.0	23.3
1960	17.8	15.9	14.7	22.6	19.1	24.9	23.5
1961	17.4	15.8	14.0	20.9	17.5	23.8	22.7
1962	16.7	15.7	12.9	19.6	16.2	22.4	21.9
1963	16.4	16.9	13.1	19.0	15.7	21.2	21.4
1964	16.1	17.1	13.1	18.1	15.2	19.7	20.8
1965	15.3	16.4	13.1	17.4	14.6	18.4	20.9
1966	14.9	15.6	13.6	16.7	14.3	18.2	20.2
1967	15.0	15.1	14.6	16.3	27.1	17.4	19.5
1968	17.0	15.1	15.1	16.3	26.3	17.3	18.9

* From United Nations publications (Demographic Yearbook, Population and Vital Statistics Report, Monthly Bulletin Statistics).

Table 1. Legal abortions to some extent simply replace criminal abortions. The actual increase in the total number of abortions is reflected in the reduction of the birth rate in countries with liberal abortion laws.

1950 and 1952. The liberalization coincided with the introduction of similar abortion laws in other East European countries. However, the impact of the new laws upon birth rate was most profound in Hungary (Table 1).

In 1970 a detailed analysis of the relevant data was published by Klinger[9] from the Central Bureau of Statistics in Budapest. His report presented a comprehensive exposition of the numerous demographic factors in connection with artificially induced legal abortion (Tables 2–12).

The effect of legalized abortion upon the rate of premature births in Hungary was analyzed by Pohanka and Török[14] and Lampé.[11] They noted a gradual rise in the rate of premature births following 1953 (Fig. 1). Others reported evidence of a significant increase in the rates of abortion,[4] placenta previa, abruption of the placenta and low birth weight infants[2,13,15] (Fig. 2). Concomitantly, the total number of obstetric events (i.e., all reported gestations) nearly doubled. A part of this increase presumably was due to the fact that most of the estimated annual 94,000 criminal abortions of the preceding years became legal and were therefore reported. However, the rest of the rise reflected an increase in the number of unwanted pregnancies after the liberalization of the law. A high percentage of the induced abortions occurred among unmarried, nulliparous teenagers.

Table 2. Reported Induced Abortions, 1955–1968.

	NO. OF ABORTIONS (THOUSANDS)				
YEAR	BULGARIA	CZECHO-SLOVAKIA	HUNGARY	POLAND	YUGO-SLAVIA
1955	1.1	2.1	35.4	1.4	—
1956	—	3.1	82.4	18.9	—
1957	30.9	7.3	123.3	36.4	—
1958	37.5	61.4	145.6	44.2	—
1959	45.6	79.1	152.4	79.0	54.5
1960	54.8	88.3	162.6	158.0	76.7
1961	68.8	94.3	170.0	155.3	104.7
1962	76.7	89.8	163.7	199.4	—
1963	83.3	70.5	173.8	190.0	—
1964	91.5	70.7	184.4	177.5	150.0
1965	96.5	79.6	180.3	168.1	—
1966	101.4	90.3	186.8	156.7	—
1967	98.2	96.4	187.5	146.1	210.9
1968	85.2	99.9	200.8	121.7	—

Table 2. The number of legal abortions in five East European countries. (Tables 2–12 are published by courtesy of Dr. András Klinger and the Editor of Internat. J. Gynaec. Obstet.)

Table 3. No. of Reported Induced Abortions per 100 Live Births.

YEAR	BULGARIA	CZECHO-SLOVAKIA	HUNGARY	POLAND	YUGO-SLAVIA
1955	—	1	17	0	—
1956	—	1	43	2	—
1957	22	3	74	5	—
1958	27	26	92	6	—
1959	33	36	101	11	13
1960	39	41	111	24	18
1961	50	43	121	25	25
1962	57	41	126	33	—
1963	63	30	131	32	—
1964	69	29	140	32	37
1965	75	34	136	31	—
1966	76	40	135	30	—
1967	79	44	126	28	54
1968	60	47	130	23	0

Table 3. The abortion: live birth ratios in Eastern Europe following liberalization of the abortion laws.

Table 4. Abortion Rates and Ratios by the Age of Women.

AGE GROUP	HUNGARY			CZECHOSLOVAKIA		
	1960	1964	1968	1960	1964	1968*
	No. of induced abortions per 1000 women					
15–19	23	32	34	9	7	12
20–24	102	120	137	33	26	49
25–29	126	145	134	50	37	56
30–34	102	118	121	47	37	45
35–39	63	66	73	34	29	31
40–49	12	14	12	6	7	6
15–49	65	74	76	28	22	29
	No. of induced abortions per 100 live births					
15–19	43	76	66	20	15	—
20–24	64	84	84	17	13	—
25–29	120	143	133	37	25	—
30–34	192	243	221	73	52	—
35–39	254	343	369	116	97	—
40–49	338	415	516	141	180	—
15–49	111	140	130	40	29	46

* Estimation.

Table 4. Note the increasing rate of induced abortion among teenage girls under liberal abortion legislation.

Table 5. Abortion Rates and Ratios by the Marital Status of Women.

MARITAL STATUS	HUNGARY			CZECHOSLOVAKIA		
	1960	1964	1968	1961	1966	1968
Induced abortions per 1000 women 15–49 years old						
Married	81	91	91	34	31	34
Nonmarried*	21	33	43	—	16	19
Single	20	31	40	—	—	—
TOTAL	65	74	76	28	22	29
Induced abortions per 100 live births						
Married	106	123	115	—	35	—
Nonmarried*	199	346	412	—	141	—
Total	111	140	130	—	40	—

* Single, divorced, and widowed.

Table 5. Note the increasing incidence of pregnancies among unmarried women during the years of liberal abortion laws. There was no significant change in the availability of birth control methods during the same period of time.

Table 6. Abortion Rates and Ratios by the Number of Living Children of Women (Hungary)

NO. OF LIVING CHILDREN	NO. OF INDUCED ABORTIONS PER 1000 WOMEN 15–49 YEARS OLD			NO. OF INDUCED ABORTIONS PER 100 LIVE BIRTHS		
	1960	1964	1968	1960	1964	1968
0	23	35	36	28	42	40
1	74	84	95	108	147	129
2	91	95	100	283	430	437
3	105	106	102	315	377	415
4+	106	111	102	182	221	204
TOTAL	65	74	76	111	140	130

Table 6. Note the increasing ratio of abortion among nulliparous women.

Table 7. Induced Abortions by Number of Previous Induced Abortions.

	PERCENTAGE OF INDUCED ABORTIONS BY NUMBER OF PREVIOUS INDUCED ABORTIONS			
NO. OF PREVIOUS INDUCED ABORTIONS	HUNGARY			CZECHO— SLOVAKIA
	OCT. 1960	APR. 1964	1968	(1968)
0	47	40	42	56
1	27	29	26	28
2	14	15	15	10
3+	12	16	17	6
TOTAL	100	100	100	100

Table 7. Note the increasing ratio of women with multiple abortions.

Pohánka et al.[13,15] suggested that the rise in the rate of premature births was causally related to the increased number of previously induced abortions in the general population. Furthermore, they noted that between 1950 and 1953 the reported rate of spontaneous abortion was high in Budapest, but low in the rural counties and postulated that this difference was related to the easy availability of criminal abortion in the capital city (in contrast to its unavailability and social unacceptability in rural Hungary). They considered this circumstance responsible for the fact that the prematurity rate was relatively high even before the liberalization of abortion in Budapest as compared to that in the rural counties. After the introduction of the new legislation, this picture soon changed. By 1964, the percentages of all diagnosed pregnancies reported as terminated by induced abortion were as

Table 8. Abortion Rates and Ratios by Economic Activity and Socio-economic Status of Women (Hungary).

ECONOMIC ACTIVITY AND STATUS	INDUCED ABORTIONS PER 1000 WOMEN 15–49 YEARS OLD		INDUCED ABORTIONS PER 100 LIVE BIRTHS	
	1960	1968	1960	1968
Economically inactive women	73	71	90	124
Economically active women	60	80	151	135

Table 9. Distribution by Subjective Motive of Women Undergoing Induced Abortion.

MOTIVE	HUNGARY			CZECHO-SLOVAKIA	RUSSIAN SFSP. (1959)	
	OCT. 1960	APR. 1964	1965-1968	(1968)	TOWNS	COUNTRY
Sanitary and biologic	10	8	17	22	6	5
Do not want to have more children	31	33	23	26	33	44
Economic or financial problems	19	16	19	8	10	11
Housing problems	15	16	12	11	14	4
Family problems or other subjective causes	25	27	29	33	37	36
Total	100	100	100	100	100	100

**Table 10. Distribution by Cause of Pregnancy in
Surgically Aborted Women Who Were Regular
Contraceptive Users (Hungary).**

	%	
CAUSE OF PREGNANCY	OCT. 1960	APR. 1964
Negligence in prevention	63	44
Improper use of contraceptive	21	27
Defective contraceptive	4	13
Other	2	3
Unknown	10	13
Total	100	100

follows: in Budapest-72 percent; in Baranya-Zala County—58 percent; in
Szabolcs-Szatmar—49.5 percent; and in Hajdu-Bihar—48 percent. The rate
of premature births appeared to increase in direct proportion to the increasing acceptance of legal abortion by the population in all counties and
leveled off finally at approximately 11 percent (Fig. 3).

More recently Klinger[10] demonstrated that the likelihood of subsequent
premature births in any patient increased exponentially according to the
number of preceding pregnancy terminations (Tables 13 and 14). The same

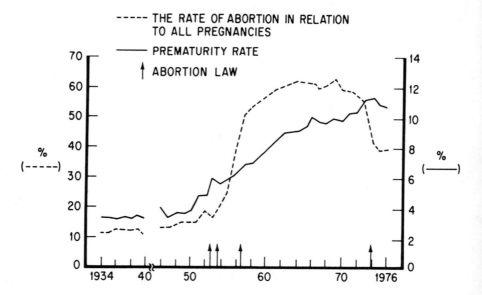

Fig. 1. Correlation between the rate of abortions (in relation to all diagnosed pregnancies) and
the rate of prematurity in the general population.[14]

Table 11. Rates on Induced Abortions by Age on the Basis of the Hungarian TCS-66 Study.

NO. OF WOMEN PER 100 AT THE DATE OF THE STUDY

AGE	HAD INDUCED ABORTIONS			HAD ABORTION AND USED CONTRACEPTION ALSO	HAD ABORTION ONLY	USED CONTRACEPTION ONLY
	REPORTED	"UNKNOWN"	TOTAL REPORTED AND "UNKNOWN"			
15–19	13	—	13	9	4	40
20–24	21	1	22	18	4	52
25–29	34	8	42	35	7	43
30–34	35	28	63	50	13	26
35–39	33	39	72	58	14	15
40–44	27	46	73	52	21	11
45–49	17	52	69	42	27	10
Total	29	29	58	44	14	26

Table 11. Note that by the end of their reproductive lives more than 2/3 of all women had had induced abortion previously. Thus, the aborters in Hungary represent the general population and not a special "sub-group".

Table 12. Attitude Toward Birth Control by the Age Group of Women.

EVIDENCE OF ATTITUDES TOWARD BIRTH CONTROL	PERCENTAGE IN AGE GROUP				
	15–19	20–29	30–39	40–49	TOTAL
Control by means of contraceptives	40	47	20	11	26
Control by means of induced abortion	13	34	68	71	58
Use of induced abortion exclusively	4	6	13	20	13
Use of contraception also	9	28	54	48	44
Use of sterilization and induced absorption	—	0	1	3	1
Sterilization	—	0	2	5	2
Noncontrol, sterile	47	19	10	13	14
Control never used	47	19	6	5	10
Sterile	—	0	4	8	4
Total	100	100	100	100	100

Table 12. Note that teenage girls were more likely to rely on abortion for birth control than were women of higher age groups.

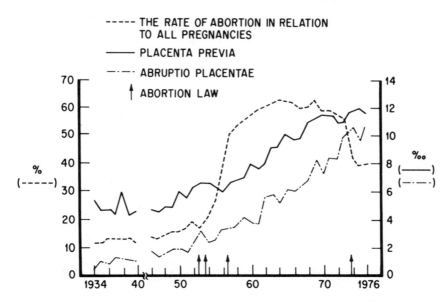

Fig. 2. Correlation between the rate of abortions, placenta previa and placenta accreta.[14]

study suggested that previous parity—particularly that of teenagers—was also a contributory factor. The statistics suggested srongly that only about 50 to 60 percent of all women were willing to admit their previous abortion experience,[5] a fact which affects the validity of the controls in Tables 13 and 14. Interestingly, similar observations were made previously in Japan.[12]

According to official estimates, by the year 1972, more than 70 percent of all women in Hungary had had at least one induced abortion during their reproductive lifetimes. The data indicate that unmarried women were 4 times more likely to seek artificial abortion than were married women and that one of every six aborters was childless. Due to the high rate of prematurity, the neonatal mortality following induced abortion was found to be increased by 75 percent following a single episode, by 100 percent after two or three and by 200 percent after four or more.[10]

In the early 1960's, Árvay et al.[1] analyzed the obstetric history of 946 multigravidas with premature birth and compared them with a group of matched controls. The results indicated that the history of patients with premature births and spontaneous abortions included a high incidence of induced abortions (Figs. 4–6). The same authors demonstrated by preoperative and postoperative hysterography that the majority of the patients developed cervical incompetence after abortion by D & E (Fig. 7). These findings support Klinger's calculations[10] indicating that the relative

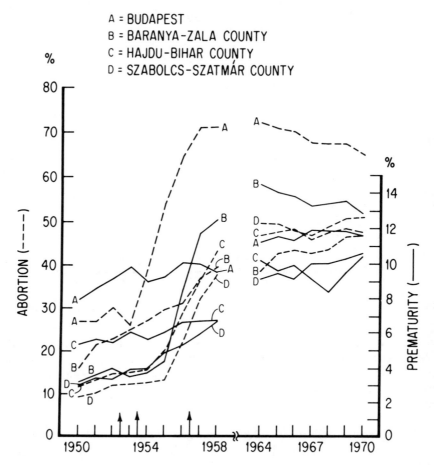

A = BUDAPEST
B = BARANYA-ZALA COUNTY
C = HAJDU-BIHAR COUNTY
D = SZABOLCS-SZATMÁR COUNTY

Fig. 3. Changes in the relative rate of induced abortions (in relation to all diagnosed gestations) and the rate of premature births in 4 geographic areas: A. Budapest, B. Baranya -Zala County, C. Hajdu - Bihar County, D. Szabolcs - Szatmar County. Note that with increasing spread of induced abortion in the rural areas the initially low prematurity rates increased to the level of the metropolitan area.[14]

prevalence of induced abortions is high in the background of premature births (Figs. 8 and 9). The data of the Central Bureau of Statistics in Budapest indicate that manual work and smoking are contributory predisposing factors to prematurity. In addition, the statistics show that all obstetric events, not only induced abortions, predispose to subsequent prematurity. Thus, the difference between the impact upon future childbearing of induced abortion and of undisturbed term gestation is quantitative rather than qualitative.

Table 13. Hungarian Statistics Concerning Existing Correlations Among Birth Weight, Maternal Age and the Number of Previous Induced Abortions.

MATERNAL AGE	BIRTH WEIGHT	NO PRECEDING INDUCED ABORTION		TOTAL OF PRIMI, AND MULTIPARAE	NUMBER OF PRECEDING INDUCED ABORTIONS						ALL CASES TOGETHER
		PRIMIPARAE	MULTIPARAE		1	2	3	4	5	UN-KNOWN	
-19	- 999	14	12	26	4	—	—	—	—	—	30
	1000–1499	40	4	44	9	1	—	—	—	—	54
	1500–1999	96	27	123	13	2	—	—	—	—	138
	2000–2499	276	52	328	19	3	1	—	—	—	351
	–2499	426	95	521	45	6	1	—	—	—	573
	2500-x	3182	536	3718	157	16	5	—	—	—	3898
	TOTAL:	3608	631	4239	202	22	6	—	—	—	4469
20–29	- 999	34	51	85	41	22	8	1	5	—	162
	1000–1499	75	108	183	93	39	14	6	4	—	339
	1500–1999	148	172	320	140	40	18	5	4	—	527
	2000–2499	490	403	893	231	85	27	19	9	—	1264
	–2499	747	734	1481	505	186	67	31	22	—	2292
	2500-x	7973	6916	14889	2794	849	185	55	55	5	18832
	TOTAL:	8720	7650	16370	3299	1035	252	86	77	5	21124
30–39	- 999	6	27	33	12	7	5	2	1	—	60
	1000–1499	7	43	50	19	15	7	3	2	—	96
	1500–1999	17	80	97	33	30	7	5	7	—	179
	2000–2499	39	168	207	83	48	20	3	12	—	373
	–2499	69	318	387	147	100	39	13	22	—	708
	2500-x	374	2330	2704	699	347	155	55	61	—	4021
	TOTAL:	443	2648	3091	846	447	194	68	83	—	4729

Table 13. (Cont.)

MATERNAL AGE	BIRTH WEIGHT	NO PRECEDING INDUCED ABORTION			NUMBER OF PRECEDING INDUCED ABORTIONS						ALL CASES TOGETHER
		PRIMIPARAE	MULTIPARAE	TOTAL OF PRIMI. AND MULTIPARAE	1	2	3	4	5	UN-KNOWN	
40–x	– 999	—	2	2	1	—	—	1	—	—	4
	1000–1499	—	4	4	3	4	—	1	—	—	12
	1500–1999	—	7	7	2	—	1	1	2	—	13
	2000–2499	5	11	16	6	3	1	—	3	—	29
	–2499	5	24	29	12	7	2	3	5	—	58
	2500–x	35	150	185	55	10	15	—	10	—	275
	TOTAL:	40	174	214	67	17	17	3	15	—	333
All ages together	– 999	54	92	146	58	29	13	4	6	—	256
	1000–1499	122	159	281	124	59	21	10	6	—	501
	1500–1999	261	286	547	188	72	26	11	13	—	857
	2000–2499	810	634	1444	339	139	49	22	24	—	2017
	–2499	1247	1171	2418	709	299	109	47	49	—	3631
	2500–x	11564	9932	21496	3705	1222	360	110	126	5	27024
	TOTAL:	12811	11103	23914	4414	1521	469	157	175	5	30655
	UNKNOWN:	32	76	108	14	14	6	1	—	12	155
	GRAND TOTAL:	12843	11179	24022	4428	1535	475	158	175	17	30810

Courtesy of Dr. András Klinger.

Table 14. Correlations Among Birth Weight, the Age of the Mother and the Number of Previous Induced Abortions 20 Years After the Introduction of Liberal Abortion Laws in Hungary (%).

| MATERNAL AGE | BIRTH WEIGHT | NO PRECEDING INDUCED ABORTION | | | NUMBER OF PRECEDING INDUCED ABORTIONS. | | | | | ALL CASES TOGETHER |
		PRIMIPARAE	MULTIPARAE	TOTAL OF PRIMI AND MULTIPARAE	1	2	3	4	5(+)	
-19										
	- 999	0.4	1.9	0.6	2.0	—	—	—	—	0.7
	1000–1499	1.1	0.6	1.1	4.5	4.6	—	—	—	1.2
	1500–1999	2.7	4.3	2.9	6.4	9.1	—	—	—	3.1
	2000–2499	7.6	8.3	7.7	9.4	13.6	16.7	—	—	7.8
	–2499	11.8	15.1	12.3	22.3	27.3	16.7	—	—	12.8
	2500–x	88.2	84.9	87.7	77.7	72.7	83.3	—	—	87.2
	TOTAL:	100.0	100.0	100.0	100.0	100.0	100.0	—	—	100.0
20–29										
	- 999	0.4	0.7	0.5	1.2	2.1	3.2	1.1	6.5	0.7
	1000–1499	0.9	1.4	1.1	2.8	3.8	5.6	7.0	5.2	1.6
	1500–1999	1.7	2.2	1.9	4.3	3.9	7.1	5.8	5.2	2.5
	2000–2499	5.6	5.3	5.5	7.0	8.2	10.7	22.1	11.7	6.1
	–2499	8.6	9.6	9.0	15.3	18.0	26.6	36.0	28.6	10.9
	2500–x	91.4	90.4	91.0	84.7	82.0	73.4	64.0	71.4	89.1
	TOTAL:	100.0	100.0	100.0	100.0	100.0	100.0	100.0	100.0	100.0
30–39										
	- 999	1.4	1.0	1.1	1.4	1.6	2.6	2.9	1.2	1.3
	1000–1499	1.6	1.6	1.6	2.3	3.4	3.6	4.4	2.4	2.0
	1500–1999	3.8	3.0	3.1	3.9	6.7	3.6	7.4	8.4	3.8
	2000–2499	8.8	6.4	6.7	9.8	10.7	10.3	4.4	14.5	7.9
	–2499	15.6	12.0	12.5	17.4	22.4	20.1	19.1	26.5	15.0
	2500–x	84.4	88.0	87.5	82.6	77.6	79.9	80.9	73.5	85.0
	TOTAL:	100.0	100.0	100.0	100.0	100.0	100.0	100.0	100.0	100.0
40–x										
	- 999	—	1.2	0.9	1.5	—	—	33.3	—	1.2
	1000–1499	—	2.3	1.9	4.5	23.5	—	33.4	—	3.6
	1500–1999	—	4.0	3.3	3.0	—	5.9	33.3	13.3	3.9
	2000–2499	12.5	6.3	7.5	8.9	17.7	5.9	—	20.0	8.7
	–2499	12.5	13.8	13.6	17.9	41.2	11.8	100.0	33.3	17.4
	2500–x	87.5	86.2	86.4	82.1	58.8	88.2	—	66.7	82.6
	TOTAL:	100.0	100.0	100.0	100.0	100.0	100.0	100.0	100.0	100.0
All ages together:										
	- 999	0.4	0.8	0.6	1.3	1.9	2.8	2.5	3.4	0.8
	1000–1499	1.0	1.4	1.2	2.8	3.9	4.5	6.4	3.4	1.6
	1500–1999	2.0	2.6	2.3	4.3	4.7	5.5	7.0	7.5	2.8

Table 14.   (Cont.)

MATERNAL AGE	BIRTH WEIGHT	NO PRECEDING INDUCED ABORTION			NUMBER OF PRECEDING INDUCED ABORTIONS.					ALL CASES TOGETHER
		PRIMIPARAE	MULTIPARAE	TOTAL OF PRIMI AND MULTIPARAE	1	2	3	4	5(+)	
	2000–2499	6.3	5.7	6.0	7.7	9.2	10.4	14.0	13.7	6.6
	–2499	9.7	10.5	10.1	16.1	19.7	23.2	29.9	28.0	11.8
	2500–x	90.3	89.5	89.9	83.9	80.3	76.8	70.1	72.0	88.2
	TOTAL:	100.0	100.0	100.0	100.0	100.0	100.0	100.0	100.0	100.0

Courtesy of Dr. András Klinger.

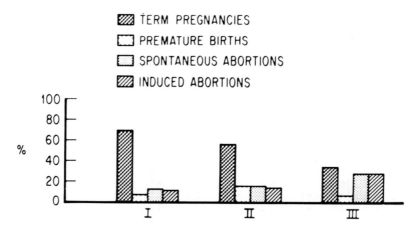

Fig. 4. Group I = term deliveries
Group II = premature births
Group III = imminent abortion
The outcome of all previous pregnancies in relation to that of previous gestations. Note the increased incidence of induced abortions in the backgrounds of premature births and spontaneous miscarriages.[1]

The suction apparatus was not introduced into Hungary until recently. It has been suggested, therefore, that a more general adoption of this method might reduce the extent and severity of cervical damage and its consequences, since the vacuum aspiration procedure requires less extensive cervical dilatation than does evacuation with the ovum forceps and/or by curettage.[15]

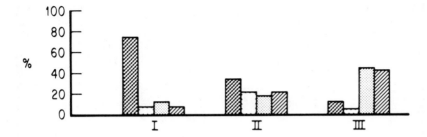

Fig. 5. Group I = term deliveries
    Group II = premature births
    Group III = imminent abortions
    The outcome of the last preceding pregnancy in relation to that of the last gestation.
    Note the high rate of induced abortions immediately preceding premature births and
    spontaneous miscarriages.[1]

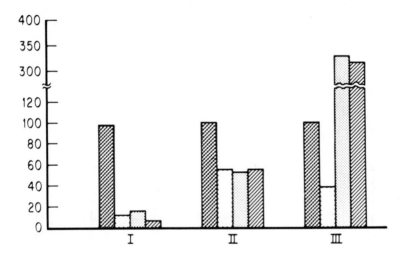

Fig. 6. Group I = term deliveries
    Group II = premature births
    Group III = imminent abortions
    The number of previous term deliveries, premature births and induced abortions in
    relation to the outcome of the last gestation. The data have been pro-rated to 100 cases
    in each category.[1]

Biostatisticians often point out the effect of demographic factors, such
as social, nutritional and educational status, etc., upon the rate of
prematurity in various populations. Undoubtedly, since 1950, all of these
conditions have ameliorated or improved substantially in Hungary. It
should be emphasized that in accordance with the operation of a socialistic

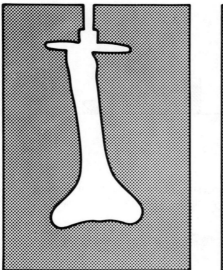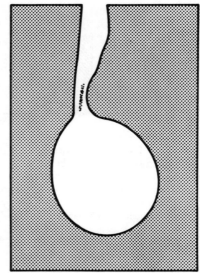

Fig. 7. A. Cervico-hysterography in a primigravida immediately before the interruption of a
first trimester gestation by dilatation and evacuation by ovum forceps and curettage.
B. Cervico-hysterography in the same patient 8 weeks after the abortion procedure.
Note the loss of the original structure of the isthmus suggesting cervical incompetence.[1]

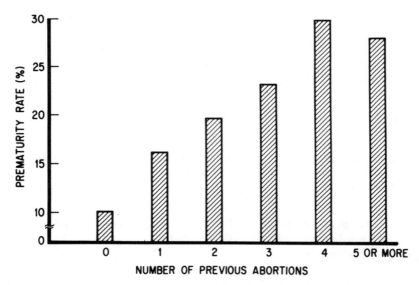

Fig. 8. Note the increase of the relative frequency of premature births following multiple induced abortions.[10]

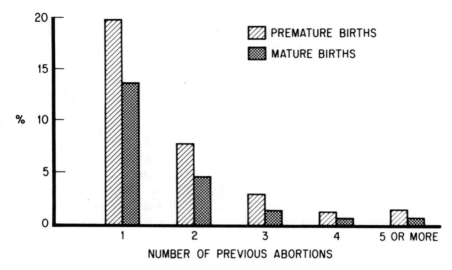

Fig. 9. Interpretation: Of all premature births reviewed, about 20 percent had one, 8 percent had two, 2 percent had three, 1 percent had four and just over 1 percent had five or more previous induced abortions. The respective figures for term deliveries were 14, 5, 1, ½ and ½ percent, respectively.[10]

system such as that prevailing in Hungary during the last quarter-century, one aim was to reduce the socioeconomic differences of its citizens. Accordingly, it would have been impractical to divide the Hungarian population into subgroups on the basis of socioeconomic differences. Indeed, the fact that such factors have been largely eliminated makes the Hungarian population a favorable experimental model for studying the impact of legalized abortion upon perinatal statistics.

The applicability of the above-quoted developments to the reproductive events following induced abortion in the U.S. is conditioned by the following factors:

a) The use of the suction apparatus requires less cervical dilatation than does D & E.

b) The Hegar dilators used in Europe increase by 1/2 mm increments and are therefore less traumatic than the Hegar instruments used in the U.S. which augment almost invariably by 1 mm increments. (Some American clinics use the Pratz dilators which are not more traumatic than the Hegars used in Europe.)

c) By law, abortions have been restricted in Hungary to the first trimester in contrast to the 20-week limit in the U.S. Theoretically, second trimester abortions carried out after dilation of the cervix[6] are more likely to cause cervical imcompetence than are first trimester abortions.[8]

It is a unique feature of the Hungarian abortion experience that the majority of the pregnant women voluntarily participated in it. Thus, there is little likelihood that the results would reflect the reproductive performance of women following elective rather than induced abortion. Another interesting feature of the Hungarian abortion experience[7] is that between 1953 and 1973 abortion was considered the most economical form of birth control. Accordingly, alternative modern methods, such as the "pill" and the "IUD" were virtually unavailable. Since other techniques such as the diaphragm, the condom and the rhythm method had been generally used both before and following liberalization of the law, the reported results could not be influenced by relevant modifying factors.

The statistical data quoted above are of obvious interest for perinatologists who seek identification of all risk factors conducive to reproductive losses. Thus, a more thorough study of the relevant American data appears warranted in light of the information that has become available from abroad.

ACKNOWLEDGMENTS

Some of the presented data and illustrations have been taken from:
L. Iffy et al.: The Effect of Liberalized Abortion Law Upon Perinatal Statistics: The International Experience. *In* T. W. Hilgers: Abortion and Social Justice. The authors wish to record their gratitude to the editor and publisher of that volume for the use of the quoted material.

REFERENCES

1. Árvay, A., Görgey, M. and Kapu, L. La relation entre les avortements (interruptions de la grosses) et les accouchements prématurés. *Rev. Franç, Gynec. Obstet.* **62:** 81, 1967.
2. Barsy, G. and Sárkány, J. A müvi vetélések hatása a születések és a csecsemö halálozás számára. Demográfia (Budapest) **6:** 427, 1963.
3. Bognár, Z. and Czeizel, A. Mortality and morbidity associated with legal abortions in Hungary, 1960–1973. *Amer. J. Publ. Health* **66:** 568, 1976.
4. Czeizel, A., Bognár, Z., Tusnády, G. and Révész, P. Changes in mean birth weight and proportion of low birth weight births in Hungary. *Brit. J. Prev. Soc. Med.* **24:** 146, 1970.
5. Demographic Research Institute. The concealment of induced abortion: an estimate of induced abortions. Survey Techniques in Fertility and Family Research: Experience in Hungary. Budapest, Central Bureau of Statistics, 1969, pp. 110–118.
6. Grimes, D. A. and Cates, W., Jr. Gestational age limit of twelve weeks for abortion by curettage. *Amer. J. Obstet. Gynecol.* **132:** 207, 1978.
7. Iffy, L. Abortion laws in Hungary. *Obstet. Gynecol.* **45:** 115, 1975.
8. Iffy, L. and Patel, R. Gestational age limit for abortion by "D&E." *Obstet. Gynecol.* (In press.)
9. Klinger, A. Demographic consequences of the legalization of induced abortion in Eastern Europe. *Int. J. Gynaecol. Obstet.* **8:** 680, 1970.

10. Klinger, A. Personal communication, 1978.
11. Lampé, L. Az elsö terhesség. *Orv. Hetil. (Budapest)* **119:** 1331, 1978.
12. Moriyama, Y. and Hirokawa, O. The relationship between artificial termination of pregnancy and abortion on premature birth. *In* Family Planning Federation of Japan: Harmful Effects of Induced Abortion. Tokyo, 1966.
13. Pohánka, Ö., Balogh, B. and Rutkovszky, M. Az abortusok hatása az ujszülöttek testsúlyának alakulására. *Orv. Hetil. (Budapest)* **34:** 1983, 1975.
14. Pohánka, Ö. and Török, I. A gestatiós esemeńyek alakulása és a koraszülés-kérdés összefüggése hazánkban 1934 és 1970 között. *Orv. Hetil. (Budapest)* **116:** 243, 1975.
15. Pohánka, Ö., Török, I., Balogh, B. et al. Az idö elötti burok-repedés összefüggése a cervicális elégtelenséggel koraszülésekben. *Orv. Hetil. (Budapest)* **117:** 965, 1976.

28

Teenage Pregnancy

JOSEPH F. RUSSO, M.D.

DIMENSIONS OF THE PROBLEM

The number of pregnancies among adolescents is increasing throughout the world. In the United States the fertility rate in adolescents is among the world's highest. Only Romania, New Zealand, Bulgaria, and East Germany have higher rates.[1] Regardless of the teenage fertility rate in any single country, there is a significant increase in the teenage fertility rate compared with the fertility rate in older women.

Denmark, which has a relatively low teenage fertility rate in comparison with that of other countries, has had a 100 percent increase in the number of teenage births per 1000 women during the past twenty years. On the other hand, women ten years older exhibited a steady decline.[2] The United Kingdom, which has a moderate teenage fertility rate and until the mid-1950's had fewer than 200 mothers under the age of 16 per year, has had a steady rise in the number of births and abortions among teenagers during the past several years.[3] In the United States birth rates among teenagers have declined. However, the decrease has been limited to the older adolescent and the young adult. There has been no decline in the birth rate in the 14 to 17-year-old age group. Actually, it rose among girls younger than 14.[1] The rising teenage fertility rate is nationwide.

Parkland Memorial Hospital in Dallas, Texas reported a threefold increase in the number of patients under 15 years of age who gave birth to first infants; the overall pregnancy rate had more than doubled for this group.[4] Grady Memorial Hospital of Atlanta, Georgia reports a 51 percent increase in the number of births among 13 to 16-year-olds compared to a 10 to 20 percent increase among 17 to 19-year-olds.[5]

Until recently, teenage pregnancies were considered to be a problem confined primarily to the nonwhite, lower income, inner city teenager. It is now clear that pregnancy during the teenage years increasingly involves middle class individuals in both rural and suburban settings. In Arizona during 1971, 18.9 percent of all births involved teenaged gravidas who were under 16 years of age; 63 percent were white and of the middle class.[6]

The national and international trend of increasing numbers of adolescent pregnancies occurring at younger ages is clear. Teenage pregnancies have reached epidemic proportions and affect every level of society. Furthermore, there is a 50 percent likelihood that a second pregnancy will occur within two years following the first.[7,8]

In the United States there are 21 million teenagers, an estimated 11 million of whom are sexually active; one million will become pregnant and 600,000 will give birth. This accounts for one-fifth of the total births in the United States.[1]

ETIOLOGY

Many investigators have attempted to discover why there has been this sharp increase in the number of teenage pregnancies. Apparently, many factors are involved.

In the past, the extended family constituted a primary source of values and information considered basic to the integration of the adolescent in the adult world. It exerted considerable control over the behavior of young people. With the emergence of the nuclear family and emphasis upon the youth culture, there was a decline in the influence of the traditional sources of control and management of behavior. The decline was accelerated by the promotion of popular youth culture models by the mass media.[9]

Evidence from a number of studies indicates that the level of sexual activity has been increasing among adolescents. An overall increase of 30 percent in the level of premarital sexual activity has been reported among 15 to 19 year-old-women during the period 1971 to 1976.[10] The greatest increase in premarital sexual activity was among 15 to 17-year-olds. By the age of 19 more than 50 percent of unmarried teenage women had engaged in premarital sexual intercourse.

A downward trend for the age at menarche has been noted in a number of Western countries. The decrease has been estimated at about four months per decade. In the United States the age at menarche was 14 years of age in the early 1900s as compared to 12.5 years of age in the mid-1950's.[11] With decreasing age at menarche the possibility of pregnancy occurring at a young age is increased.

The above-cited changes in societal behavior might explain the increase in the population-at-risk but they do not explain the sharp increase in the actual number of teenage conceptions.

Psychological factors are important. There are teenagers who consciously desire to become pregnant; this type represents about one-third of the pregnancies.[1] What are the conscious and unconscious motivations of these young women?

Three specific personality syndromes have been observed by one group of investigators who worked in a free public youth clinic with more than 150 adolescent women who requested counseling for unwanted pregnancies. The first syndrome is called the "Angel Syndrome." These girls are the attractive, intelligent, popular female teenagers who are uncomfortable with their sexual maturity and the contest of their parents' insistence upon retaining them as angelic little girls. The second syndrome is the "Parent-Expectation Syndrome" which is found among adolescents whose parents are preoccupied with the pregnancy of a sibling which is unconsciously perceived by the adolescent as an expectation that she should do the same. The third syndrome is the "Unloved Syndrome." This type of adolescent is emotionally deprived and expresses the need to receive love from someone—namely the infant.[12]

Three groups of typical personality profiles have been reported by other investigators. Group I consists of very young, inexperienced, passive girls who submit to intercourse under the pressure of an older persuasive male. Group II are the young girls who, in their attempt to form a heterosexual relationship, experiment with sex and engage in intercourse before they are fully aware of the consequences. Group III are the emotionally disturbed teenagers in marked conflict with their parents. They use premarital intercourse as a pathological behavior pattern to fulfill unsatisfied emotional needs.[13]

Another investigator emphasizes the need to understand the differences in psychological development between the early, middle and late stages of adolescence in attempting to understand the motivations of the pregnant adolescent. The *early stage* of adolescent psychological development is marked by ambivalence toward parents. The adolescent dependence upon the family is in conflict with the growing need to be independent. The teenager usually lacks information about conception and birth control methods. Her primary motivation involves a wish to draw closer to her own mother by becoming a mother herself; secondarily she is motivated by the need to see if her body works. She employs the mechanism of denial regarding the pregnancy and is likely to seek an abortion rather than delivery at term. The baby-fetus is perceived as an "it" and is represented pictorally as a stick figure which represents a lifeless image.

The hallmark of the *middle stage* of adolescent psychological development is the self-centered and dramatic behavior of the adolescent. She knows how to prevent pregnancy and understands her role in contraception. Her primary motivation is to compete with her mother for the love of her father (re-emergence of the oedipal struggle). A secondary motivation is a desire to be autonomous by having something of her own. The baby-fetus is perceived as larger than life, a perception representing the baby's dependency needs which are in conflict with the young woman's own dependency needs. The middle stage adolescent has a difficult time deciding between abortion and delivery. Usually the adolescent's mother raises the baby if the teenager decides to continue the pregnancy.

During the *late stage* of adolescence there is a resolution of love and work identity commitments. These young women are usually realistic and aware. They know how to prevent pregnancy and understand their role in the pregnancy. They usually have a personal regard for the putative father. Their primary motivation concerns the need to elicit a commitment from a reluctant boyfriend. The baby-fetus is perceived of in mother-child terms.[14]

Another investigator sees teenage pregnancy as the outcome of psychological conflicts against which the teenager attempts to defend herself. The intra-family relationships are seen as the primary cause of the pregnancy. If there is hostility in the parents' marriage, a satisfactory identification of the adolescent with the mother does not take place. If the teenager is alienated from the mother, she will have low self-esteem. In an effort to compensate for the latter, she engages in unprotected intercourse from which she derives an impression of being sought after.

If there is a seductive father-daughter relationship, anxiety is produced in the teenager because of its incestuous overtones. These feelings lead to a compulsive use of sex with other men so as to place a barrier between herself and her father.[15]

All of the investigators have theories to explain the conscious or unconscious motivations behind a "wanted" pregnancy in adolescents. Superficially, the theories appear vastly different from one another. There is a common theme, however, shared by all of the theories. Many teenagers become pregnant in attempts to resolve conflicts in normal psychological development.

Etiological Factors in Unwanted Pregnancies

What about the teenager whose pregnancy is not desired? These pregnancies account for approximately two-thirds of the adolescent pregnancies.[1]

The most recent data available indicate that the proportion of sexually active adolescent girls who use contraception is relatively small.[9] It has been found, however, that the older the teenager is at the time of first intercourse, the greater is the likelihood that she will commence contraception at the same time. Furthermore, there is no evidence to suggest that the time interval between the age at first intercourse and the age at first use of contraception has narrowed between 1971–1976.[10] Why do sexually active teenagers avoid using contraception when they do not desire pregnancy?

A survey was conducted in 1971. Six reasons were given by adolescent females 15 to 19 years of age for not using contraception. Three-quarters of the responses reflected a lack of understanding of reproductive physiology or about the capacity to conceive.[16] Another study showed that the percentage of never-married women 15 to 19 years of age who correctly perceived the time of greatest risk within the menstrual cycle has increased by only 3 percent in the period between 1971 to 1976. There was no increased understanding among 15 and 16-year-olds. This continued high level of misinformation and ignorance is surprising in the light of the attention given to sex education in recent years.[10]

There are other reasons for the avoidance of contraception, and lack of information about birth control methods and services is one. Many young women ask: "What are the methods? How are they used? When are they used? Where can you get them?"

Misinformation about birth control methods is another. Patients consistently state that The Pill causes cancer or the coil causes infection, bleeding and pain. Some have called birth control pills "junk" and are not aware that birth control methods include a variety of alternatives.

Some adolescents have anxieties about obtaining contraceptives. They express fear of "being hassled" if they seek contraception through medical channels or fear of needing parental consent. There may be a conflict regarding sexual activity, and the use of contraception may appear to be entirely too premeditated and a commitment to engage in sexual intercourse.

Finally, there are not enough family planning services available to meet the need for these services. About 2,300,000 never-married young women between 15 and 19 years of age are in need of family planning services. Of these, 460,000 are being served by organized family planning services—which represents only one-fifth of the need being met.[17]

CONSEQUENCES

The detrimental effects of becoming pregnant during the adolescent developmental years are considerable. Many aspects of the young woman's health are affected. It is a time of psychological as well as biological stress. Furthermore, childbirth at a young age has serious socioeconomic consequences.

Psychological Effects

The psychological impact of pregnancy upon the adolescent female may be more detrimental to her lifetime well-being and that of her child than are the effects of biologic immaturity.[18] In order to understand the psychological stresses faced by an adolescent gravida, it is necessary to understand the normal stages of adolescent psychosocial development.

Three stages of normal adolescence have been identified. They are again designated early, middle and late adolescence and they do not relate directly to specific chronologic ages. During *early adolescence* the young woman faces the onset of puberty with all of the accompanying physiologic, endocrinologic and emotional changes. It is a time when she becomes deeply involved with her girlfriends and loosens her attachment to her mother. The hallmark of this stage is an ambivalence which represents a conflict between the obvious dependency and the growing need to be independent. Assuming that the challenges of early adolescence are negotiated, the young woman proceeds to the next stage. The *middle adolescent* female is stereotypically self-involved and subject to considerable emotional lability. Conflicts with Mother for the love and attention of Father emerge. Daughter is able to negotiate this stage when heterosexual dating begins. During *late adolescence,* the resolution of the love and work identities occur with the formation of a more stable ego. A firm sense of self and purpose develops. The individual is more comfortable in loosening the ties with her family.[14]

If a young woman becomes pregnant during this period of psychosocial development, additional challenges stress her. She must now develop her role as a mother-to-be and must make adjustments to the physical and emotional changes that accompany pregnancy. Furthermore, a school-age pregnant adolescent will sense personal failure through the shocked looks on her parent's faces which express sorrow, anger and a sense of their own failure. Often she is rejected by the boy involved. She sees herself as the cause of serious disruption in the lives of all of those around her. Since there was an emotional need to be involved with a male, the parental rejection of the boy will result in a conflict in the young woman between filial allegiance and love for the baby's father.

The younger the girl, the more likely she will be considered too young to make correct decisions and she becomes the object of manipulations designed to help her without considering her wishes, allowing her to explore options, or supporting her in the choices she makes. If she disagrees with them, she risks rejection by those individuals upon whom she is dependent emotionally and she worries about having made a serious error.[19]

The transition from childhood to adulthood is stressful even in the absence of pregnancy. Adding the stress of pregnancy results in severe conflict, confusion, and disruption at a time when the young woman has to make important decisions (Figures 1 and 2).

Physical Effects

Young age is a negative factor in regard to physical readiness for pregnancy. Girls younger than 17 years who become pregnant before cessation of their own growth may have nutritional requirements greater than that of adult women. Under these circumstances, pregnancy creates a dual growth demand. Furthermore, many adolescent girls restrict their caloric intake in order to lose weight, and have poor dietary habits.

Even though the requirements for dual growth demand are evident, it has been pointed out that by the age of 12.5 years (average age of menarche), both height and weight increments diminish rapidly and addi-

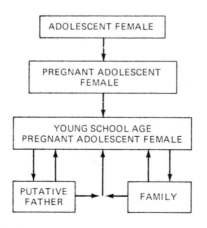

Fig. 1.

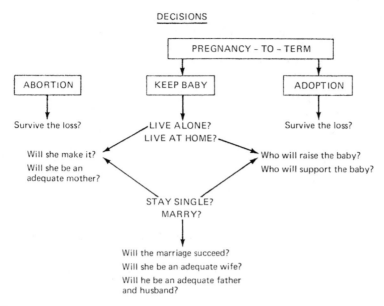

DECISIONS

Fig. 2.

tional nutritional requirements are likely to be negligible after the age of 14. At the ages when the incidence of pregnancy is rising steeply, growth normally has almost ceased. Although our knowledge is incomplete, it is likely that any biologic damage associated with pregnancy in adolescence is largely confined to the group of early maturing girls. If they become pregnant while still in the active phase of anabolic demands, the pregnancy may compromise the ultimate adult stature.[20] Since the rate of fertility has increased among young girls under 14 years of age, the issue of dual growth demand may become a critical health problem.

Although diet during pregnancy is an important consideration, the lifelong nutritional status of the adolescent is the critical determinant of her reproductive performance.[18] The important variables which affect the dietary intake of an individual are education, food habits, availability, economics and the nutritional adequacy of the foods consumed.[21] Therefore, pregnant adolescents need nutritional services in order to correct or support previous dietary patterns.

Many studies have been published which describe the nutritional status and dietary intake of pregnant adolescents.[22-27] They show that about one-half have good diets, one-quarter have fair diets and the remaining one-quarter have poor diets with commonly deficient intakes of calcium, ascorbic acid, vitamin A, protein, and iron. All studies show a high intake of snack foods and soft drinks. It was evident from these studies that the lower the socioeconomic level, the poorer the dietary intake.

Studies in which serum vitamin levels have been measured show decreased levels of vitamin B_6, folate, niacin, vitamin A, thiamin, and vitamin B_{12}. Folate and vitamin B_6 are decreased in all pregnant women regardless of age, race, or socioeconomic condition, probably as a result of altered metabolism and not necessarily from low intake. However, the decreased levels of the other vitamins do suggest a low intake.

One study, in which intensive nutritional counseling was provided for the pregnant adolescents and in which repeat dietary histories were taken, showed little improvement in intake during the pregnancy; the (iron and multivitamins) supplements were not taken on a regular basis by many gravidas.[28] However, these patients were unsupervised, lived at home, and attended an outpatient care facility. The results were better in a study conducted in a special school for pregnant girls in which daily attendance was required and breakfast and lunch were provided. The dietary histories showed improved food intake and a mild decrease in only two vitamins (B_6 and folate).[29]

The nutritional status of the majority of pregnant adolescents is inadequate prior to pregnancy. Pregnancy serves to increase the nutritional demands of the woman, thus furthering nutritional depletion. Efforts need to be directed toward changing dietary habits prior to conception as well as providing the means to improve dietary intake during pregnancy.

OBSTETRICAL EFFECTS-COMPLICATION RATES

Many studies have been published which describe the detrimental obstetrical consequences associated with early childbearing. It is generally accepted that babies born to teenagers are more likely to be premature and of low birth weight than are babies born to older women. Not only is the infant of a teenage mother at greater risk of death, defect and illness, but the teenage mother herself is more likely to die or suffer illness or injury. What is not clear is why young gravidas have more complications than their older sisters have.

Table 1 lists those major studies which have established the basis for the previous statements and their important variables: year and size of the study, race and economic level of the patients, quality of prenatal care and control group, if any. Table 2 lists the same studies with their most significant complications—preeclampsia, anemia and prolonged labor, the cesarean section rate and its association with cephalopelvic disproportion, and the prematurity and perinatal death rates. Studies with different variables come to completely different conclusions with regard to the rate

Table 1.

	YEAR	SIZE	AGE	RACE (% BLACK)	SOCIO-ECONOMIC	PRENATAL CARE		CONTROL GROUP
Marchetti (30)	1945-47	634	12-16	99	Low	Fair-Good	No	Entire service
Briggs (31)	1951-60	201	12-16	7	High	Excellent	Yes	> 21 y/o Primigravidas
Clark (32)	1957-68	1104	10-15	99	Low	Mixed	No	Entire service
	1957-59	291	,,	,,	,,	Poor		
	1960-65	400	,,	,,	,,	Good		
	1966-67	413				Good		
Dwyer (33)	1966-71	231	12-16	72	Low	Fair-Good	No	Other studies
	,,	37	12-14	86	,,	,,		
	,,	194	15-16	69	,,	,,		
Youngs (34)	1973-75	202	12-17	89	Low	Good	No	Other studies
Webb (35)	1967-71	204	< 18	68	Low	Good	No	
Israel								
Woutersz (36)	1958	3995	12-19	52	Mixed	?	No	Entire service?
Dott (37)	1972	414	10-14	82	Mixed	Mixed	No	Age specific rates
Coates (38)	1961-66	137	12-14	99	Low	Poor	Yes	> 14 y/o Primigravidas
Battaglia (39)	1951-60	291	11-14	88	Low	Poor-Fair	Yes	15-19 y/o nonwhite Primigravidas
Duenhoelter (40)	1968-72	471	< 15	76	Low	Poor	Yes	19-25 y/o Primigravidas Matched
Mellor (England) (41)	1963-72	178	11-15	7	Low	Fair	No	Other studies
Zackler (42)	1965-67	2404	11-15	100	Low	Good		MIC
,,	,,	4403	,,	,,	,,	Poor		Non MIC
Claman (Canada) (43)	1964	224	13-15	2	Low	Poor-Fair	Yes	21-25 y/o

Table 1. (Cont.)

	YEAR	SIZE	AGE	RACE (% BLACK)	SOCIO-ECONOMIC	PRENATAL CARE	CONTROL GROUP	
Hassan (44)	1955–62	159	12–15	28	Mixed	Good-Excellent	No	22 y/o Primigravida
Israel (45)								
Deutschberger	1964	491	11–15	46	Low	Poor-Fair	No	Age specific rates
Hulka (46)	1957–62	139	12–15	85	Low	Poor-Fair	Yes	19–21 y/o Matched
Aznar (47)	1953–59	1083	12–16	80	Low	Poor	No	Older primigravidas

Table 2.

	TOXEMIA %	ANEMIA %	PROLONGED LABOR (%)	AV. HRS	CESAREAN SECTION %	PERINATAL DEATH RATE (PER 1000)	PREMATURITY (PER 1000)	COMMENT
Marchetti (30)	20	—	—	13	< 1	38	119	
Briggs (31)	3	—	0(> 24 hr)	12	4	15	70	
Clark (32)	16	2	—	—	1.3	—	139	
	22	—	—	—	< 1	—	206	
	13	1.2	—	—	< 1	—	105	
	13	4.1	—	—	1.4	—	126	
Dwyer (33)	1	4	0(< 24 hr)	—	3	21	160	
	3	(6)	—	—	(5)	0	—	# Small
	< 2	4	—	—	2	26	—	No significance
Youngs (34)	10	7	3(> 24 hr)	—	10	—	170	
Webb (35)	4	18	6(> 20 hr)	10	5	—	75	
Israel								
Wountersz (36)	6	(17)	(5)(> 20 hr)	?	4	25	128	
Dott (37)	—	—	—	—	—	56	150	
Coates (38)	15	20	0.7(?)	10	4	66	190	
Battaglia (39)	28	—	5(< 30 hr)	13	3	82	234	
Duenhoelter (40)	35	8	—	—	10	30	105	
Mellor								
(England) (41)	14	9	9(> 24 hr)	?	1	56	150	
Zackler (42)	5.1	—	—	—	2.7	—	135	
,,	—	—	—	—	—	—	192	
Claman								
(Canada) (43)	36	2	12(> 30 hr)	12	< 1	—	70	Rates peak 14 y/o
Hassan (44)	9	—	3(> 30 hr)	11	3	25	107	

Table 2. (Cont.)

	TOXEMIA %	ANEMIA %	PROLONGED LABOR (%)	AV. HRS	CESAREAN SECTION %	PERINATAL DEATH RATE (PER 1000)	PREMATURITY (PER 1000)	COMMENT
Israel Deutschberger (45)	—	—	6(> 20 hr)	?	2	43	224	Stillbirth = Neonatal
Hulka (46)	11	4	5(?)	10	4	67	136	,,
Aznar (47)	10	16	7.8(> 24 hr)	12	2	50	187	,,

of a given complication, even though they imply that the cause is age-specific.

The period of time during which the study was performed is an important variable. Table 3 lists three studies by decade, all of which have matched controls. Therefore, a given complication rate should be age-related. Furthermore, the ages of the patients included in each study, as well as the racial distribution and socioeconomic level of the patients, are the same. Battaglia and Frazer[39] conclude that adolescents have perinatal death and prematurity rates 2½ -times greater than the national average. By contrast, Duenhoelter et al.[40] conclude that the rates of these two complications are about the same as the national average. Coates' study[38] quotes moderately elevated rates. By looking at the decade during which the studies were performed, it is apparent that the more recent the study, the lower the rates for these two complications. Therefore, the complication rates are not age-specific. It is probable that the lower rates are related to improvement in both antenatal care and in neonatal intensive care, or to changes in the character of the population, with more middleclass young women served during recent years, or as a result of greater governmental intervention for disadvantaged young women.

The effects of income, race, and quality of prenatal care can be seen by comparing the prematurity and perinatal death rates quoted by Battaglia[39] and Briggs[31] (Table 4). These studies were performed in the same decade (1951–1960), and both of them had matched controls. One could expect that the complication rate would be age-specific. However, the complication rates were much higher in Battaglia's than in Briggs' study. The differences can be explained by pointing out that Battaglia's patients were inner-city, poor black women who received fair to poor prenatal care, whereas Briggs' patients were mostly white middleclass women who lived in a home for unwed mothers where diet, activity and prenatal care were controlled. Therefore, it is probable the health of the young woman prior to conception and the quality of prenatal care is more important than the age of the patient at the time when conception occurs.

Table 3.

		YEAR	PREMATURITY RATE (per 1000)	PERINATAL DEATH RATE (per 1000)
Battaglia	(39)	1951–60	234	82
Coates	(38)	1961–66	190	66
Duenhoelter	(40)	1968–72	105	30

Table 4.

		YEAR	RACE (% BLACK)	SOCIOECONOMIC	PRENATAL CARE	PREMATURITY RATE (per 1000)	PERINATAL DEATH RATE (per 1000)
Battaglia	(39)	1951–60	88	Low	Poor-Fair	234	82
Briggs	(31)	1951–60	7	High	Excellent	70	15

Most studies had too few patients from which to draw valid conclusions. Furthermore, if a study included patients above 16 years of age, the data concerning younger women would be diluted by the far greater numbers of older pregnant adolescents. If there are age-specific complications due to inherent biologic hazards of physical immaturity, these complications would be found among the smaller number of very young pregnant women. Therefore, the data should be broken down to yearly groups rather than reported on a 5-year basis as is the current practice.

Some of the studies had control groups, while others did not and compared the complication rates with national statistics, the results of other studies, or age-specific rates for the institution. Hence they included many variables in addition to age. Even in studies with matched controls, it is doubtful that age was the only variable noted when the decades during which a study was performed were compared.

Preeclampsia was the most common complication. Twenty-one studies reported it, eleven concluded that the rate was higher for adolescents than for adults. A total of fifteen studies showed a rate greater than the national average. However, the cause of preeclamptic toxemia is not known, nor are the criteria for diagnosis consistent from study to study. The form of the disease was almost always of the late-onset type and mild, with good fetal and maternal outcomes. Comparison of Clark's[32] with Briggs'[31] study (Table 5) indicates that the better the prenatal care, and the better the socioeconomic condition, the lower the rate of preeclamptic toxemia.

There was no evidence to indicate that anemia was an age-related complication. Dietary habits prior to conception and diet during pregnancy, which reflect socioeconomic conditions as well as the quality of prenatal care, appear to be more important than age.

Of the thirteen studies which referred to the duration of labor, six concluded that labor was prolonged in adolescents. Many different definitions, however, were used to define prolonged labor (greater than 20, 24, or 30 hours) and all of the studies had a 10 to 13-hour average. Therefore, there is little evidence that prolonged labor is a significant complication. Further-

Table 5.

	SOCIOECONOMIC	PRENATAL CARE	TOXEMIA (%)
Clark	Low	Poor	22
(32)	Low	Good	13
	Low	Good	13
Briggs	High	Excellent	3
(31)			

more, older primiparas may be more likely to be delivered early by cesarean section, if labor appears prolonged, than are younger primiparas for whom the fact of a cesarean section scar could be socially detrimental.

Several of the studies have recorded a high incidence of pelvic inlet contraction in the very young pregnant adolescent suggesting that the bony pelvis had not reached its mature size at the time of delivery. One study showed that the majority appeared immature on X-ray film, with lack of fusion of the femoral epiphysis and a contracted inlet.[48] The clinical significance of these findings is questionable since no study reported an increase in the rate of cesarean section or of cephalopelvic disproportion.

The second most commonly reported complication was prematurity; 22 studies reported it and 16 showed a high prevalence. The cause of premature labor is unknown. In reported series with rates below the national average, there is evidence of good to excellent prenatal care and favorable socioeconomic status. The weight of the premature babies was consistent with gestational age, suggesting no reduction of fetal growth due to the young age of the mother. Thus, low birth weight is due more to unfavorable socioeconomic conditions and lack of prenatal care than to maternal physical immaturity.

Some contend that adolescents have an increased perinatal death rate, suggesting that age itself is a causal factor. The perinatal mortality rate is the number of fetuses who die in utero per 1000 births (stillbirth rate) plus the number of infants who die during the first four weeks of life per 1000 births (neonatal death rate). In view of the fact that the stillbirth rate was not increased whereas the neonatal death rate was, the perinatal mortality rate was probably related to the increased incidence of prematurity, which usually reflects socioeconomic conditions and the quality of prenatal care.

All investigators agree that the young pregnant adolescent is at risk, but the data indicate that prenatal care and socioeconomic conditions are more important determinants of outcome than is the age of the patient. The better the health of the mother prior to and during pregnancy, the better the fetal and maternal outcome.

Socioeconomic Effects

Pregnancy is the most frequent known cause for a young woman to discontinue her education. As a result, many intelligent individuals do not develop marketable job or social skills and have lifelong difficulty because of a single act. The majority of young, school-age pregnant women have poor performance in school prior to pregnancy. Interest and success in school, apparently, contribute to more cautious heterosexual experimentation. A study of pregnant adolescents from 13 to 16 years of age indicated that a pregnancy-to-term group had more problems in school, with lower grades and less desire for formal education than did the nonpregnant controls.[49] The majority of school systems do not deal with the problem of pregnancy in that they either excuse or exclude the young woman by providing home instruction or high-school classes. The detrimental effect of this approach is obvious. It was found in another study that of 20 girls under 14 years of age, only 4 continued their education while the rest did not and went on to have repeated pregnancies.[32] In contrast, the young pregnant women in a special education facility completed school, with the majority maintaining or improving their grades.[50]

The number of years in school has an important effect upon labor force participation and wage level.[51] The job experience is not an adequate substitute.[52] Therefore, the lower the number of the years in school, the lower the wage rate, and the less likely an individual will be motivated to find work. In short, the likelihood of poverty rises substantially as the age at which a woman first becomes pregnant decreases. Among women who have a first child at ages of 13–15, 16–17, and 18–19 years is a 2.6, 2.0, 1.4 times greater incidence of poverty, respectively, than among those who do so when they are 20 years old.[53]

The risk of separation and divorce rises as age of parenting falls. The incidence of divorce for women under 17 years of age is 2.6 times greater than for women at age 20.[54] Furthermore, young mothers have larger families in that they give birth to 1.3 times more children than do their older counterparts.[55]

The effects of early childbearing involve educational and economic deprivation as well as detrimental sociologic patterns of living. These effects are perpetuated from one generation to the next (Fig. 3).[56]

CONCLUSIONS

Throughout the industrialized world increasing numbers of adolescents are becoming pregnant. The problem cannot be ignored. The reasons for this phenomenon must be understood if the trend is to be reversed.

Society has changed; families are small and move frequently, weakening the traditional sources of behavioral control—family, community and church. Sexual activity at younger ages is increasing at a time when the age of fecundity has decreased, resulting in a larger population-at-risk. Many young women become pregnant as an attempt to resolve conflicts in normal adolescent psychosocial development, whereas others do not use or have available to them contraceptive methods. Communication between the teenager, family, community, church, school and medical services must be improved and must lead to complementary rather than competitive care

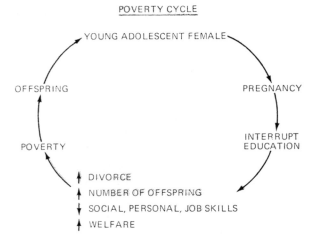

Fig. 3. Poverty Cycle.

and education. What is needed is a family life education program which goes beyond traditional concepts of sex education and covers contraception, the problems of family life and parenthood, and the ethical questions involved in interpersonal relationships and reproductive behavior. Furthermore, services must be offered as a comprehensive, coordinated program including health, educational, and social services in order to be effective in the prevention of early pregnancy and childbearing.

When a very young woman becomes pregnant, many aspects of her health are affected—psychological, biological and socioeconomic. The psychological stress of pregnancy will affect her future psychosocial development, interfering with her ability to cope with the responsibilities of adulthood. The teenage mother and her child have an increased biological risk of death, injury, or illness. Since pregnancy interrupts her education, the young mother has less social, personal, and job skills. She is more likely to be unemployed and live in poverty which may well involve her child. Prenatal care must be provided in a special setting where nonjudgmental professional and staff members are interested and skilled in relating to pregnant teenagers as people rather than as problems. Psychological, nutritional and social work services should be an integral part of obstetrical care. Follow-up care for the young mother and child must combine vocational, educational, and social work services. Easy access to nonjudgmental professionals, who will provide ongoing care and assist in handling common adjustment problems, is essential if one expects to interrupt the usual devastating effects of early childbearing.

REFERENCES

1. Planned Parenthood Federation of America. 11 Million Teenagers, New York, The Alan Guttmacher Institute, 1976.
2. Braestrup, A. Teenage pregnancy in Denmark, 1940–71. *J. Biosocial Science* **6:** 471, 1974.
3. Editorial. School Pregnancies. *Brit. Med. J.* **2:** 545–6, 1976.
4. Duenhoelter, J. H., Jimenez, J. M. and Daumann, G. Pregnancy performance of patients under fifteen years of age. *Obstet. Gynecol.* **46:** 1, 49, 1975.
5. Klein, L. Early teenage pregnancy, contraception, and repeat pregnancy. *Am. J. Obstet. Gynecol.* **120:** 249, 1974.
6. Youngs, D. and Niedyl, J. Adolescent pregnancy and abortion. *Med. Clin. N. Amer.* **59:** 1419, 1975.
7. Currie, J., Jekel, J. and Kerman, L. Subsequent pregnancies among teenager mothers enrolled in a special program. *Am. J. Publ. Health* **62:** 1606, 1972.
8. Drillien, C. School disposal and performance for children of different birthweight born 1953–1960. *Arch. Dis. Childhood* **44:** 562, 1969.
9. Pregnancy and Abortion in Adolescence, Report of a WHO Meeting. *WHO Technical Report Series* **583:** 1, 1975.
10. Zelnik, M. and Kanter, J. Sexual and Contraceptive Experience of Young Unmarried Women in the United States, 1976 and 1971. *Family Planning Perspectives* **9:** March/April, 1977.
11. Tanner, J. M. Growth at Adolescence (2nd Ed.) London, Blackwell Scientific Publications, 1962.
12. Gispert, M. and Falk, R. Sexual experimentation and pregnancy in young black adolescents. *Am. J. Obstet. Gynecol.* **126:** 459, 1976.
13. Perez-Reyes, M. G. and Falk, R. Follow-up after therapeutic abortion in early adolescence. *Arch. Gen. Psychiat.* **28:** 120, 1973.
14. Hatcher, S. L. Understanding adolescent pregnancy and abortion. *Primary Care* **3:** 407, 1976.
15. Abernathy, V. Prevention of unwanted pregnancy among teenagers. *Primary Care* **3:** 399, 1976.
16. Shah, F., Zelnik, M. and Kantner, J. F. Unprotected intercourse among unwed teenagers. *Fam. Plan. Persp.* **7:** 32, 1975.
17. Morris, L. Estimating the need for family planning services among unwed teenagers. *Fam. Plan. Persp.* **6:** 2, 1974.
18. The Working Group on Nutrition and Pregnancy in Adolescence. Relation of nutrition to pregnancy in adolescence. *Clin. Obstet. Gynecol.* **14:** 376, 1971.
19. McDonald, T. F. Teenage pregnancy. *JAMA* **236:** 598, 1976.
20. Thomson, A. M. Pregnancy in Adolescence. *In* (Mckigney, J. I. and Munro, H. M., Eds.) Nutrient Requirements in Adolescence. Cambridge, Mass., M.I.T. Press, 1976, pp. 245–256.
21. Hyck, M. I. Nutrition services for pregnant teenagers. *J. Am. Diet. Assoc.* **69:** 60, 1976.
22. McGamty, W. J., Little, H. M. et al. Pregnancy in the adolescent: I. Preliminary summary of health status. *Am. J. Obstet. Gynecol.* **103:** 773, 1969.
23. Smith, A. F. Dietary habits of girls pregnant at 16 and under. *Pub. Health Rep.* **84:** 213, 1969.
24. King, J. C., Chenour, S. H. et al. Assessment of Nutritional Status of Teenage Pregnant Girls. I. Nutrient Intake and Pregnancy. *Am. J. Clin. Nutr.* **25:** 116, 1972.
25. Osofsky, H. J., Rizk, P. T. et al. Nutritional status of low income pregnant teenagers. *J. Reprod. Med.* **6:** 29, 1971.

26. Serler, J. M. and Fox, H. M. Adolescent pregnancy, association of dietary and obstetric factors. *Home Econ. Res. J.* **1:** 188, 1973.
27. Thompson, M. F., Morse, E. H. and Merrow, S. B. Nutrient intake of pregnant women receiving vitamin-mineral supplement. *J. Am. Diet. Assoc.* **64:** 382, 1974.
28. Kaminetzky, H. A., Langer, A. et al. The effect of nutrition in teenage gravidas on pregnancy and the status of the neonate. I. Nutritional Profile. *Am. J. Obstet. Gynecol.* **115:** 639, 1973.
29. Hansen, C. M., Brown, M. L. and Trontell, M. Effects on pregnant adolescents of attending a special school. *J. Am. Diet. Assoc.* **60:** 538, 1976.
30. Marchetti, A. A. and Menaker, J. S. Pregnancy in the adolescent. *Am. J. Obstet. Gynecol.* **59:** 1013, 1950.
31. Briggs, R. M. and Herren, R. R. Pregnancy in the young adolescent. *Am. J. Obstet. Gynecol.* **84:** 436, 1962.
32. Clark, J. F. Adolescent obstetrics - obstetric and sociologic implications. *Clin. Obstet. Gynecol.* **14:** 1026, 1971.
33. Dwyer, J. F. Teenage pregnancy. *Am. J. Obstet. Gynecol.* **118:** 373, 1974.
34. Youngs, D., Niebyl, J. et al. Experience with an adolescent pregnancy program. *Obstet. Gynecol.* **50:** 212, 1977.
35. Webb, G. A comprehensive adolescent maternity program in a community hospital. *Am. J. Obstet. Gynecol.* **113:** 511, 1972.
36. Israel, S. L. and Woutersz, T. B. Teenage obstetrics. *Am. J. Obstet. Gynecol.* **85:** 659, 1963.
37. Dott, A. D. and Fort, A. T. Medical and social factors affecting early teenage pregnancy. A literature review and summary of the finding of the Louisiana Infant Mortality Study. *Am. J. Obstet. Gynecol.* **125:** 532, 1976.
38. Coates, J. B. Obstetrics in the very young adolescent. *Am. J. Obstet. Gynecol.* **108:** 68, 1970.
39. Battaglia, F. C. and Frazer, T. M. Obstetrical and pediatric complications of juvenile pregnancy. *Pediatrics* **32:** 902, 1963.
40. Duenhoelter, J. H., Jimenez, J. M. and Daumann, G. Pregnancy performance of patients under fifteen years of age. *Obstet. Gynecol.* **46:** 49, 1975.
41. Mellor, S. and Wright, J. D. Adolescent pregnancy. *Practitioner* **215:** 77, 1975.
42. Zackler, J. and Adelman, S. The young adolescent as an obstetrical risk. *Amer. J. Obstet. Gynecol.* **103:** 305, 1969.
43. Claman, D. and Bell, H. Pregnancy in the very young teenager, *Am. J. Obstet. Gynecol.* **90:** 350, 1964.
44. Hassan, H. M. and Fall, F. H. The young primipara - A clinical study. *Am. J. Obstet. Gynecol.* **88:** 256, 1964.
45. Israel, S. L. and Deutschberger, J. Relation of mother's age to obstetrical performance. *Obstet. Gynecol.* **24:** 411, 1964.
46. Hulka, J. F. and Schaaf, J. T. Obstetrics in adolescents: A controlled study of deliveries in mothers 15 and under. *Obstet. Gynecol.* **23:** 678, 1954.
47. Aznar, R. and Bennett, A. Pregnancy in the adolescent girl. *Am. J. Obstet. Gynecol.* **81:** 934, 1961.
48. Aiman, J. X-ray pelvimetry of the pregnant adolescent. Pelvic size and the frequency of contraction. *Obstet. Gynecol.* **48:** 281, 1976.
49. Gispert, M. and Falk, R. Sexual experimentation and pregnancy in young black adolescents. *Am. J. Obstet. Gynecol.* **126:** 459, 1976.
50. The Webster School - A District of Columbia Program for Pregnant Girls. *Children's Bureau Research Reports*, 1968.

51. Bowen, W. and Finegan, T. A. The Economics of Labor Force Participation. Princeton, N. J., Princeton University Press, 1969.

52. Trussell, T. J. Economic consequences of teenage childbearing. *Fam. Plan. Perspect.* **8:** 180, 1976.

53. Bacon, L. A. Early motherhood, accelerated role transition and social pathology. *Social Forces,* Mar., 1974.

54. Ross, H. L. and Sawhill, I. V. Time of Transition: The Growth of Families Headed by Women. The Urban Institute, Washington, D.C., 1975.

55. Bonham, G. S. and Placek, P. J. The impact of social and demographic, maternal and infant health factors on expected family size: Preliminary findings from the 1973 National Survey of Family Growth and the 1972 National Natality Survey. Population Association of America, Apr., 1975.

56. Johnson, C. L. Adolescent pregnancy: Intervention in the poverty cycle. *Adolescence* **9:** 391, 1974.

29

The Life and Work of Ignatz Philipp Semmelweis

ANDREW J. BAEDER, M. D.

In a number of biographies which have dramatized Semmelweis' life, he has been glorified to such an extent that he appears more a victim in a Greek tragedy than a great scholar and scientist. The research conducted during recent decades has provided a more realistic picture of him as a human being and a scientist. At the same time, these investigations have cleared up many of the mysteries regarding his illness and death.

Recent research has concentrated on two relevant areas, namely his mental disease and the rather obscure circumstances pertaining to his last days and death. Schurer von Waldheim, an Austrian historian, was the first to notice (1905) the many contradictory statements regarding the latter. It was clear that he had died of septicemia, but there was no way to determine whether or not he was mentally ill. At any rate, if he was, the insufficient and contradictory data do not offer reliable information as to the nature of his mental illness. Some distinguished professionals have suggested that his delirious state was caused by sepsis rather than insanity. His hospital chart, which might bring an end to the controversy, could not be found.

Eventually, Dr. Istvan Darvas, an elderly independent Semmelweis researcher, found out that this chart did in fact exist. We shall never know how he learned about it because he took the secret to his grave. However, in 1967 he handed over his correspondence to the Dean of the Budapest School of Medicine, and these letters proved that Darvas was on the right track. The most important document was a letter written to Darvas in 1961 by the Viennese medical historian Dr. Marlene Jantsch stating that Semmelweis' chart did exist but was securely locked away. Without asking for permission, she sent excerpts of its content to Darvas. As it turned out later, she had done a good job of passing on all relevant data except the diagnosis of Semmelweis' mental illness and the treatment he had received.

In answer to his inquiry Darvas also received a letter in 1963 from Dr. W. Podhajsky, Director of the Vienna Psychiatric Hospital, stating that in Austria the release of Semmelweis' chart or its copy would be unlawful. In the fall of the same year Darvas was refused access to the chart by the Vienna City Council. Hungarian officials, backed by Darvas' evidence, made several unsuccessful attempts to examine this record. Dr. Endre Reti, director of the Budapest Medical Library, spoke to Dr. Jantsch in an attempt to get the record. She admitted having a copy but stated that the Dean of the Vienna University had threatened her with disciplinary action if she released it. The Hungarian authorities were informed by the Vienna City Council that the chart had disappeared during the 1963 reconstructions and that for legal reasons it could not have been released anyway. As an additional complication, Dr. Erna Lasky, Director of the Vienna Institute of Medical History, stated that the original document no longer existed. Thus the struggle to obtain the chart reached a deadlock.

In 1976 a German gynecologist of Hungarian extraction, Dr. George Sillo-Seidl, started an independent Semmelweis research. He discovered that contrary to all previous statements, Semmelweis was never in Dobling but was admitted to the Lower Austria State Hospital on July 30, 1865. In the last 100 years this hospital was three times relocated and eventually demolished, hence the disappearance of the chart was explained. Nonetheless, he did not give up his search and found out that the original chart was in the Vienna Institute of Pathology and that the Vienna Civil Authorities were holding one copy. After many frustrating attempts, Dr. Sillo finally wrote to Dr. Stacher, the new chairman of the Vienna Civil Authorities, pointing out that under the existing Austrian law the release of the chart was legal. Thus, he suggested that if the Austrian authorities kept on refusing to release the record, this would then indicate that Semmelweis died under obscure and possibly criminal circumstances, leading the Austrian authorities to withhold this vital information.

This letter got things moving. Sillo's timing was also good, because the elderly officials who had opposed the release of the copy had died or retired and their successors found no valid reason for withholding the copy. Dr. Stacher instructed Podhajsky's successor, Dr. Solms, to make a photocopy of Semmelweis' chart and send it on to Dr. Sillo. After receiving the documents on February 26, 1977, Dr. Sillo handed them over to the Semmelweis Museum of Medical History on March 2, 1977 to be checked and studied. (As this copy was barely legible, the museum requested and received a more legible microfilm from Vienna in May 1977).

The documents made available were:

(1) One medical certificate (parere) signed by three Hungarian physicians. According to Austrian Law, nobody could be committed to a psychiatric institution without such certificate (Table 1).

(2) One three-page medical history written by Dr. Bokai (Geschichtliche Mitteilung über den Krankhaften Zustand des Dr. Semmelweis).

(3) The hospital chart itself containing the progress report and the result of the autopsy report written in German with Gothic symbols, and the autopsy report written in Latin (Table 2).

HISTORICAL DATA

Semmelweis was born in Buda in 1818, the son of a well-to-do Hungarian family. He graduated from Vienna Medical School in 1844, and in 1846 became the clinical assistant to the chief of Obstetrics and Gynecology at

Table 1.

MEDICAL CERTIFICATE

We the undersigned herewith certify that Dr. Ignaz Semmelweis university professor in Pest has been suffering since three weeks from troubles of his frame of mind, which requires both removal from his present environment and employment and appropriate supervision and medical treatment, which can be best carried out in an institute for melancholics. Therefore we the undersigned recommend that he be accommodated in an Imperial State Hospital.

Pest, July 29, 1865

Dr. Wagner   Dr. Balassa

Professor of Internal   Professor of Practical
Medicine   Surgery

Dr. Bokai

DIRECTOR
Children's Hospital

Table 2.

"DIAGNOSE

Hyperaemia meningum. Hyperaemina et atrophia cerebri cum hydrocephal. chron. Myelitis acuta gangraena digiti medii manus dextr. articulationem ejus interphalangeam ultimam perforans. Metastases in tela cellulosa subcutanea extremitatum et abscessus metastaticus intermusculum pectoral. major et minor sinistr. Thoracem perforans susequente pyopneumothorace sinistro circumscriptio (aere nempe externodato orto) - Metastases, renis sinistr. Pyaemia -''

the Allgemeines Krankenhaus in Vienna. This Hospital had been founded by the liberal Emperor Joseph II and was apparently the most humane institution of the time. Women, mostly unmarried girls, were admitted as early as the fourth month of their pregnancy without disclosing their names. Following the birth, the mother could decide whether she wanted to stay in the hospital with her infant, be placed as a wetnurse or be discharged. If the child was left behind, it was taken care of by the state. However, these women paid a high price for this humane treatment. Their mortality rate was appallingly high, for example in October 1843 one out of three (29.3%) fell victim to childbed fever. In April 1847 the mortality rate was 18 percent. The authorities did not seem to be alarmed, because the situation was no better in other European maternity hospitals The fatalities were explained by "contagion" or by mysterious meteorological influences.

   However, Semmelweis initiated a systematic study of patient records to find the cause of this high mortality since the existing theories were of no help in explaining the large number of fatalities. Eventually, his capacity for critical observation led him to the etiology of puerperal fever.
He was impressed by two facts:
(1) The much higher mortality rate on the teaching wards than on the adjacent non-teaching wards run by midwives.
(2) The low mortality rate among women who gave birth on filthy streets or in slums and were admitted *only after* the birth.

   A tragic accident provided the answer to this puzzle. A friend of Semmelweis', Koletschka, a pathologist, died as a consequence of an injury sustained during an autopsy. When studying his autopsy report, Semmelweis was astonished to learn that the findings were exactly the same as those in women who died of puerperal fever. In addition, the postmortem examination revealed a well known clinical entity: septicemia. Semmelweis postulated that there had to be some relationship between these findings and childbed fever. First he assumed that childbed fever was caused by some poisonous substance produced by corpses. This poison was then transmitted into the system of the parturients by the physician who had performed autopsies and thereafter examined the women. This theory provided the answer to the question of why the number of fatalities was low on wards run by midwives and in women hospitalized *following* delivery: neither group was examined by a physician. In concurrence with Professor Klein, Semmelweis instructed al physicians to wash their hands in chlorine water before entering the ward. The validity of his theory was proven by the decline of childbed fever.

For reasons of his own, he didn't publish his results for two years and propagated his views in informal conversations only. Apparently, in so doing he antagonized his colleagues by spreading his views by force rather than by persuasion. He paid no attention to the opinions of others, nor did he spare his superiors. This led to interpersonal conflicts. At that time, between 1848–49 there was unrest and revolution involving the monarchy; this atmosphere intensified the personal and professional controversy.

In spite of the prophylactic procedures, the fatalities on Semmelweis' ward increased again. His adversaries seized upon this fact, but he did not give up until he had found the cause: a woman with a necrotic cervical cancer. Two months later a patient with a suppurative knee joint who was on the same ward and was treated by the same physicians as the parturient women caused another outbreak. It was this very event that made him expand his theory, indicating that not only corpse poison but also any "decaying animal material" could cause childbed fever.

Semmelweis' theory was readily accepted by enthusiatic young people and by some of his personal friends. Hebra, a dermatologist, compared the importance of Semmelweis' discovery with the smallpox inocculation. In January of 1849, Skoda, a prominent physician on the faculty of the Vienna Medical School gave a report of Semmelweis' activities. It was decided that a committee be sent to investigate his results. However, the committee was never formed. On the contrary, Semmelweis' appointment was terminated by his superior, Dr. Klein, who was apparently afraid that the rebellious younger generation might replace him with Semmelweis. Thus in March, 1849 Semmelweis lost his job.

His application to be appointed "Dozent" was first rejected. Then with the backing from Rokitansky he was given the title, but with the restriction that he could teach only on phantoms. For a while Semmelweis tried to prove the etiology of childbed fever with animal experiments in a laboratory. However, Semmelweis was not adept at laboratory research. He wanted to work on human subjects. Soon he discontinued the experiments.

He felt ignored and isolated in Vienna and in October, 1849 moved to Budapest. He was given a cordial welcome, but the general public and the profession did not show much interest in him. He was offered five small rooms and the position of honorary consultant under the supervision of the Chief Surgeon at the St. Rocus Hospital. Even though his working conditions were unfavorable, puerperal mortality on his wards fell to 0.85 percent, which was unique at that time. This success may have earned him the professorship of obstetrics at Budapest University (1855).

The fatalities due to puerperal fever were as high as 26 percent in Wuertzburg, 15 percent in Christiania and 12.4 percent in the Maternité in Paris. Yet hardly anybody acknowledged the validity of Semmelweis' theory. Even his famous book "Die Aetiologie, der Begriff und die Prophylaxis des Kindbettfiebers" was given very little attention. The majority of obstetricians belittled his results or considered them accidental.

Thereupon he became increasingly desperate and wrote his well known open letters in medical journals to outstanding European obstetricians such as Spaeth, Siebold and Scanzoni calling them murderers for failing to comply with his instructions. Even though Semmelweis had a valid point, these letters only increased the controversy. Sinclair had good reason to say at the unveiling of the Semmelweis statue in 1906: "Had Semmelweis had Holmes' human trait he would have convinced the whole world with his etiology in twelve months."

Unfortunately, Semmelweis had a difficult personality.

According to his friend Dr. Bokai, Semmelweis was a sincere and forthright man with brusque manners. He could not tolerate being contradicted, and would consider anyone an enemy who was not in unconditional agreement with him. He often tyrannized his own family.

His open letters written in 1860 and 1861 reflect an obsessive argumentativeness. Although this behavior exceeded the limits of normal behavior it could not be characterized as insanity.

There is no doubt that his personality played a decisive role in the reluctance with which his theory was received. In 1862 some young physicians in St. Petersburg gave a favorable account of his theory and in England, Simpson, Queen Victoria's accoucheur, his former foe, became his most devoted advocate. On the Continent, however, except for Michaelis, Lange and Chiari few joined forces with him. In the American literature, however, Oliver Wendell Holmes, another authority on the prevention of puerperal fever, mentions in his publication (1855) a Viennese physician by the name of "Senderein"—he probably meant Semmelweis.

According to earlier biographies, it was the negative response to his theory that made Semmelweis antisocial and quarrelsome. However, recent research shows that it was after a comparatively calm and productive period (1861–65) that he suddenly showed symptoms of insanity. We do not know exactly when this occurred, but by the summer of 1865 he was under observation. Doctor Balassa hired two physicians to take care of him. He was not seen by a psychiatrist so the only evidence available is Dr. Bokai's medical records. This indicates that Semmelweis was physically healthy, but drowsy to such an extent that he often fell asleep even when in cheerful company. Until mid-June of 1865 he appeared normal mentally. Thereafter, he paid less and less attention to his appearance, had trouble sleeping, spent money freely and made grandiose scientific plans. Although previously he had eaten moderately, he began to eat and drink excessively. There was another striking change in his personality, namely the previously prudish Semmelweis became sensuous and obscene. His bizarre behavior was mentioned in Fleischer's memorial speech (1872), and much later by his widow. Finally his outrageous behavior could no longer be tolerated. In 1865 his family and his physicians committed him to an insane asylum pretending that they were taking him to Graefenberg to the hydrotherapy institute of his friend Hebra.

Semmelweis researchers have been trying to find an explanation for the contradictory circumstances relating to his admittance to the hospital. Although, in 1865 there were many good psychiatrists and a psychiatric hospital of good reputation in Budapest, he was never seen by a psychiatrist (the physicians who signed his commitment papers were not psychiatrists). The reason for his commitment to a state hospital outside the country and not to a Budapest psychiatric hospital is not clear. A possible explanation is provided by Istvan Beuedck, a distinguished Semmelweis researcher. In 1865 mental illness was a disgrace; they tried to cover it up, and for that reason did not want him to be seen by a psychiatrist for fear that his insanity would become known. He was taken to Austria to hide his "disgraceful illness" from his acquaintances and the general public. The physicians committing him tried to minimize the situation by stating that he had "troubles of his frame of mind."

According to the hospital notes and to the autopsy report, the direct reason for his death was septicemia. At the autopsy severe injuries of his wrists were found, and the 1963 exhumation revealed a well-healed fracture of the humerus. The old humerus fracture is of no significance and the wrist injuries simply relate to the methods used for patients' restraint in the state hospital. These data do not confirm the speculation that Semmelweis fell victim to violence in the hospital.

The septicemia originated from a finger injury, but we do not know when, where or how it was caused. Long after his death his widow furnished the following information: While treating a patient, he injured the middle finger of his right hand. An infection followed which he treated by soaking his finger overnight. The "scratch on the finger" was not mentioned in his commitment papers, but was referred to in Dr. Bokai's history. The physician who took care of his admission at the hospital described a blue and red lesion on the radial side of his right middle finger which he diagnosed as a contusion or gangrene. As to its origin, the patient (Semmelweis) stated that it appeared "without any reason." There is another interesting comment, "Neither did he get infected at that scandalous delivery three weeks ago." As there is no "scandalous delivery" mentioned in Bokai's report the admitting physician taking the history could only have heard it from Semmelweis' wife or the accompanying physician (Dr. Bathory).

During Semmelweis' two-week stay in the hospital (July 31, 1965-August 13, 1965) the finger infection and its spread was mentioned only twice (August 4 and 7) in addition to the dates of the admission and the death. These superficial notes do not reflect the severe open injuries and suppurating wounds "going down to the bone" that were found at the autopsy. There is also no indication of any treatment other than the application of wet compresses. Could this negligence have been the reason for the refusal by the Austrian authorities to release the record for 112 years?!

As to his mental status, Semmelweis was very restless at the time of the admission to the hospital. He would lie naked on the floor, he wrestled with his guard and tried to jump out of the window. During the days that followed he was agitated and talked much; his speech was slurred and his steps were uncertain. Because of his restlessness he was kept in restraint. On August 5th an old friend, Dr. Skoda, came to visit. Semmelweis recognized him and told him about his grandiose plans: as the world's greatest obstetrician he would apply for membership in the Academy. On August 13th he no longer recognized anybody, was short of breath and died amid increasing convulsions. The clinical diagnosis was "Tobsucht" (rage) which at that time was considered a mental disease.

The day after his death an autopsy was performed by Rokitansky, or by his assistant, Dr. Scheuthauer who published the protocol in the Hungarian Medical Weekly as early as 1865. The pathologic and histologic examination of the central nervous system revealed two different abnormalities: acute changes, which account for Semmelweis' septic delirium and cerebral and spinal changes which indicated that Semmelweis suffered from a chronic central nervous system disease. It might have been progressive paresis but there is inadequate evidence to confirm this diagnosis.

Semmelweis died in the prime of his life at the age of 47. He was buried in Schmelz, Austria. A eulogy appeared in the Hungarian Medical Weekly, but foreign medical journals either ignored his death or wrote only a short note in the *Personal News*.

After Semmelweis' death his name and work were all but forgotten. Lister, the proponent of surgical antisepsis never mentioned Semmelweis in his lectures or publications, although some of his principles were based on Semmelweis' discovery. When asked why Semmelweis was not cited, he said he had not known about him. Lister made four trips to Hungary, lectured there and met with prominent physicians, but no one ever mentioned Semmelweis to him.

Why did the world forget Semmelweis so quickly? The strongest opposition was probably generated by Virchow, the famous pathologist who considered puerperal fever a thrombosis and stated that Semmelweis' theory was based on false premises. Eventually, physicians became interested in other problems as the incidence of puerperal fever decreased throughout the world due to improvement in preventive procedures. Finally, and this may have been the decisive factor, the decades after Semmelweis' death were marked by significant progress in microbiology; the discoveries of Pasteur, Roux and others distracted physicians' attention from such outdated definitions as "decaying animal material." Until the beginning of this century Semmelweis was hardly mentioned in the professional literature. To the professional community Oliver Wendell Holmes and not Semmelweis was the central figure in the struggle against childbed fever. Many years went by until it became recognized that Semmelweis was the most accurate investigator to describe the causes of childbed fever and that his "Prophylaxis" was a most effective way to save the mothers' lives. Apparently all this was not enough to make him universally famous. As late as 1932 Paul de Kruif in his well known book wrote the following: "During the past year, out of ten intelligent doctors I have asked about Semmelweis only one had more than a foggy recollection of that strange Hungarian's name . . . "

Semmelweis' life was tragic. For a long time posterity did not respect his memory. Nonetheless, this lack of gratitude does not change the fact that his fundamental contribution in saving so many lives provides a place for him among the most outstanding physicians of all time.

Subject and Author Index